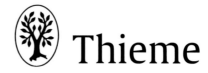

FRCR 2B Viva:
A Case-Based Approach

Paul S. Sidhu, BSc (Hons.), MBBS (Hons.), MRCP, FRCR, DTM&H
Professor of Imaging Sciences
King's College London
Consultant Radiologist
King's College Hospital
Denmark Hill, London
United Kingdom

Suzanne M. Ryan, MRCPI, FRCR
Consultant Gastrointestinal and Abdominal Radiologist
King's College Hospital
Denmark Hill, London
United Kingdom

Phillip F. C. Lung, BSc (Hons.), MBBS, MRCS, FRCR
Subspeciality Fellow in Gastrointestinal Radiology
King's College Hospital
Denmark Hill, London
United Kingdom

409 illustrations

Thieme
Stuttgart • New York

Library of Congress Cataloging-in-Publication Data is available from the publisher.

Important note: Medicine is an ever-changing science undergoing continual development. Research and clinical experience are continually expanding our knowledge, in particular our knowledge of proper treatment and drug therapy. Insofar as this book mentions any dosage or application, readers may rest assured that the authors, editors, and publishers have made every effort to ensure that such references are in accordance with **the state of knowledge at the time of production of the book**.

Nevertheless, this does not involve, imply, or express any guarantee or responsibility on the part of the publishers in respect to any dosage instructions and forms of applications stated in the book. **Every user is requested to examine carefully** the manufacturers' leaflets accompanying each drug and to check, if necessary in consultation with a physician or specialist, whether the dosage schedules mentioned therein or the contraindications stated by the manufacturers differ from the statements made in the present book. Such examination is particularly important with drugs that are either rarely used or have been newly released on the market. Every dosage schedule or every form of application used is entirely at the user's owwn risk and responsibility. The authors and publishers request every user to report to the publishers any discrepancies or inaccuracies noticed. If errors in this work are found after publication, errata will be posted at www.thieme.com on the product description page.

© 2013 Georg Thieme Verlag KG
Rüdigerstrasse 14, 70469 Stuttgart, Germany
http://www.thieme.de
Thieme Medical Publishers, Inc., 333 Seventh Avenue,
New York, NY 10001, USA
http://www.thieme.com

Cover design: Thieme Publishing Group
Printed in Germany by AZ Druck und Datentechnik GmbH, Kempten

ISBN 978-3-13-166291-0
eISBN 978-3-13-166361-0

Some of the product names, patents, and registered designs referred to in this book are in fact registered trademarks or proprietary names even though specific reference to this fact is not always made in the text. Therefore, the appearance of a name without designation as proprietary is not to be construed as a representation by the publisher that it is in the public domain.

Dedications

Thanks must go to my wife, Monica, and children, Francesca and Gianluca, for their remarkable tolerance.

Paul S. Sidhu

Thanks to my supportive family, Niall, Ruby, and Evie.

Suzanne M. Ryan

I wish to thank my wife, Elaine, for being my inspiration, and my family, Raphael, Amy, Andrew, and James, for their unending encouragement.

Phillip F. C. Lung

Contributors

Section 1: Gastrointestinal Imaging

Phillip F. C. Lung, BSc (Hons.),
MBBS, MRCS, FRCR
Subspeciality Fellow in Gastrointestinal Radiology
Department of Radiology
King's College Hospital
Denmark Hill, London
United Kingdom

Suzanne M. Ryan, MRCPI, FRCR
Consultant Gastrointestinal and Abdominal
Radiologist
Department of Radiology
King's College Hospital
Denmark Hill, London
United Kingdom

Section 2: Chest Imaging

Joseph Jacob, BSc, MBBS (Hons.),
MRCP, MRCS, FRCR, DTM&H
Specialist Registrar in Radiology
Department of Radiology
King's College Hospital
Denmark Hill, London
United Kingdom

Sujal Desai, MBBS (Hons.),
MD, FRCP, FRCR
Senior Lecturer
King's College London

Consultant Thoracic Radiologist
Department of Radiology
King's College Hospital
Denmark Hill, London
United Kingdom

Section 3: Musculoskeletal Imaging

Ounali S. Jaffer, MBBS, MRCP, FRCR
Specialist Registrar in Radiology
Department of Radiology
King's College Hospital
Denmark Hill, London
United Kingdom

Imran Khan, MBBS, MRCS, FRCR
Specialist Registrar in Radiology
Department of Radiology
King's College Hospital
Denmark Hill, London
United Kingdom

David A. Elias, BSc, MRCP, FRCR
Consultant Musculoskeletal Radiologist
Department of Radiology
King's College Hospital
Denmark Hill, London
United Kingdom

Section 4: Neurological Imaging

Aarti Shah, MA, BM, BCh, MRCP, FRCR
Specialist Registrar in Radiology
Department of Radiology
King's College Hospital
Denmark Hill, London
United Kingdom

Nagachandar Kandasamy, MBBS, DMRD, FRCR
Consultant Neuroradiologist
Department of Neuroradiology
King's College Hospital
Denmark Hill, London
United Kingdom

Section 5: Urogynaecological Imaging

Diana Bosanac, MBBS, FRCR
Specialist Registrar in Radiology
Department of Radiology
King's College Hospital
Denmark Hill, London
United Kingdom

Dean Huang, BMedSci, BMBS, MRCPCH, FRCR, EBIR
Consultant Radiologist in Genitourinary and
Interventional Radiology
Department of Radiology
King's College Hospital
Denmark Hill, London
United Kingdom

Section 6: Paediatric Imaging

Preena Patel, BSc, MBBS, FRCR
Specialist Registrar in Radiology
Department of Radiology
King's College Hospital
Denmark Hill, London
United Kingdom

Maria E. K. Sellars, MBBS, FRCR
Consultant Paediatric Radiologist
Department of Radiology
King's College Hospital
Denmark Hill, London
United Kingdom

Section 7: Radionuclide Imaging

Simon M. Y. Wan, MA, MB, BChir, MRCP, FRCR
Specialist Registrar in Radiology
Department of Radiology
King's College Hospital
Denmark Hill, London
United Kingdom

Nicola Mulholland, MBBS, MSc, MA (Cantab), FRCR, FRCP
Consultant Radiologist and Nuclear Medicine Physician
Department of Radiology
King's College Hospital
Denmark Hill, London
United Kingdom

Foreword

This book is an excellent collection of cases ideal for the preparation of FRCR 2B Viva examinations. There is a great variety of cases with a wonderful section on tips for candidates appearing for the examination. This has been constructed from a continuum of knowledge gained over three decades from consultants who have experience of examining candidates and specialist registrars who have passed the examination. The cases span the spectrum of diseases commonly brought to the examination by generations of examiners. When I read the book it became obvious that it is a vital link in the teaching portfolio because it demonstrates how to approach each case, pick up the radiological signs, and formulate an answer. There are notes related to the disease and a short bibliography. The contents cover gastrointestinal, chest, musculoskeletal, neuroradiology, urogynaecological, paediatrics, and radionuclide imaging. This book is modern, up to date, and is based on organ imaging. I believe it will also prove to be an excellent revision book that will not become obsolete and is well worth owning.

Professor Philip Gishen, MB, BCh, DMRD, FRCR
Imperial College Healthcare NHS Trust

Preface

There are several Fellowship of the Royal College of Radiologists (FRCR) Part 2B examination books on the market at present, detailing cases in a manner that will test the candidate. These books are of course an invaluable source of information and allow for self-testing. Here, we have designed a book for the FRCR 2B Viva examination not to test the candidate's knowledge, but to demonstrate the approach to the case and formulation of the ideal answer. The purpose of this book is not to test but to allow construction of the most suitable response in the examination.

The vast majority of candidates for the FRCR 2B examination are well prepared, with an extensive and comprehensive knowledge of the subject. The expression of this knowledge in the formal setting of the examination may, however, be a problem for some of the candidates. There is no point in knowing everything if you cannot demonstrate this to the examiner. Our aim is to establish a formula to allow the candidate to achieve this; we have detailed the best approach to an image, and the response to further questions, in a manner that is succinct and clearly responds to the situation. Each case has a model answer, with all the relevant background information needed to confidently assess and detail an appropriate explanation of a film. The cases presented are classics in each section; the answers are models to build on; the background knowledge and bibliography are to be read and understood.

Each section is authored by a specialist registrar who has recently passed the FRCR 2B examination, supervised by an experienced consultant with a sub-specialty interest, all of whom have at some time been teachers on the King's College Hospital FRCR 2B course. To this effect, we believe we have produced an ideal approach to assimilating the response desired by the examiner and providing success in the examination.

Paul S. Sidhu
Suzanne M. Ryan
Phillip F. C. Lung

Acknowledgements

As with any book, a large number of people make contributions, which are often unacknowledged in the final manuscript. Without their contributions, success would not have been possible, particularly with a book like this that requires many teaching cases. We wish to thank the entire Department of Radiology at King's College Hospital, London.

Paul S. Sidhu
Suzanne M. Ryan
Phillip F. C. Lung

Contents

Introduction to the FRCR 2B Viva

A medical career is littered with numerous examinations, a necessity for climbing further up the ladder of specialisation and for the eventual attainment of a goal, in this case attainment of a postgraduate qualification and career in radiology. Very few people enjoy an examination, particularly an examination that involves "face-to-face" confrontation with two examiners; the "viva voce" beloved by purveyors of examinations. However, there is no substitute for this type of examination, stressful as it is for the candidate; the viva examination has from time immemorial been the best method of assessing skills of processing information and formulating an opinion. It is here to stay.

The candidate for the FRCR 2B examination is subject to a viva and will need to be fully prepared for this process. There is no reason why the candidate should be anything but fully confident in this process and be ultimately successful. But candidates will not pass the examination if they have not put in years of toil, reviewing all manner of images and building up a "databank" of knowledge. There is no substitute for hard work. Examinations are also a game, played out to achieve a result. Play the game right and you will pass. Once the knowledge has been attained by candidates, displaying all they have learned in a meaningful manner is the winning game.

A breakdown of the components will give a better understanding of the process.

The Candidate. After many years as a medical student, postqualification ward work, and often 3 years of basic grounding in radiology, the examination is tackled. At this stage, the candidate should have reviewed thousands of "examination" style films, in all imaging modalities, and have read around the subject every time a new disease or abnormality is encountered. Very often the presentation of a disease process is faced while "on call," when there is pressure to come to a diagnosis, a process that will reinforce any knowledge gained—do not underestimate the importance of emergency work.

The entire working life of a candidate up to the examination is a learning process, and the ability or desire to accumulate knowledge is the candidate's own responsibility. If the hours of work and accumulation of knowledge have not been achieved, the candidate will not pass the examination. Nobody can teach this; this is an attitude that should be acquired from early in the candidate's career. Poor knowledge is very quickly spotted by the examiner. Do not blame others in your department for your failure—it is your responsibility to seek out, acquire, and consolidate knowledge. Teaching guides and directs you to the correct manner in which to use the knowledge you acquire by reading and experience.

Nevertheless, even the most prepared candidate will be a nervous wreck on examination day. The ability to process the knowledge and formulate an intelligent answer needs to be implicit—this is the "game." The game is not won without knowledge, but the presentation of the self-acquired knowledge in a meaningful manner can be taught. This is where pre-examination teaching is important; sit with your senior colleagues and practise the viva technique. Never go into an examination without being fully prepared as you will not succeed. Candidates need to have a rigid formula to present their knowledge in a manner that cannot be faulted.

The Examiner. Spare a thought for this poor soul—unpaid, unloved, and subject to 5 or more gruelling days of listening to anxious, nervous individuals who are often incoherent, all in a room 6 foot (or less) square, with no natural light. If this sounds cruel, it is, but the examiners keep coming back. The examiner has previously been a candidate and will understand the anxiety. The examiner will not only be knowledgeable, but most importantly will know exactly what is on the film being shown and will know the final diagnosis. The candidate will not. This is often the only differentiating factor between candidate and examiner, as often the breadth of knowledge is greater in the candidate.

The examiner is not out to fail the candidate. All the examiners are selected and trained to be decent, respectable examiners; they will do their utmost to settle the candidate, tease out knowledge, and try to get the candidate through the examination. No examiner will lead the candidate in the wrong direction or try to humiliate the candidate. But if candidates have poor knowledge, they will not succeed.

Two examiners are present, and both will assess the candidate and each other—if one examiner has been harsh in judging the candidate, the other will note this. The examiners are not out to fail a candidate—candidates fail because they were not good enough. The examiners have homes, families, and work places to go to after the examination period is over; they will be courteous and fair to all the candidates and will not single anyone out for "rough" treatment. The capability of the candidate is usually obvious at the end of the viva, as is whether the candidate has been successful. Rarely is a candidate subject to a review at the end of the process and there is disagreement.

The Examination. Confined in the small room are two examiners and a candidate, so pay attention to your personal hygiene. Dress in a presentable and nonprovocative manner. Be pleasant but not overly friendly; do not address the examiners by their first name. Do not rush to the examination hall but arrive with plenty of time to spare. Sit and have a cup of tea or coffee with colleagues, and go to the bathroom before the viva! Do not try to learn something new before going into the examination, as this is a waste of time and will push up your state of anxiety.

The examiner is likely to start off with a simple and straightforward film to ease you into the examination and to calm you down. You will not be given the "prize-winning" set of films of the rarest case for your first set of examination questions. Look at the film carefully, look at review areas, and think about the film. If you have worked hard, listened to your senior colleagues, read around the subject, been "on call," you will have encountered a similar film in the past. Do not blurt out an answer you cannot retract. Count to 5, and then describe what you see. Give the diagnosis if it is an "Aunt Minnie" (often this will be the case with the first film) and wait for the examiner to reply. This is not a dinner party or social occasion where you as the host need to keep a conversation going. Shut up when there is nothing more to say and let the examiner take you on to the next stage with a question. If you are correct, the film will be removed; if more is needed, a question will be asked. The examiner not involved in asking questions is the one doing the marking. No examiner is supposed to show films in their own sub-specialty, and the other examiner will note this.

The number of films viewed in the course of the examination is no indication of your success: if you have reviewed only one complex case and have got it correct, you have passed. Normally, there is plenty of time to show many cases. Never argue with the examiner, as it will get you nowhere and you will be likely to fail. All the films are vetted before the examination, and there are no films that are "'wrong"—you do not have more insight than the panel of examiners. If the examiner tells you something that you disagree with, move on with the case or move to the next case. At the end of the examination, thank both examiners in a brief and professional manner. There is no place for a hug if you think you have done well.

After the Examination. There is a gap between the end of the examinations and the availability of the results; this is the time to "brag." Every candidate has been shown the worse possible combination of "sneaky" films designed to "trip up" innocent candidates and fail them outright. Nevertheless, the candidate, with incredible foresight and intelligence, has spotted this trap set by the evil examiners, designed to foil career progression, and spun out an incredible answer that could not be faulted, has undoubtedly shown the examiners to be clowns, and has secured a pass. It was even said that the President of the College had heard about this incredible candidate and had asked to personally meet to offer congratulations; a standing ovation among the examiners would precede this meeting.

It is true that candidates pass because they are good enough—candidates fail because they were not good enough. The tendency is often to dwell on the "missed" aspects of the films and forget the correct diagnosis made. This is a natural tendency, and it is best to wait for the result rather than agonise over the possibilities. Discussion after the examination is good for all; it lets off all that accumulated anxiety, so do it and embellish all you like as it does no harm.

So, in summary:
1. Knowledge is gained only by hard work.
2. Teaching is desirable but is no substitute for reading and working.
3. A well-prepared candidate will not fail.
4. Teaching of examination technique is mandatory prior to the examination.
5. The examiners are not out to fail the candidate—lack of knowledge is easily evident.
6. Think before you speak in the examination—you cannot retract what you have said.

The ability to formulate a suitable response forms the basis of the chapters of this book.

Paul S. Sidhu

1 Introduction to Gastrointestinal Imaging

Phillip F. C. Lung and Suzanne M. Ryan

Good knowledge and understanding of gastrointestinal imaging is essential for success at radiological examinations. However, this can be difficult at a time when fluoroscopic techniques are on the wane and use of MRI on the rise; examinees are caught in the middle of changing clinical practice. Examiners tend to display barium studies (prized films kept as important teaching examples) that many candidates may not have experienced outside of educational examination courses.

While there is no substitute for experience, there are pointers that may make the interpretation easier.

❶ Plain abdominal films may be difficult to read, but can be broken down into "bite-size" chunks:
- Bowel. The study has usually been performed to look at the bowel, in particular the bowel gas pattern. Unless there is an obvious abnormality elsewhere that immediately catches your eye, you should first assess the bowel; gaseous distension, constipation, absence of gas, dilatation, and abnormal wall are all important.
- Intra-abdominal free gas. This should be excluded in all films in spite of whatever clinical details you have. Rigler's sign and retroperitoneal free gas outlining the kidney must be specifically checked for.
- Solid organs. Are they enlarged or atrophic? Is there any associated calcification? Are they outlined by gas? Is there any gas within the structure (biliary or portal venous in the liver, gas within the bladder)?
- Bone and joint degenerative disease is common, and bony destruction from tumour may be a pointer to the reason the film was shown.
- Review areas. Look at the lung bases and hernial orifices.

❷ Be methodical and you will pick up the vast majority of lesions. Difficult films are there to identify candidates who are not methodical.

❸ Barium studies remain a staple of the examination, despite the fact that fewer such examinations take place in routine clinical practice. As a result, it is unlikely that the candidate will be shown a subtle case, but the candidate should have good knowledge of the following types of cases:
- Cancers of any part of the gastrointestinal tract must be searched for and excluded.

- Emergencies include volvulus and megacolon.
- Inflammatory bowel disease: Always look out for gallstones, sacroiliitis, and malignancy.
- Target lesions may be subtle and multiple.
- Changes may be seen in the overall fold pattern, as in coeliac disease and scleroderma.
- "Aunt Minnies": Achalasia, candidiasis, linitis plastica, and so on may all occur.

❹ Take your time to look at all of the opacified lumen. Always check the background chest or abdomen, as well as the bones. At the end of every review of a barium study, you must say that you would like to view the entire series as an important detail may be on a view that you have not yet seen.

❺ CT and MRI are currently viewed on hard copies in the viva. As a result, there will be multiple images on each film, and the technique for viewing these is different from that of scrolling on a computer. This will alter in due course, with computer-based examinations being introduced; however, accumulation of sufficient examination cases will take time.
- Have a quick look at the film to see if an obvious abnormality is apparent. Use the clinical information that is available to direct this.
- If no overt abnormality is seen on the initial survey, concentrate on a single organ before moving to another organ. This will allow you to build up a picture and exclude abnormalities as you progress. If you try to look at every organ on one image before moving to another one, you will spend overall more time and may miss details.
- There will often be several abnormalities on the film, and you need to pick them all up. Once you have picked up one abnormality, think about the clinical context to direct your search. For example, if the liver looks cirrhotic, make sure you exclude hepatocellular carcinoma, and look for portal vein thrombosis, varices, and ascites.

❻ All your cases should end by discussing the management options. Try to remember what you do at your institution. Local multidisciplinary clinical meetings are the ideal environment to pick up these details. In your preparation, you should always know what the management is for any particular case. If you do not know, ask.

1.1 Achalasia

Clinical History

A 42-year-old woman presents with a history of dysphagia (**Fig. 1.1.1**).

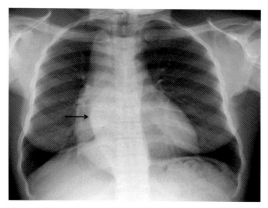

Fig. 1.1.1

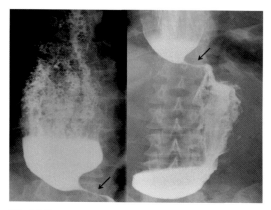

Fig. 1.1.2

Ideal Summary

This is a frontal chest radiograph of a woman. There is a double right cardiac contour with a right paravertebral opacity that extends below the level of the hemidiaphragm (**Fig. 1.1.1**, arrow). No air–fluid level is seen. There is no bony destruction or loss of disc space in the adjacent thoracic spine. The lungs and pleural spaces are clear. The hila appear unremarkable, and the aortic knuckle is to the left of the midline. I would like to compare this with any previous films. Given the clinical history, the opacity is most likely due to a dilated oesophagus. Causes for this include achalasia and malignancy. I would confirm this with a barium swallow examination.

These are two images from a barium study on the same patient (**Fig. 1.1.2**).

These are selected images from a contrast swallow study. A grossly distended oesophagus is seen overlying the mediastinum. There is a transition point in the region of the gastro-oesophageal junction (**Fig. 1.1.2**, arrow) with smooth narrowing into a "bird's beak" (also known as a "rat's tail"). Contrast is seen distally within the stomach. No mucosal abnormalities are identified. I would like to review the remainder of the series. The most likely diagnosis is achalasia, and I would recommend that this patient be referred to the gastroenterology team.

Examination Tips

- Always ask for the full series of films if it is available.
- Check the outline of the oesophagus, and if there is massive dilatation of the oesophagus, consider either achalasia or previous oesophageal resection and colonic bypass.
- Comment on the outline of the oesophagus
  - If it is smooth, consider achalasia.
  - If there is focal irregularity, consider oesophageal malignancy.
  - If diffuse irregularity is present, candidiasis may produce oesophageal dilatation with aperistalsis.
- Always check the stomach as primary gastric carcinoma with gastro-oesophageal stricture may produce a similar appearance.
- Comment on the gastro-oesophageal junction. If it is patulous, this may be from scleroderma or drugs; if it is narrowed, this may indicate achalasia, malignancy, postinflammatory or extrinsic compression.
- Look at the lung fields for evidence of aspiration.

Differential Diagnosis

The imaging appearances shown in **Fig. 1.1.2** are classic for achalasia. However, important differential diagnoses to consider in a case of oesophageal narrowing include:

- Oesophageal malignancy:
  - There is likely to be an irregular contour of the distal oesophagus with possible shouldering present.

- The narrowed distal segment may produce a rat's tail appearance.
- It may occasionally produce imaging findings similar to those of achalasia with a smooth symmetrical narrowing and aperistaltic dilated proximal oesophagus.
- Inflammatory stricture at the gastro-oesophageal junction:
  - Typically, there is smooth narrowing of a short segment of distal oesophagus.
  - Peristalsis is maintained, and the degree of oesophageal dilatation is less than that found in achalasia.
  - Ulcers and thickened mucosal folds may suggest an inflammatory component.

Notes

- Achalasia is a motility disorder with failure of relaxation of the lower oesophageal sphincter.

- Primary achalasia occurs in the 30- to 50-year age group.
- Primary achalasia is an idiopathic process, while secondary achalasia may be caused by malignancy, inflammatory strictures, and scleroderma. The oesophageal dilatation in secondary achalasia (< 4 cm) is typically less than that found in primary achalasia (> 4 cm). The narrowing of the distal oesophagus in secondary achalasia may be irregular, reflecting the underlying cause.
- Primary peristalsis is absent in classic achalasia.
- There is an increased risk of squamous cell carcinoma of the order of 2 to 7%.

Bibliography
Cole TJ, Turner MA. Manifestations of gastrointestinal disease on chest radiographs. Radiographics 1993;13(5):1013–1034
Jang KM, Lee KS, Lee SJ, et al. The spectrum of benign esophageal lesions: imaging findings. Korean J Radiol 2002;3(3):199–210

1.2 Acute Appendicitis

Clinical History

*A 23-year-old man presents with right-sided abdominal pain (**Fig. 1.2.1**).*

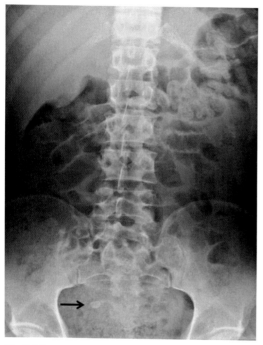

Fig. 1.2.1

Ideal Summary

This is a plain film abdominal radiograph of an adult. Two calcific densities can be seen in the right hemipelvis (**Fig. 1.2.1**, arrow). They do not have the central lucency typical of phleboliths. There are no dilated bowel loops or any evidence of free intraperitoneal gas. The appearances are nonspecific, but, given the clinical history, an important differential diagnosis to consider would be an appendicolith. I would perform an ultrasound examination to assess the right iliac fossa to see if an abnormal appendix could be identified.

*These are two images from the ultrasound examination on the same patient (**Fig. 1.2.2**).*

These are ultrasound images of a blind-ending viscus, likely the appendix, with high reflectivity

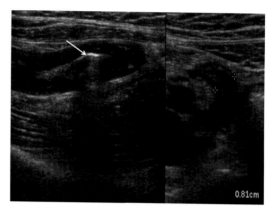

Fig. 1.2.2

centrally (**Fig. 1.2.2**, arrow) and posterior acoustic shadowing that may represent an appendicolith or gas. There is thickening of the appendix wall, with a combined wall thickness greater than 7 mm in diameter (0.81 cm between the callipers). No free fluid is seen. The imaging findings are in keeping with acute appendicitis, and I would urgently refer the patient to the surgical team for consideration for an appendicectomy.

*These are further images from the same patient; a CT examination was performed (**Figs. 1.2.3** and **1.2.4**).*

These are selected axial images of a contrast-enhanced CT examination. There is a calcified appendicolith (**Fig. 1.2.3**, arrow) seen at the base of the appendix, and the appendix itself is distended with fluid

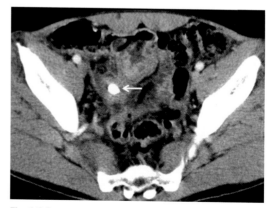

Fig. 1.2.3

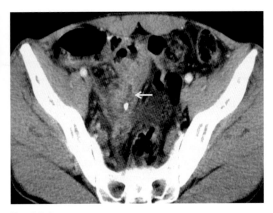

Fig. 1.2.4

(**Fig. 1.2.4**, arrow). There is fat stranding around the appendix with free fluid in the pelvis. There is no evidence of a mass at the appendix level or free gas to suggest a perforation.

Examination Tips

If you are shown a case of appendicitis, be aware of the specific findings within and the limitations of each modality:

- Plain film:
  - Only 5 to 10% of appendicoliths are visible on a plain abdominal film.
  - Appendicitis may result in small bowel obstruction.
  - An appendiceal mass may displace bowel loops away from it and appear as an ill-defined area of increased density.

- Ultrasound:
  - The appendix should be seen as blind-ending and arising from the caecum. It is best seen using a high-frequency linear transducer, especially in children.
  - An appendicolith may be seen as intraluminal high reflectivity with posterior acoustic shadowing, although gas may produce a similar finding.
  - An inflamed appendix is noncompressible, with a combined wall thickness measuring greater than 7 mm; associated free fluid may also be seen.
- CT scanning:
  - Fat stranding and free fluid are often the first clues to locating the abnormality.
  - Always check for adjacent extraluminal free gas.

Differential Diagnosis

In a patient with the features demonstrated above, no differential diagnoses need to be offered.

Notes

- Classic clinical symptoms are periumbilical pain moving to the right iliac fossa. However, atypical signs are seen in one-third of patients.
- Around 95% of patients with acute appendicitis have a raised white blood cell count.

Bibliography

Gaitini D. Imaging acute appendicitis: state of the art. J Clin Imaging Sci 2011;1:49

1.3 Carcinoid Tumour

Clinical History

*A 55-year-old man presents with a history of watery diarrhoea (**Figs. 1.3.1** and **1.3.2**).*

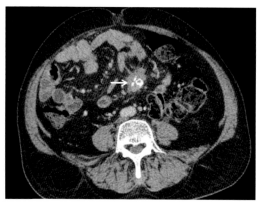

Fig. 1.3.1

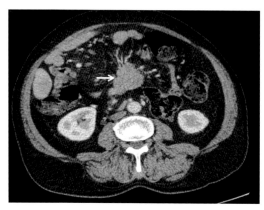

Fig. 1.3.2

Ideal Summary

These are axial CT images through the abdomen with intravenous contrast enhancement. There is a spiculated soft tissue mass, lying centrally, seen within the mesentery and containing focal areas of calcification (**Fig. 1.3.1**, arrow). A desmoplastic reaction is centred on the mesenteric soft tissue (**Fig. 1.3.2**, arrow) with tethering of several small bowel loops. The bowel appears unremarkable. Hazy fat stranding of the adjacent mesentery is also present. The most likely diagnosis is a carcinoid tumour. Given the clinical history, I would like to examine the liver to assess the patient for liver metastases and also look for a possible primary tumour in the bowel.

*Here is further imaging performed on the patient (**Fig. 1.3.3**).*

This is an octreotide nuclear medicine study taken at 24 hours. Several focal areas of increased uptake are seen within the centre of the abdomen, corresponding to the mesenteric mass seen on the CT examination. A smaller focus of increased uptake is seen within the anterior liver. No other sites of abnormal increased uptake are seen. The findings are consistent with a mesenteric carcinoid tumour and liver metastasis. I would like to assess the liver on a biphasic CT.

Examination Tips

When dealing with a mesenteric mass, comment on the following:
- Is the lesion well-defined or irregular?
- Is there spiculation to suggest a desmoplastic reaction?
- When multiple mesenteric masses are present, necrotic change is more in keeping with infection with tuberculosis.
- Calcification may represent treated disease and may be either lymphoma or tuberculosis.
- Look for complications associated with a carcinoid tumour:
  - Tethered small bowel loops, which may cause adhesional small bowel obstruction.
  - Small bowel ischaemia related to mesenteric vessel infiltration.
  - Intussusception with a carcinoid tumour as the lead-point.

Differential Diagnosis

There is no differential diagnosis for the above imaging appearances.

Notes

- Carcinoid tumours are most common in patients aged 50–60 years, and are twice as common in men.

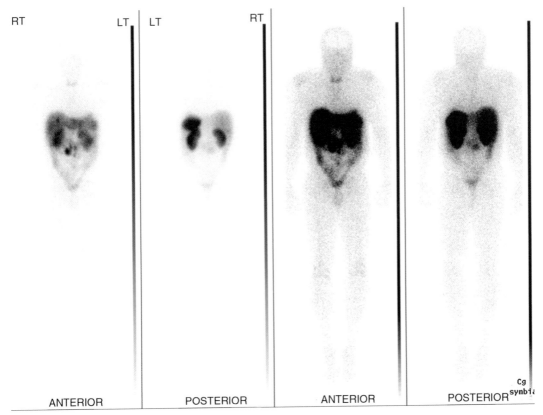

RT · LT · LT · RT

ANTERIOR · POSTERIOR · ANTERIOR · POSTERIOR

Fig. 1.3.3

- Patients with carcinoid tumours are most commonly asymptomatic.
- Carcinoid syndrome occurs in 10% of patients, in the presence of liver metastases, and the patient may experience flushing, watery diarrhoea, and bronchial constriction.
- Carcinoid syndrome is associated with cardiac abnormalities in two-thirds of patients, including pulmonary/tricuspid stenosis or regurgitation; there may be right heart enlargement.
- A total of 30% of carcinoid tumours are multiple.
- The primary gastrointestinal carcinoid tumour is submucosal, and a barium follow-through examination was historically used to detect this, although this was associated with a poor sensitivity when the primary was less than 2 cm in size.
  - Carcinoid tumours may appear as smooth intraluminal defects and may appear as a "target" lesion if there is ulceration.
  - There may be thickening of the mucosal folds caused by the primary tumour.
- With mesenteric involvement and a desmoplastic reaction, there may be tethering and angulation of the small bowel loops.
- A small bowel carcinoid tumour is better depicted on triphasic CT enterography with negative (or neutral) oral contrast, as the submucosal masses are highly vascular.
- Liver metastases are also highly vascular and must be assessed on both arterial and portovenous phase CT imaging.
- Iodine 131-MIBG may be used to detect neuroendocrine tumours such as carcinoid tumours, pheochromocytoma, and neuroblastoma.
- Indium 111-octreotide has a sensitivity of 75% and a specificity of 100% in the detection of carcinoid tumours.

Bibliography

Horton KM, Kamel I, Hofmann L, Fishman EK. Carcinoid tumors of the small bowel: a multitechnique imaging approach. AJR Am J Roentgenol 2004;182(3): 559–567

1.4 Cirrhosis

Clinical History

*A 54-year-old man presents with a history of abdominal pain (**Figs. 1.4.1** and **1.4.2**).*

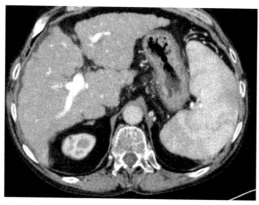

Fig. 1.4.1

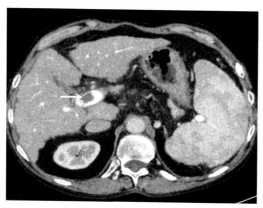

Fig. 1.4.2

Ideal Summary

These are selected axial portal venous phase images through the upper abdomen. The contour of the liver is irregular throughout, and the parenchyma is heterogeneous, but there are no focal intrahepatic lesions. I can see a filling defect within the main portal vein (**Fig. 1.4.2**, arrow) in keeping with a portal vein thrombus. The spleen appears enlarged, but I would like to see a coronal reformat to confirm this. A small volume of ascites is present in a perihepatic distribution. I can see no evidence of variceal formation. The features are in keeping with decompensated liver cirrhosis with portal vein thrombosis. I would refer the patient to the hepatologists for further management.

Examination Tips

In any patient with suspected cirrhosis, look for the following:
- Irregular hepatic contour
- Enlargement of the caudate lobe
- The presence of biliary duct dilatation, which raises the possibility of primary sclerosing cholangitis
- Focal hepatic lesions: hepatocellular carcinoma is a recognised complication
- Portal vein thrombus: also look for a portal vein cavernoma following thrombosis
- Sequelae of portal vein hypertension:
  - Left gastric and oesophageal varices; recanalisation of the umbilical vein within the falciform ligament; venous collaterals in the anterior abdominal wall
  - Mesenteric oedema due to raised venous pressure
  - Splenomegaly
- The presence of ascites, which is suggestive of liver function compromise and decompensation

Differential Diagnosis

There is no differential diagnosis for the above imaging appearances.

Notes

- The liver margin may be smooth, nodular, or lobular; however, this does not correspond to the underlying cause of the cirrhosis.
- The presence of a mass, focal increased arterial enhancement, with portal venous washout and arterio-portal shunt are all suggestive of a hepatocellular carcinoma.

● A transjugular intrahepatic portosystemic stent-shunt will divert flow from the portal venous circulation and into the hepatic vein. This will improve portal hypertension and has a role in the treatment of variceal bleeding.

Bibliography

Brancatelli G, Federle MP, Ambrosini R, et al. Cirrhosis: CT and MR imaging evaluation. Eur J Radiol 2007; 61(1):57–69

1.5 Colorectal Cancer

Clinical History

*A 70-year-old man presents with a history of weight loss (**Figs. 1.5.1** and **1.5.2**).*

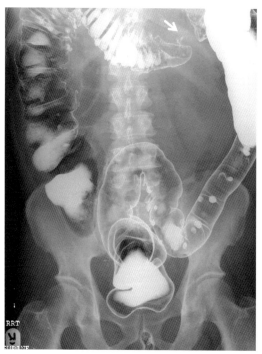

Fig. 1.5.1

Ideal Summary

These are selected images from a barium enema series. There is a short segment of irregular circumferential narrowing in the mid-transverse colon with an "apple core" appearance (**Figs. 1.5.1** and **1.5.2**, arrow). Multiple diverticula are seen throughout the colon. No other lesions are seen in the remainder of the visualised colon, and there is no proximal bowel dilatation present to suggest bowel obstruction. The most likely diagnosis is colorectal carcinoma. I would urgently refer the patient to the surgical team and arrange a staging CT examination.

*This is another case from a different patient, with CT colonoscopy images (**Figs. 1.5.3** and **1.5.4**).*

This is an axial CT colonography image through the abdomen with a three-dimensional intraluminal view. There is a polypoid mass in the right colon (**Fig. 1.5.3**,

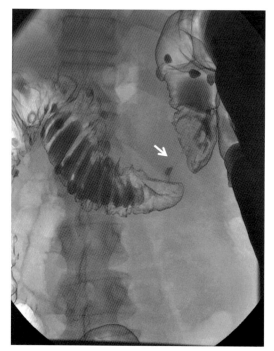

Fig. 1.5.2

arrow), which exhibits a "saddle-shape" morphology on the three-dimensional image (**Fig. 1.5.4**, arrow). I cannot see any soft tissue extending beyond the muscularis propria or enlarged mesenteric or retroperitoneal lymph nodes. I would like to review the remainder of the images. The findings are suspicious for a polyp malignancy. I would ensure a staging CT was performed. At my institution, I would refer the patient for a same-day endoscopy examination and discuss this further at the multidisciplinary meeting.

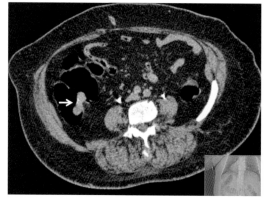

Fig. 1.5.3

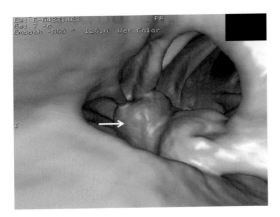

Fig. 1.5.4

Examination Tips

- When assessing a stricture on a barium enema series, look at:
  - The site of the lesion.
  - The configuration of the colon. Has there been previous surgery? Is the site of stricture at an anastomosis?
  - Is it in a watershed area? This raises possibility of ischaemia.
  - Length. Malignant strictures tend to be shorter in length. A longer length stricture may be secondary to colitis, diverticulitis, or ischaemia.
  - Is the stricture smooth or irregular?
  - Are the ends of the stricture tapered or shouldered?
  - Assess for the presence of diverticula.
- In a primary colonic malignancy, look specifically for a synchronous lesion (5%) and polyps (30%).
- Always check for and comment on complications: obstruction, perforation, or invasion into adjacent organs.
- Assess the bones (on the correct window settings) for metastases.
- On CT colonography, polyps that demonstrate the following morphology are suspicious for malignancy:
  - Saddle-shaped lesions
  - Polyps with a central depression
  - Flat polyps: you are unlikely to have this in the examination as it is a difficult lesion to identify.

Differential Diagnosis

There are no differential diagnoses for the above appearances. However, the differentials for a colonic stricture include the following:

- Ischaemic colitis
  - This usually occurs in watershed areas, and there may be evidence of "thumb-printing."
  - A smooth stricture on barium enema with tapered margins may be seen in chronic cases.
- Diverticulitis
  - This is most often seen in the sigmoid colon and is usually a long (> 5 cm) segment of luminal narrowing on a background of multiple diverticula.
- Extrinsic pathology
  - There is smooth narrowing making obtuse angles with bowel wall, usually on the anti-mesenteric border of the colon.
  - Causes for this include endometriosis and ovarian malignancy.

Notes

Around 25% of colorectal carcinoma occurs in the sigmoid colon, 20% in the rectum, and 15% in the transverse and ascending colon.

Regarding colorectal cancer screening in the UK:

- Offered to men and women aged 60 to 69 years every 2 years (extending up to 75 years in some areas).
- If there is a positive faecal occult blood test, the individual is referred for colonoscopy.
- CT colonography is offered when:
  - Colonoscopy has been incomplete
  - The patient is unfit or unsuitable for colonoscopy
  - The patient refuses colonoscopy.

CT Colonography

- Look for a rectal insufflation tube to confirm the type of study.
- Depending on the institution, the study may involve a low radiation dose with or without intravenous contrast.
- Oral contrast produces a "faecally tagged" study.
- Reconstruction of the CT data may be used to produce a three-dimensional volume-rendered intraluminal image – "virtual endoscopy."

Bibliography

Dighe S, Swift I, Brown G. CT staging of colon cancer. Clin Radiol 2008;63(12):1372–1379

http://www.cancerscreening.nhs.uk/bowel/index.html (accessed Nov 2012)

1.6 Crohn's Disease

Clinical History

A 33-year-old man presents with abdominal bloating and pain (**Fig. 1.6.1**).

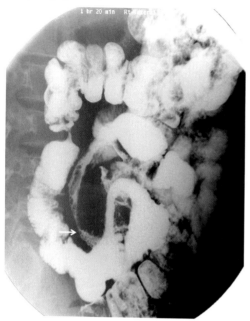

Fig. 1.6.1

Ideal Summary

This is a selected image from a barium follow-through study. There are several loops of abnormal distal small bowel that are narrowed with "cobble-stoning" and linear ulceration (**Fig. 1.6.1**, arrow) separated by shorter distended loops of ileum. The distal ileal loops show separation. No definite fistulas are seen. The appearances of the right colon are suggestive of previous resection with a short segment of narrowing at the ileocolonic anastomosis, although contrast is seen within the colon. The features are consistent with active Crohn's disease. I would like to assess the remainder of the series and any old films.

Examination Tips

In a case with Crohn's disease, comment on:
- Location. Although Crohn's disease can occur anywhere along the gastrointestinal tract, there is usually involvement of the terminal ileum with small bowel involvement. Describe where exactly the abnormalities are: proximal, mid, or distal small bowel, terminal ileum, or colon
- Distribution. Are there skip lesions, and are the abnormalities aymmetrical?
- Luminal narrowing. Is there any contrast downstream of the narrowing; is there any pre-stenotic bowel dilatation?
- Ulceration. Are there aphthous ulcers that appear as target lesions, linear ulcers that cross perpendicular to the folds, fissuring, or cobble-stoning?
- Fistula formation: enteroenteric, enterocolonic, or enterocutaneous
- Bowel loop separation
- Obstruction: upstream bowel dilatation
- Evidence of previous operations
- Associations with Crohn's disease: gallstones or sacroiliitis; comment if these are present on the barium image.

Differential Diagnosis

No differential diagnoses should be given in a case of classic Crohn's disease. However, if there is only isolated terminal ileal abnormality, the following should be considered:
- Lymphoma
- Tuberculosis
- "Backwash" ileitis with ulcerative colitis
- Ischaemia

Notes

- There is an equal male to female distribution.
- Two peaks in incidence occur at ages 15 to 25 and 60 to 70 years.
- Small bowel follow-through was historically frequently used in the diagnosis of Crohn's disease, but this is now being replaced by CT and MR enterography
  - A small bowel follow-through and CT enterography are able to detect mucosal abnormalities.
  - A small bowel follow-through and MRI cine loops help provide functional and dynamic information such as peristalsis and the presence of small bowel adhesions.
  - It may help estimate the extent of the disease and the length of remaining bowel.

- It may be used to map small bowel fistulas associated with Crohn's disease.

Bibliography

Nolan DJ, Gourtsoyiannis NC. Crohn's disease of the small intestine: a review of the radiological appearances in 100 consecutive patients examined by a barium infusion technique. Clin Radiol 1980;31(5):597–603

Sinha R, Murphy P, Hawker P, Sanders S, Rajesh A, Verma R. Role of MRI in Crohn's disease. Clin Radiol 2009;64(4):341–352

1.7 Focal Nodular Hyperplasia

Clinical History

*A 35-year-old asymptomatic woman (**Fig. 1.7.1**).*

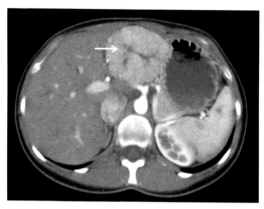

Fig. 1.7.1

Ideal Summary

This is a selected axial arterial-phase CT image through the upper abdomen. There is an enhancing lesion in the left lobe of the liver, with a central low-density scar and radiating septa (**Fig. 1.7.1**, arrow). There are no other liver lesions. There are no features to suggest liver cirrhosis. The most likely diagnosis is focal nodular hyperplasia (FNH), and other differential diagnoses would include hepatic adenoma and hepatic malignancy. I would like to ask if there is any venous-phase imaging to confirm my diagnosis.

*This is the venous-phase CT image at the same level (**Fig. 1.7.2**).*

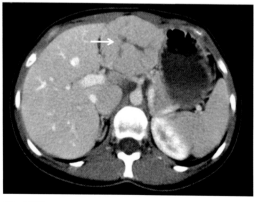

Fig. 1.7.2

The venous-phase CT image demonstrates an enhancement pattern within the lesion, which is isodense or slightly hypodense to the liver. The central scar remains of low density with no evidence of enhancement (**Fig. 1.7.2**, arrow). The features are consistent with a diagnosis of FNH.

Examination Tips

When dealing with liver lesions, ask yourself the following questions:
- Is it single or multiple? Multiple lesions will favour metastatic disease, while a single lesion is more likely hepatic adenoma, FNH, or fibrolamellar hepatocellular carcinoma (HCC).
- Is there homogeneous or heterogeneous enhancement? Homogeneous lesions include FNH or smaller hepatic adenoma, while malignancy must be excluded in heterogeneous enhancing lesions.
- Is there a scar? If so, it is more likely to be FNH or fibrolamellar HCC.
- Is there background hepatic cirrhosis? If yes, HCC should be the primary diagnosis, unless there is strong evidence to suggest otherwise.
- What is the enhancement pattern?
  - Arterial phase: FNH, hepatic adenoma, HCC, and neuroendocrine metastases are hyperenhancing. Other metastases are usually hypodense to liver.
  - Portal venous phase: hepatic adenoma and FNH are usually isodense compared with liver; malignancies are usually hypodense to liver.
  - Delayed phase: FNH and fibrolamellar HCC are isodense to liver; hepatic adenoma, HCC, and metastases are hypodense compared with liver.
  - Is there disruption to (haemorrhage of) the lesion? This favours hepatic adenoma or HCC.
  - Extrahepatic primary tumour: look specifically for this.

Differential Diagnosis

The diagnostic possibilities for an arterial-phase enhancing lesion include:
- Hepatic adenoma:
  - Heterogeneous enhancement on arterial phase
  - Variable enhancement on portal venous phase
  - May be associated with disruption (haemorrhage)

- Fibrolamellar HCC:
  - Usually very large and heterogeneous
  - Presence of metastatic deposits in 70% of cases
- Metastases:
  - Usually multiple and in an older population
  - Washout during the portal venous phase
- "Flash" haemangioma: a lesion that fills rapidly and not visibly from the periphery:
  - Should continue to enhance on delayed-phase imaging

Notes

- Focal nodular hyperplasia is the second most common benign liver tumour.
- There is usually only a single lesion in 80% of cases.
- Oral contraceptives do not cause FNH but have a positive effect on its growth.
- The lesion contains both hepatocytes and non-communicating biliary structures.
  - Gadolinium BOPTA (gadobenate dimeglumine) is excreted by the biliary epithelium.
  - It produces delayed and persistent enhancement on MRI.
  - This may help differentiate FNH from hepatic adenoma, which will typically not enhance on a hepatocyte-specific phase with gadolinium BOPTA.

- Approximately 20% of FNHs are atypical.
  - This includes telangiectatic FNH, which does not have a central scar, demonstrates persistent enhancement, and exhibits a high T1 and T2 signal on MRI.
  - However, atypical FNH still comprises biliary epithelium, and gadolinium BOPTA scanning may help in differentiating.
- Ultrasound findings:
  - It is homogeneous and isoechoic to liver, with a hypoechoic central scar.
  - It may demonstrate a "spoke-wheel" pattern on colour Doppler imaging.
  - Contrast-enhanced ultrasound demonstrates the classical "spoke-wheel" pattern and persisting enhancement into the late portovenous phase.
- MRI findings:
  - Tumour parenchyma: T1 $\downarrow$/$\leftrightarrow$, T2 $\uparrow$/$\leftrightarrow$
  - Central scar: T1 $\downarrow$, T2 $\leftrightarrow$
  - Postcontrast: hyperintense on the arterial phase, and then isointense on the venous phase.

Bibliography

Kehagias D, Moulopoulos L, Antoniou A, et al. Focal nodular hyperplasia: imaging findings. Eur Radiol 2001;11(2):202–212

1.8 Gallstone Fistula

Clinical History

*A 49-year-old woman presents with a history of abdominal pain and vomiting (**Fig. 1.8.1**).*

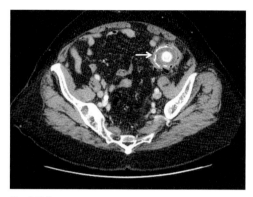

Fig. 1.8.2

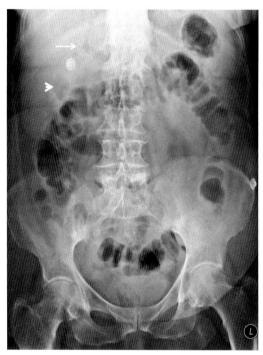

Fig. 1.8.1

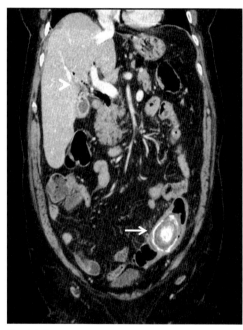

Fig. 1.8.3

Ideal Summary

This is a plain abdominal film. I can see branching lucencies projected over the liver centrally that are likely biliary in origin (**Fig. 1.8.1**, arrow). There is also an ovoid lucency more laterally and may represent gas within the gallbladder (**Fig.1.8.1**, arrowhead). There are no dilated loops of small bowel, and the colon is gas-filled and of normal calibre. There is no free gas. I cannot see any focal calcification that would correspond to a gallstone. The differential diagnoses for biliary gas include previous intervention and gallstone fistula. Are there any old films available for comparison? I would discuss the case with the referring team, and an abdominal CT may be necessary to confirm the diagnosis.

*These are two images from the abdominal CT examination (**Figs. 1.8.2** and **1.8.3**).*

These are axial and coronal images of a venous-phase CT through the abdomen. A large, calcified gallstone is seen in the region of the proximal sigmoid colon, with surrounding fat stranding (**Figs. 1.8.2** and **1.8.3**, arrows). The colon and small bowel upstream of this are not distended. There is no free gas. On the coronal image, there is gas within the biliary system without overt biliary duct dilatation (**Fig. 1.8.3**, arrowhead). Some fluid is seen around the gallbladder, but there is no associated fat stranding. The pancreas appears unremarkable. The findings are in keeping with a biliary fistula secondary to a gallstone. I would inform the surgical team of these results.

Examination Tips

Rigler's triad of small bowel obstruction, biliary gas, and ectopic radiopaque gallstone is rarely seen, and the candidate will usually be shown two of the three signs on a plain abdominal film. When gas is identified within the liver, it is important to differentiate biliary gas from portal venous gas, as the implications for the patient are substantial. Gas in the biliary tree is typically near the hilum, carried there by the flow of bile, in contradistinction to portal venous gas, which is peripheral:

- Aerobilia: recent endoscopic retrograde cholangiopancreatography (ERCP), sphincterotomy, biliary stent, biliary surgery (such as hepaticojejunostomy)
- Portal venous gas: ischaemic bowel, or occasionally secondary to pneumatosis coli

Differential Diagnosis

Gas within the biliary system may arise from several different causes:

- Sphincterotomy: from previous ERCP
- Surgical intervention: hepaticojejunostomy may result in biliary gas

- Emphysematous cholecystitis: from gas-forming organisms within the biliary tract. The patient will present with a septic clinical picture.
- Biliary fistula

Notes

- Gallstones are found in 8% of the population, most commonly in the 40- to 60-year-old age group.
- Around 10% of gallstones can be visualised with conventional radiographs.
- Approximately 95% of all gallstones can be identified by ultrasound, while CT has a sensitivity of only 80 to 85%.
- Gallstones can occasionally erode through the gallbladder wall and create a fistulous tract, usually into the duodenum, although the stomach and colon may be involved. Gas may enter the biliary system via the fistulous connection, giving rise to the branching linear lucencies.
- Large gallstones are often trapped at the ileocaecal valve, causing obstruction, but obstruction may occur at any point along the bowel.

Bibliography

Chou JW, Hsu CH, Liao KF, et al. Gallstone ileus: report of two cases and review of the literature. World J Gastroenterol 2007;13(8):1295–1298

Summerton SL, Hollander AC, Stassi J, Rosenberg HK, Carroll SF. US case of the day. Gallstone ileus. Radiographics 1995;15(2):493–495

1.9 Gastric Carcinoma

Clinical History

A 65-year-old man presents with a history of dyspepsia (Fig. 1.9.1).

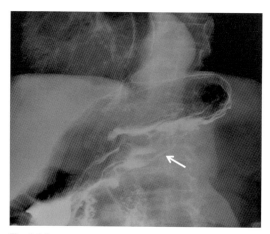

Fig. 1.9.1

Ideal Summary

This is a selected image from a barium meal series. There is mucosal irregularity and nodularity, with thickened folds involving the gastric antrum and body, along the greater curvature (**Fig. 1.9.1**, arrow). The stomach does not distend in this region, and contrast passes distally into the proximal duodenum. The gastro-oesophageal junction appears to be spared. There is no destructive bony abnormality. The appearances are in keeping with a diagnosis of linitis plastica, most likely related to gastric carcinoma. I would like to review the rest of the barium series, and I would recommend an endoscopy and a staging CT examination.

This is a CT image from the same patient (Fig. 1.9.2).

This is a selected axial image from a venous-phase CT examination. There is nodular thickening of the gastric wall posteriorly at the level of the body of the stomach (**Fig. 1.9.2**, arrow). There is surrounding fat stranding, but no definite peritoneal nodularity is seen. There is evidence of lymph node enlargement around the aorta. There are several enlarged lymph

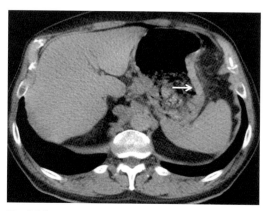

Fig. 1.9.2

nodes adjacent to the lesser curve. An area of low density is seen peripherally in the left lateral lobe of the liver, which likely represents focal fatty infiltration. The stomach abuts the spleen, but there is no definite evidence of involvement on this image. These findings are consistent with a diagnosis of gastric adenocarcinoma with nodal involvement. I would like to review the rest of the CT series to look for evidence of metastatic disease.

Examination Tips

When reviewing the stomach on CT, look for the following:

- Is the abnormality a discrete mass or diffuse thickening? If this is an exophytic mass, think of a gastrointestinal stromal tumour; if there is marked diffuse mural thickening, consider lymphoma.
- Which part of the stomach is the abnormality centred on? If it involves the gastro-oesophageal junction, is there oesophageal dilatation; if it involves the pylorus or antrum, is there gastric outlet obstruction?
- Is there evidence of direct invasion of the adjacent organs or abdominal wall? Look specifically for involvement of the aorta, adrenals, pancreas, spleen, and bowel.
- Is there metastatic disease or peritoneal disease? Look for peritoneal nodularity and thickening, best seen on CT coronal reformats.

Differential Diagnosis

Although scirrhous gastric adenocarcinoma is the most likely cause of linitis plastica, other less common differential diagnoses include:

- Breast and lung metastases
- Lymphoma
- Radiotherapy

Notes

Gastric adenocarcinoma accounts for over 95% of malignant tumours of the stomach.

Bibliography

Hargunani R, Maclachlan J, Kaniyur S, Power N, Pereira SP, Malhotra A. Cross-sectional imaging of gastric neoplasia. Clin Radiol 2009;64(4):420–429

1.10 Gastrointestinal Stromal Cell Tumour

Clinical History

A 55-year-old woman presents with abdominal pain (**Figs. 1.10.1** and **1.10.2**).

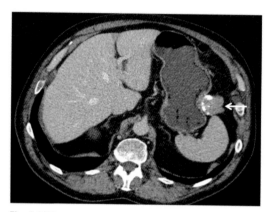

Fig. 1.10.1

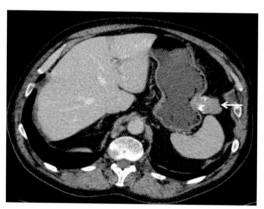

Fig. 1.10.2

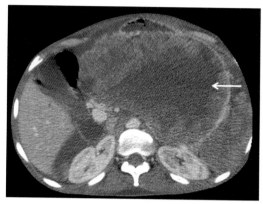

Fig. 1.10.3

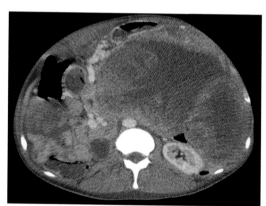

Fig. 1.10.4

Ideal Summary

These are selected postcontrast CT images through the upper abdomen. There is an exophytic soft tissue mass arising from the greater curve of the body of the stomach (**Figs. 1.10.1** and **1.10.2**, arrows). There are multiple foci of calcification within the mass, and the adjacent stomach wall is slightly thickened. I cannot see any enlarged lymph nodes in the region of the mass or around the coeliac axis. There are no focal intrahepatic lesions. The most likely differential is a gastrointestinal stromal cell tumour (GIST). I would like to review the rest of the CT images for

evidence of distant disease, and I would refer the patient for discussion at a gastrointestinal multidisciplinary meeting.

These are images from another patient with an abdominal mass (**Figs. 1.10.3** and **1.10.4**).

These are selected postcontrast CT images through the abdomen. There is a large, well-circumscribed mass taking up most of the abdominal cavity (**Fig. 1.10.3**, arrow). The mass is centred on the left upper quadrant and is causing mass effect, displacing the bowel. The mass itself is heterogeneous, being predominantly necrotic centrally with peripheral soft tissue density. No focal calcification is present. Inferiorly, the mass appears to be lobulated. There is ascites. The bowel is mostly collapsed. I cannot see any enlarged mesenteric lymph nodes. I would like to review the remainder of the CT images for evidence of distant disease. The imaging findings are of a large intra-abdominal mass arising from the left upper quadrant. The differential diagnosis includes GIST and lymphoma. I would like to correlate this with any previous images and the clinical history. I would take this further by offering percutaneous biopsy of the abnormal mass.

Examination Tips

When dealing with a large intra-abdominal mass, consider the following:
- Try to identify the area of the abdomen the mass appears to be centred on or arising from. Is the mass arising from the pelvis? Are the bowel loops pushed to one side? Are the retroperitoneal structures lifted anteriorly?
- Once you have localised the mass, think about the structures that lie there anatomically:
  - Bowel. If there is evidence of bowel obstruction, think of bowel malignancy.
  - Solid organs. Look at the contour for distortion.
  - Lymph nodes. Look for multiple enlarged masses with possible central necrosis.
  - Mesenchymal origin, that is, sarcomas. These are rare, but you need to consider this diagnosis if you are uncertain about the origin of the mass.
  - Vascular. Is the mass an aortic aneurysm? Look closely at the vascular structures, particularly if this is not an image from the arterial-phase CT examination.
- Describe the mass in detail: size, homogeneity, calcification, enhancement, and relationship to other structures.

- Complications of masses:
  - Compressive effect: on bowel, vessels, ureters, and other abdominal structures.
  - Invasion of adjacent structures.
- Metastatic disease, look for evidence of a primary or suggest that this may be the cause if the intra-abdominal mass is indeterminate.

Differential Diagnosis

- Lymphoma: expect to see enlarged abdominal lymph nodes.
- Pancreatic pseudocyst: look for pancreatic calcification as a marker for previous pancreatitis.
- Sarcoma arising from the retroperitoneum should be considered.

Notes

GIST:
- Is a mesenchymal neoplasm and is distinct from leiomyomas.
- Affects patients aged over 45 years.
- Occurs in the stomach in two-thirds of patients.
- GIST is associated with metastases to the liver and lungs, but not with regional lymph nodes. If enlarged regional lymph nodes are present, GIST is unlikely.

Bibliography

Chourmouzi D, Sinakos E, Papalavrentios L, Akriviadis E, Drevelegas A. Gastrointestinal stromal tumors: a pictorial review. J Gastrointestin Liver Dis 2009;18(3):379–383

1.11 Cavernous Haemangioma

Clinical History

A 52-year-old woman presents with abdominal discomfort (**Fig. 1.11.1**).

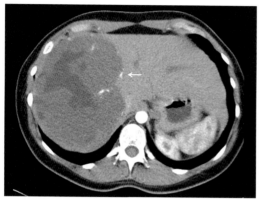

Fig. 1.11.1

Ideal Summary

This is a selected axial arterial-phase CT image through the upper abdomen. There is a large, irregularly shaped lesion taking up the majority of the right lobe. The lesion is of intermediate density with central low density and no calcification. There is peripheral nodular and discontinuous high density (**Fig. 1.11.1**, arrow). I can see no other lesions. There is no CT evidence of cirrhosis. The differential diagnosis for these appearances includes a giant haemangioma or malignancy. I would like to ask if any delayed imaging is available.

This is a delayed CT image (**Fig. 1.11.2**).

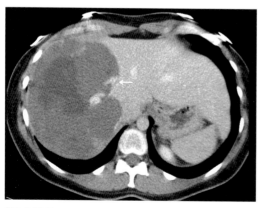

Fig. 1.11.2

This is a venous-phase CT image of the same patient. There now appears to be progressive peripheral enhancement (**Fig.1.11.2**, arrow). The most likely diagnosis is a giant hepatic haemangioma.

Examination Tips

Haemangiomas classically demonstrate centripetal "filling in" on the venous and delayed phases. However, the central scar does not enhance. It is essential that venous-phase and/or a delayed-phase CT image is obtained. You cannot conclusively say that there is "filling in" on a single phase. If there is uncertainty, ask for delayed-phase images.

Differential Diagnosis

There are no differential diagnoses for the above appearances. However, where only a single phase of imaging has been provided and it is unclear whether there is centripetal "filling in," the possibility of an atypical haemangioma may be raised (progressive centrifugal [in to out] filling on the venous and delayed phases).

Notes

Giant hepatic haemangioma:
- Is most common in postmenopausal women
- Is defined as being larger than 10 cm
- Shows calcification in only 10% of cases, this usually being in the central scar
- On MRI there is:
  - Low T1 signal: the central scar has a markedly lower T1 signal
  - High T2 signal: the central scar has a markedly higher T2 signal
  - Sometimes there are low T2 signal internal septations.
  - Progressive centripetal filling on contrast-enhanced images.
  - A nonenhancing central scar
- On ultrasound imaging:
  - Giant haemangiomas often do not demonstrate the classical increased reflectivity.
  - Colour Doppler ultrasound is disappointing as no flow is seen in the lesion.

- On contrast-enhanced ultrasound, the slow peripheral globular enhancement and "infilling" is striking and often establishes the diagnosis.

Bibliography

Caseiro-Alves F, Brito J, Araujo AE, et al. Liver haemangioma: common and uncommon findings and how to improve the differential diagnosis. Eur Radiol 2007;17(6):1544–1554

1.12 Hydatid Disease

Clinical History

*A 40-year-old woman presents with a history of abdominal pain (**Fig. 1.12.1**).*

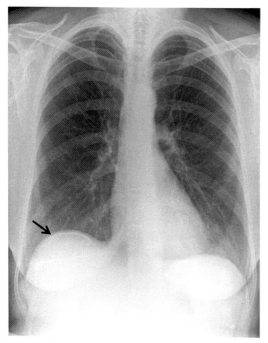

Fig. 1.12.1

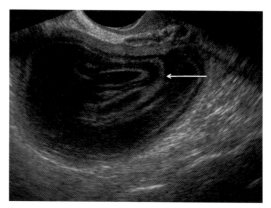

Fig. 1.12.2

*This is an image from the ultrasound examination (**Fig. 1.12.2**).*

This is an ultrasound image from a liver examination demonstrating a hypoechoic cyst with a surrounding hyperechoic wall. Multiple detached membranes (**Fig. 1.12.2**, arrow) are seen within the cyst, representing the "water lily" sign. This is pathognomonic of hydatid disease.

*This is a CT image from the same patient (**Fig. 1.12.3**).*

This is a selected arterial-phase axial image through the upper abdomen. Two well-circumscribed, rounded low-density masses are seen within the liver. Each of these masses has smaller lower density cysts along the periphery (**Fig. 1.12.3**, arrows). There is no

Ideal Summary

This is a frontal chest radiograph of a woman. There is curvilinear calcification (**Fig. 1.12.1**, arrow) seen below the right hemidiaphragm, which follows the shape of the hemidiaphragm. The right hemidiaphragm is not greatly elevated, and the right lung base is clear. No similar abnormality is seen beneath the left diaphragm, and there is no subdiaphragmatic free gas.

The curvilinear calcification is most likely related to the liver, and my primary diagnosis is a calcified wall of a cyst, with a hydatid cyst a consideration. I would like to compare this with any old films and to confirm the diagnosis with an ultrasound examination.

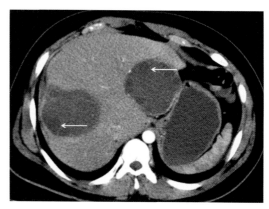

Fig. 1.12.3

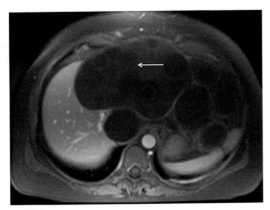

Fig. 1.12.4

lesions. If the picture is more subtle, it is easier to assess peritoneal surfaces on coronal reconstruction of the CT examination.

- Check the lungs for pulmonary lesions and also for cyst rupture into the pleural cavity.
- The cyst itself may cause a mass effect with upstream biliary duct dilatation or portal vein thrombosis.

Differential Diagnosis

The appearance of a main cyst with daughter cysts and the "water lily" sign are pathognomonic.

Notes

Hydatid disease is caused by the tapeworm *Echinococcus* spp., but negative serology does not exclude hydatid disease. There is nearly always a history of residence in an endemic area.

Ultrasound findings may vary, but include:
- A double cyst wall: two hyperechoic walls separated by a hypoechoic layer
- The presence of daughter cysts and the "water lily" sign (floating detached wall membranes), which are pathognomonic
- Daughter cysts that may be mobile and whose location can change depending on the patient's position
- An anechoic cyst with hydatid "sand" that is dependent

MR imaging findings:
- Main cyst: usually T1 intermediate/T2 high signal.
- Daughter cysts: less T1 signal intensity than the main cyst, with high T2 signal.
- Rim: low T1 and T2 signal intensity due to its fibrous nature.
- Postcontrast: enhancement of the wall and septations.

intrahepatic duct dilatation. The appearances are of hydatid disease with daughter cysts. I would like to assess the remainder of the study to look for complications known to be associated with hydatid disease.

This is an MR image from the same patient (**Fig. 1.12.4**).

This is a T1-weighted contrast-enhanced MR image of the liver. Multiple cysts are seen within the upper abdomen, with a large dominant cyst taking up most of the left lobe of the liver. The cysts are of T1 low signal, and the daughter cysts of lower T1 signal intensity (**Fig. 1.12.4**, arrow). Several cysts are seen in the left upper quadrant anterior to the spleen without definable liver parenchyma seen around them and may represent peritoneal seeding. The imaging findings are characteristic of hydatid disease.

Examination Tips

Once a diagnosis of hydatid disease is reached, it is important to assess the possible complications arising from this infection:

- Cyst rupture can occur.
- Biliary communication. This occurs in up to 90% of cases. Look for intraductal echogenic material on ultrasound and high density on CT images.
- Infected cyst. There will be low density around the cyst with irregular or ill-defined walls and possible stranding in the perihepatic fat. If the imaging findings are suggestive of acute inflammation, ask if there is a history of sepsis.
- Peritoneal seeding. Check for peritoneal nodularity. There may be large, obvious peritoneal cystic

Bibliography

Doyle DJ, Hanbidge AE, O'Malley ME. Imaging of hepatic infections. Clin Radiol 2006;61(9):737–748

Pedrosa I, Saíz A, Arrazola J, Ferreirós J, Pedrosa CS. Hydatid disease: radiologic and pathologic features and complications. Radiographics 2000;20(3):795–817

1.13 Liver Trauma

Clinical History

*A 25-year-old man who was involved in a knife stabbing (**Figs. 1.13.1** and **1.13.2**).*

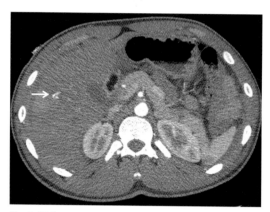

Fig. 1.13.1

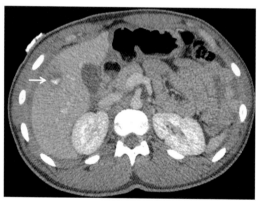

Fig. 1.13.2

Ideal Summary

These are selected axial images through the upper abdomen in both arterial and venous phases. Linear high density is seen in the right lobe on the arterial phase (**Fig. 1.13.1**, arrow), with pooling of contrast on the venous phase (**Fig. 1.13.2**, arrow). This is surrounded by low density on the venous phase, and there is perihepatic haematoma. No intraperitoneal free gas is seen. The kidneys and pancreas appear unremarkable. I would discuss this patient's case urgently with the surgical team and interventional radiologist.

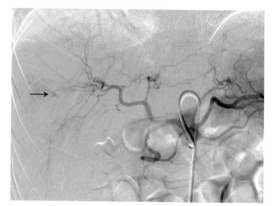

Fig. 1.13.3

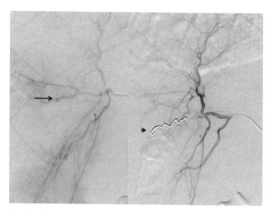

Fig. 1.13.4

*The patient was referred for angiography. These are some images from the procedure (**Figs. 1.13.3** and **1.13.4**).*

These are selected images of a digital subtraction angiogram. On the coeliac axis run, there is a small blush in the right anterior sectoral branch of the right hepatic artery (**Fig. 1.13.3**, arrow). Selective catheterisation of the right hepatic artery confirms contrast extravasation (**Fig. 1.13.4**, arrow). No evidence of ongoing haemorrhage is seen on the post-embolisation site (**Fig. 1.13.4**, arrowhead).

*This is a CT image of a different patient, a 30-year-old man, following a road traffic accident (**Figs. 1.13.5** and **1.13.6**).*

These are selected venous-phase axial CT images through the upper abdomen. I note the presence of bilateral chest drains. There is a linear

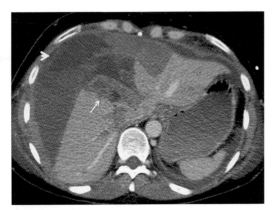

Fig. 1.13.5

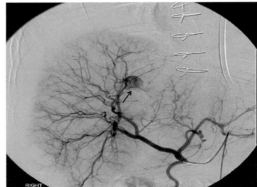

Fig. 1.13.7

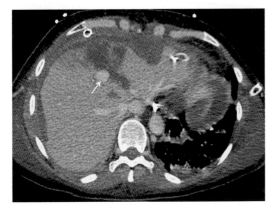

Fig. 1.13.6

laceration through the liver between the right and left lobes that extends up to the inferior vena cava (**Fig. 1.13.5**, arrow). This is associated with a large subcapsular haematoma of mixed density (**Fig. 1.13.5**, arrowhead). On the second axial image, there is a rounded enhancing opacity adjacent to the laceration (**Fig. 1.13.6**, arrow), which is suspicious for contrast extravasation, but I would like to confirm this by comparing it with the arterial-phase scan. No intraperitoneal free gas is seen. I would like to review the chest and remainder of the abdomen to identify any other injuries. I would then urgently discuss the case with the interventional radiologist for angiography with a view to embolisation.

This is an image from the angiographic procedure (**Fig. 1.13.7**).

This is an angiographic image of a coeliac axis run. A rounded opacity can be seen arising from a right lobe hepatic artery, representing ongoing haemorrhage (**Fig. 1.13.7**, arrow). No other sites of bleeding are seen.

Examination Tips

Features of liver trauma to identify include:
- Intraperitoneal blood and/or subcapsular haematoma, with effacement of the underlying liver parenchyma
- The shape and extent of the laceration: linear, branching, or stellate? Does it extend through to the opposite margin or involve the porta hepatis?
- Evidence of ongoing haemorrhage: the presence of contrast extravasation on the arterial phase, with pooling of contrast on the venous phase
- Lacerations that involve the bare area of the liver, which may be complicated by retroperitoneal haemorrhage
- Always check adjacent organs for injury and intraperitoneal free gas as a marker for bowel injury

Differential Diagnosis

There are no differential diagnoses for these imaging appearances.

Notes

The use of CT imaging before an interventional procedure is now an accepted imaging strategy with the advent of "fast" scanning times and the location of the CT scanner close to the emergency room and angiographic suites. Intervention is rarely performed without CT imaging as this localises the site and extent of the injury and allows targeted intervention.

Bibliography

Yoon W, Jeong YY, Kim JK, et al. CT in blunt liver trauma. Radiographics 2005;25(1):87–104

1.14 Lymphoma

Clinical History

*A 65-year-old man presents with a 6-month history of weight loss (**Fig. 1.14.1**).*

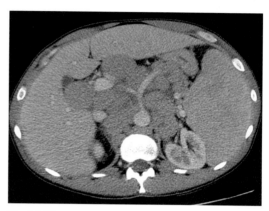

Fig. 1.14.2

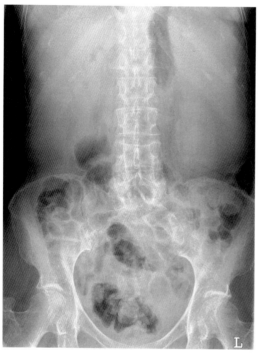

Fig. 1.14.1

*This is a CT image from the same patient (**Fig. 1.14.2**).*

This is a selected axial venous-phase CT image. Multiple enlarged lymph nodes are seen around the coeliac axis and in the retroperitoneal region. The lymph nodes do not show central low density. The spleen appears to be enlarged, with no focal lesions. These features are highly suggestive of a diagnosis of lymphoma, and I would urgently refer the patient to the haematology department. I would also ensure that the patient has had the appropriate CT neck and chest imaging for lymphoma staging.

Ideal Summary

This is a plain abdominal film of an adult. There is increased soft tissue density seen in the left upper quadrant, representing an enlarged spleen, and appearances on the right suggest that the liver may also be enlarged. There is no calcification of the liver or of the spleen. The bowel gas has been displaced inferiorly. I cannot see any bony abnormality. This is a patient with splenomegaly, and the differential diagnosis includes lymphoma, leukaemia, and myelofibrosis. I would like to ask if any old films are available for comparison. I would suggest an ultrasound for confirmation of an enlarged spleen, and would undertake a staging CT examination following referral to the haematology department.

Examination Tips

It is important to identify the sites of disease and complications in lymphoma:
- Sites—as this affects staging:
  - Enlarged lymph nodes are often the first, and sometimes only, manifestation of lymphoma in radiology.
  - However, you must always look for other sites of involvement, such as the spleen (focal lesions or diffuse enlargement), liver, bowel, and bones.
- Complications—as this affects management:
  - These include infarction (spleen, liver, and kidneys) and venous thrombosis (lower limbs and portal vein) from a mass effect.

Differential Diagnosis

The list for the differential diagnosis for splenomegaly is long, but includes:

- Myelofibrosis:
  - This is characterised by bone marrow fibrosis, extramedullary haematopoiesis, and splenomegaly. The most common imaging findings include hepatosplenomegaly, osteosclerosis, and lymphadenopathy.
- Leukaemia:
  - This may demonstrate multiple enlarged lymph nodes, but these are usually smaller than in lymphoma.
  - Look for evidence of complicating haemorrhage in the absence of trauma.
- Storage disease:
  - Gaucher's disease may produce massive splenomegaly extending into the pelvis.
- Sickle cell disease:
  - A younger age group is affected.
- Splenic sequestration produces a heterogeneous appearance with areas of infarction (hypodense) and haemorrhage (hyperdense).
  - The spleen usually infarcts and involutes with age in sickle cell disease.
- Portal hypertension:
  - This is associated with cirrhosis: look for varices, portal vein thrombosis, and ascites.

Notes

- Lymphoma is the most common malignant tumour of the spleen.
- The spleen is categorised as "nodal" in Hodgkin's lymphoma and "extranodal" in non-Hodgkin's lymphoma.

Bibliography

Thomas AG, Vaidhyanath R, Kirke R, Rajesh A. Extranodal lymphoma from head to toe. Part 2: The trunk and extremities. AJR Am J Roentgenol 2011;197(2):357–364

1.15 Pancreatic Adenocarcinoma

Clinical History

A 59-year-old man presents with a history of abdominal pain (Figs. 1.15.1−1.15.5).

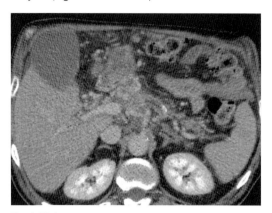

Fig. 1.15.1

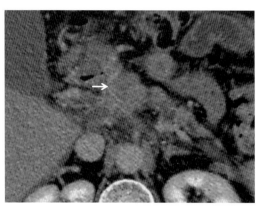

Fig. 1.15.2

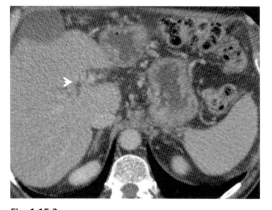

Fig. 1.15.3

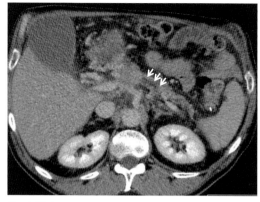

Fig. 1.15.4

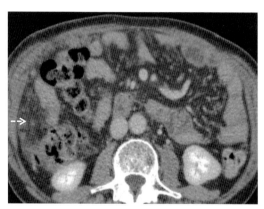

Fig. 1.15.5

Ideal Summary

These are selected axial venous-phase CT images through the upper abdomen. There is a mass in the pancreatic head of slightly lower density than the rest of the pancreas (**Fig. 1.15.2**, arrow). There is intra- and extrahepatic biliary duct dilatation (**Fig. 1.15.3**, arrowhead) and pancreatic duct dilatation to the level of the mass (**Fig. 1.15.4**, short arrows). The pancreas distal to the mass is atrophic. The portal vein is opacified, but the portosystemic confluence is effaced by the mass and multiple portosystemic varices are seen. No focal liver lesions or enlarged lymph nodes are seen. On the lower slices, there are multiple peritoneal soft tissue nodules with surrounding fat stranding (**Fig. 1.15.5**, dashed arrow). The most likely diagnosis is pancreatic malignancy with peritoneal metastatic disease. I would complete the examination by assessing the arterial-phase images and the chest for evidence of metastatic disease. I would refer the patient's case for discussion at a multidisciplinary meeting.

Examination Tips

The pancreas should be assessed in both the pancreatic (45 s) and venous (60 s) phases. There is maximal enhancement of the pancreatic parenchyma at a time intermediate to the arterial and portal venous phases. However, an arterial phase is often used in lieu of the pancreatic phase. Assessment of a pancreatic adenocarcinoma involves the following:

- Identification of the mass. The majority are hypodense relative to the pancreas, although up to 40% are isodense depending on the phase of imaging. Small tumours may be difficult to identify, and only indirect signs may be evident.
- Local effects:
  - The "double-duct sign." Dilatation of both the pancreatic and biliary ducts raises the suspicion of pancreatic adenocarcinoma. The primary tumour is not always visible, as it may be too small; indeed, the presence of the double-duct sign may be the only indicator of a small tumour, which may lead to referral for an endoscopic ultrasound examination.
  - Effacement of the portal vein. This can result in portal hypertension with portosystemic varices.
  - The "teardrop" superior mesenteric vein sign is seen where the vessel morphology has changed from a round shape to a teardrop, indicating vascular infiltration. Depending on the degree of involvement, a venous graft may be used following resection.

- Encasement and/or irregularity of the superior mesenteric artery. If this is present, it indicates that the tumour is not resectable.
- Distant disease:
  - Regional lymph node enlargement. Tumours in the body and tail drain to the splenic and retroperitoneal lymph nodes. However, enlarged lymph nodes may be reactive in nature.
  - Peritoneal deposits: soft tissue nodules and fat stranding. These are often best appreciated on coronal reformats.
  - Lung and liver metastases may be seen.

Differential Diagnosis

There is no differential diagnosis for the above appearances.

Notes

- Pancreatic adenocarcinoma carries a poor outcome due to late presentation.
- Approximately 80% of the primaries arise from the pancreatic head.
- The presence of the "double-duct" sign of common bile duct and pancreatic duct dilatation is suggestive of pancreatic adenocarcinoma. A small pancreatic head mass may not be visible on CT.

Bibliography

Smith SL, Rajan PS. Imaging of pancreatic adenocarcinoma with emphasis on multidetector CT. Clin Radiol 2004; 59(1):26–38

Wong JC, Raman S. Surgical resectability of pancreatic adenocarcinoma: CTA. Abdom Imaging 2010;35(4): 471–480

1.16 Pancreatitis

Clinical History

*A 40-year-old man presents with sudden-onset epigastric pain (**Figs. 1.16.1** and **1.16.2**).*

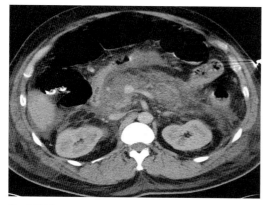

Fig. 1.16.1

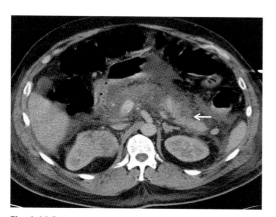

Fig. 1.16.2

Ideal Summary

These are selected axial venous-phase CT images through the upper abdomen. The pancreatic head and part of the body appear ill-defined with reduced enhancement when compared with the pancreatic tail (**Fig. 1.16.2**, arrow). There is surrounding fat stranding and free fluid. I cannot see any gallstones. There is no aerobilia, which would raise the possibility of a recent endoscopic procedure. There is no splenic vein thrombosis. The imaging findings are in keeping with necrotising pancreatitis. I would like to look at the arterial-phase CT images to evaluate

for possible pseudoaneurysm formation, and would urgently discuss the case with the surgical team.

*These are images of a different patient with known pancreatitis in haemodynamic shock (**Figs. 1.16.3** and **1.16.4**).*

These are selected axial arterial-phase CT images through the upper abdomen. There are several loculated areas of mixed density around the pancreas and spleen. A large pseudoaneurysm is seen in one of the images, surrounded by high-density haematoma (**Fig, 1.16.3**, arrow). The images findings are consistent with pseudoaneurysm formation following pancreatitis. This is a surgical emergency, and at our institution, I would discuss this with the team and arrange for urgent transcatheter embolisation.

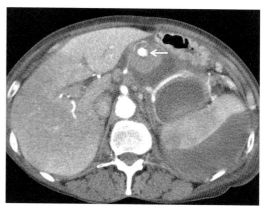

Fig. 1.16.3

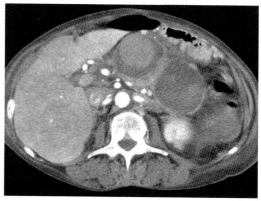

Fig. 1.16.4

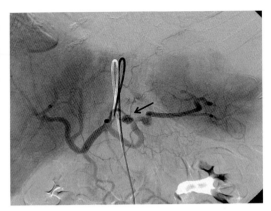

Fig. 1.16.5

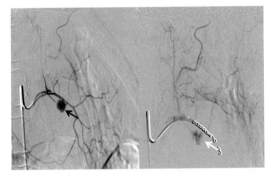

Fig. 1.16.6

*These are the images from the angiographic procedure that was performed (**Figs. 1.16.5** and **1.16.6**).*

These are selected angiogram images. On the coeliac axis and selective splenic artery images, the pseudoaneurysm arises from the splenic artery (**Figs. 1.16.5** and **1.16.6**, black arrow). On the postembolisation image, multiple embolisation coils are seen within the splenic artery. There is a minimal amount of contrast opacification within the pseudoaneurysm following embolisation (**Fig. 1.16.6**, white arrow).

Examination Tips

When dealing with acute pancreatitis, comment on:
- The presence of pancreatic enlargement (focal or diffuse) and the loss of normal lobulated contour

- Peripancreatic fat stranding or fluid
- Loss of the peripancreatic fat planes
- Enhancement characteristics of the pancreatic parenchyma. Note the phase of imaging and compare it with the rest of the pancreas. Look for evidence of pancreatic necrosis.
- Causes of the pancreatitis:
  - Gallstones
  - Evidence of cirrhosis meaning it may be related to alcohol
  - Aerobilia, which is suggestive of recent intervention, for example ERCP (endoscopic retrograde cholangiopancreatography)

Identify the potential complications of acute pancreatitis:
- Fluid collections/pseudocysts, the presence of gas being suspicious for infection
- Splenic/portal vein thrombosis
- Pseudoaneurysm formation

Differential Diagnosis

No differential diagnoses should be offered for these imaging appearances.

Notes

- Findings on a plain film may include:
  - A sentinel loop: a dilated loop of small bowel in the epigastric region
  - The "colon cut-off" sign: dilated right colon up to the splenic flexure with collapsed colon downstream
- Indications for CT imaging in acute pancreatitis include:
  - To confirm the diagnosis
  - To assess for complications
  - To evaluate and guide subsequent intervention: drainage, embolisation, or surgery

Bibliography

Bharwani N, Patel S, Prabhudesai S, Fotheringham T, Power N. Acute pancreatitis: the role of imaging in diagnosis and management. Clin Radiol 2011;66(2):164–175

1.17 Primary Sclerosing Cholangitis

Clinical History

*A 40-year-old man presents with abnormal liver function tests (**Figs. 1.17.1–1.17.4**).*

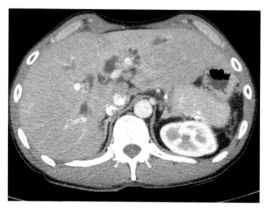

Fig. 1.17.1

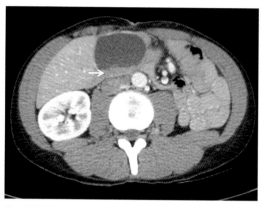

Fig. 1.17.3

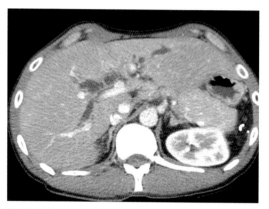

Fig. 1.17.2

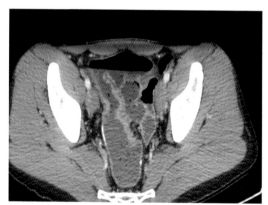

Fig. 1.17.4

Ideal Summary

These are venous-phase axial CT images of the abdomen. There are multiple dilated and narrowed intra- and extrahepatic bile ducts demonstrating a "beaded" appearance. No soft tissue masses are seen within the bile ducts. Multiple gallstones are seen within a distended gallbladder (**Fig. 1.17.3**, arrow), but no debris is seen within the bile ducts themselves. There are no focal intrahepatic lesions, and there are no features to suggest cirrhosis. The portal vein is patent. The pancreas appears normal. I also see evidence of previous colectomy and ileorectal pouch formation, most likely performed due to uncontrollable ulcerative colitis. Overall, the findings are in keeping with primary sclerosing cholangitis associated with ulcerative colitis.

*These are MR images from a different patient (**Figs. 1.17.5** and **1.17.6**).*

These are selected images of an axial HASTE (half-Fourier acquisition single-shot turbo spin-echo) sequence and a maximum-intensity projection (MIP) image of the biliary tree. There is intra- and extrahepatic biliary duct dilatation, with a beaded appearance on the MIP image. I cannot see any filling defects to suggest gallstones. The liver parenchyma is homogeneous; no T2 signal abnormalities are seen. The pancreatic duct is of normal calibre. Overall,

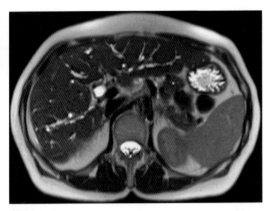

Fig. 1.17.5

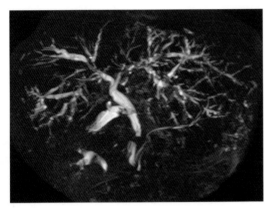

Fig. 1.17.6

the most likely differential is primary sclerosing cholangitis. I would like to ask if there is a history of inflammatory bowel disease and correlate the findings with any liver function test results.

Examination Tips

When investigating the biliary tree, comment on:

- The degree and extent of biliary dilatation. Does it involve the intra- and/or extrahepatic ducts? The duct dilatation may be very marked.
- Whether there are multiple strictures with dilated and narrowed segments, or whether there is generalised dilatation. If the latter, look for a distal transition point.
- Look for aerobilia. This implies previous intervention or possible fistula.

- Gallstones. These may occur in the gallbladder or in the ducts themselves.
- Previous surgery. Cholecystectomy or hepaticojejunostomy may have been undertaken.
- Look for evidence of ulcerative colitis in suspected primary sclerosing cholangitis: colitis, ileostomy and pan-colectomy, or an ileoanal pouch.
- Complications:
  - Intrahepatic abscesses
  - Pancreatitis
  - Cirrhosis and portal hypertension
  - Cholangiocarcinoma: associated with long strictures that may be obstructing the bile ducts. Is there a mass in the liver with focal bile duct dilatation?

Differential Diagnosis

- Pyogenic cholangitis:
  - May be difficult to differentiate on imaging from primary sclerosing cholangitis
  - Associated with a clinical history of recurrent sepsis
  - Usually associated with obstructing stricture and gallstones
- Ischaemic cholangiopathy:
  - Is there a history of surgery?
- AIDS cholangiopathy:
  - Rare: Check to elicit a history of immunosuppression
  - Imaging features may be similar to those of primary sclerosing cholangitis

Notes

- Primary sclerosing cholangitis affects the 30- to 50-year age group.
- Cholangiography may show:
  - A beaded appearance as on CT scanning
  - A "pruned tree" appearance with central duct dilatation and non/poor opacification of the peripheral ducts
  - Biliary duct diverticula

Bibliography

Vitellas KM, Keogan MT, Freed KS, et al. Radiologic manifestations of sclerosing cholangitis with emphasis on MR cholangiopancreatography. Radiographics 2000;20(4):959–975, quiz 1108–1109, 1112

1.18 Sigmoid Volvulus

Clinical History

A 65-year-old man presents with abdominal pain (**Fig. 1.18.1**).

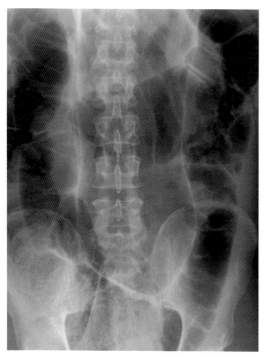

Fig. 1.18.1

Ideal Summary

This is a plain abdominal film. A large distended gas-filled viscus can be seen within the centre of the abdomen, which has a coffee-bean configuration and is arising from the pelvis. The viscus extends beyond the superior part of the film and above T12. The loop is ahaustral, and there is dilatation of the entire large bowel back to the caecum. There are no dilated small bowel loops. I cannot see any evidence of abdominal free gas. The most likely diagnosis is a sigmoid volvulus. I would urgently refer the patient to the surgeons for further clinical management.

These are the CT images of the same patient (**Figs. 1.18.2–1.18.4**).

These are selected axial images from a contrast-enhanced CT examination. There are multiple dilated

loops of large bowel. A dominant loop of large bowel is seen within the centre of the abdomen, which has a transition point (**Fig. 1.18.2**, arrow) adjacent to a "whirling" of the mesenteric vessels (**Fig. 1.18.3**, arrowhead). The rectum is collapsed,

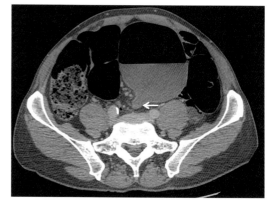

Fig. 1.18.2

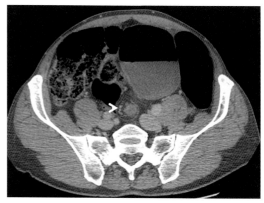

Fig. 1.18.3

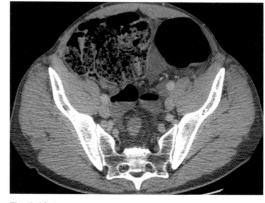

Fig. 1.18.4

and no intraperitoneal free gas is seen. The most likely diagnosis is sigmoid volvulus, and I would urgently refer the patient to the surgeons for further management.

Examination Tips

The candidate should always think of a volvulus as the cause whenever a markedly distended loop of bowel is seen. Look for and comment on the following signs that favour sigmoid volvulus; the more signs, the more likely the diagnosis:

- Gross distension of the distended loop above the level of T10, which favours sigmoid volvulus
- A distended inverted u-shaped loop, which is ahaustral
- Apex beneath the left hemidiaphragm
- Inferior convergence of the bowel loops on the left
- Left flank overlap sign: distended loop overlaps the descending colon
- Pelvic overlap sign: distended loop overlaps the left pelvic bone

In cases where there are no specific features favouring sigmoid versus caecal volvulus, play it safe (as you would in real life). The examiner is not going to fail you if you suggest a contrast enema or CT to confirm.

Differential Diagnosis

Caecal volvulus must always be considered in a case of a markedly distended loop of bowel:

- Caecal volvulus occurs in a younger population and is less common than sigmoid volvulus.
- Caecal volvulus is kidney bean–shaped with its apex in the left upper quadrant.
- It is associated with small bowel dilatation with less colonic distension. The presence of small bowel dilatation may mask the dilated caecum.

- A haustral pattern is visible in 39% of cases.
- A contrast enema may be performed to confirm the diagnosis, which will demonstrate "beaking" in the ascending colon.

Notes

- Sigmoid volvulus occurs in patients aged 60 to 70 years.
- It accounts for 60 to 75% of patients with a volvulus.
- It is the third most common cause of colonic obstruction (malignancy being the most common, followed by diverticular stricture).
- CT findings in sigmoid volvulus:
  - Severe dilatation of the sigmoid colon.
  - The presence of at least one transition point in the sigmoid colon.
  - A "whirl sign" (twisting mesentery) is present in 57 to 100% of cases.
  - The site of the "whirl" sign helps differentiate between caecal and sigmoid volvulus with an accuracy of 97%, being on the right of midline in the former and in the midline or on the left in the latter.

Bibliography

Burrell HC, Baker DM, Wardrop P, Evans AJ. Significant plain film findings in sigmoid volvulus. Clin Radiol 1994;49(5): 317–319

Levsky JM, Den EI, DuBrow RA, Wolf EL, Rozenblit AM. CT findings of sigmoid volvulus. AJR Am J Roentgenol 2010;194(1):136–143

Macari M, Spieler B, Babb J, Pachter HL. Can the location of the CT whirl sign assist in differentiating sigmoid from caecal volvulus? Clin Radiol 2011;66(2):112–117

Rosenblat JM, Rozenblit AM, Wolf EL, DuBrow RA, Den EI, Levsky JM. Findings of cecal volvulus at CT. Radiology 2010;256(1):169–175

1.19 Small Bowel Ischaemia

Clinical History

*A 70-year-old man presents with a history of abdominal pain and collapse (**Figs. 1.19.1** and **1.19.2**).*

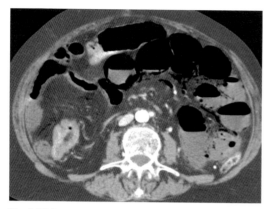

Fig. 1.19.1

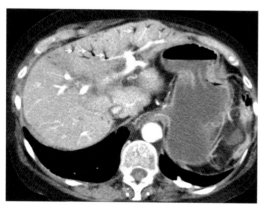

Fig. 1.19.2

Ideal Summary

These are selected arterial-phase axial CT images through the abdomen. There are multiple loops of gas and fluid-filled small bowel. There is no enhancement of the small bowel wall, and there is intramural gas, with more gas seen tracking along the mesenteric vessels. This extends superiorly with extensive portal venous gas present (**Fig. 1.19.2**, small arrows). I would like to assess the rest of the images for signs of mesenteric arterial or venous thrombosis, and in the coronal plane if available. The colon enhances normally and is collapsed. There is no intraperitoneal free gas. The appearances represent complicated small bowel ischaemia. I would refer this patient urgently to the surgeons.

Examination Tips

- In a patient with small bowel ischaemia, assess the following areas:
  - Bowel. Abnormality: is there wall thickening, absence of enhancement, mucosal enhancement, or mural gas? Distribution: is it a short or long segment, continuous or skip in nature, and is there any transition point?
  - Mesentery. Fat stranding often surrounds the abnormality; check the vessels for patency, particularly the arteries on the coronal reformats; look for gas within the vessels; assess twisting of the mesentery to suggest a closed loop obstruction.
  - Outside the gastrointestinal tract. Look at the liver for portal venous gas, other solid organs including kidneys and spleen for infarcts, and the heart for mural thrombus.

Differential Diagnosis

There is no differential diagnosis for the appearances in this case. However, it is always worth trying to discriminate between the following three types of mesenteric ischaemia:

1. Arterial mesenteric ischaemia:
   - Arterial outnumber venous causes by 9:1, and accounts for 60 to 70% of acute mesenteric ischaemia.
   - Identify filling defects along the mesenteric arterial vessels; coronal views may help.
   - The condition results in small calibre and reduced number of mesenteric vessels.
   - The bowel wall is usually thin and gas-filled.
2. Venous mesenteric ischaemia:
   - This accounts for 5 to 10% of acute mesenteric ischaemia.

- Look for mesenteric fat stranding (a "misty" mesentery).
- Congestion of mesenteric vessels will be seen.
- There is marked bowel wall thickening.

❸ Non-occlusive mesenteric ischaemia:

- This accounts for 20 to 30% of acute mesenteric ischaemia.
- The appearances are similar to those of arterial mesenteric ischaemia.
- However, where there is reperfusion, a mixed picture may be evident, with bowel wall thickening and mesenteric fat stranding.

Notes

- Small bowel ischaemia accounts for 1% of patients with an "acute abdomen."
- Approximately 50% of patients with superior mesenteric artery thrombus have associated emboli in other organs.

Bibliography

Lee R, Tung HK, Tung PH, Cheung SC, Chan FL. CT in acute mesenteric ischaemia. Clin Radiol 2003;58(4):279–287

1.20 Target Lesion

Clinical History

*A 70-year-old man presents with a history of weight loss (**Fig. 1.20.1**).*

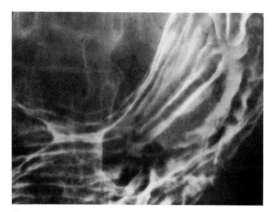

Fig. 1.20.1
Image courtesy: St. Mark's Hospital. Printed with permission.

Ideal Summary

This is a single image from a barium meal study. A relatively large "target" lesion is seen in the body of the stomach, with a central opacity surrounded by a well-defined radiolucent halo. I cannot see any additional lesions, although I would like to review the remainder of the barium meal series. The underlying bones appear normal. Given the clinical history, a "target" lesion might represent malignancy, and endoscopy referral would be appropriate. I would recommend further evaluation for staging with a CT examination if endoscopy confirms malignancy.

Examination Tips

Look for and comment on the following:
- Is there an associated soft tissue component? This could be associated with lymphoma and leiomyosarcoma.
- Are the gastric rugal folds thickened? If so, this may represent gastritis and gastric erosion.
- Underlying destructive bone lesions point to a malignant process.
- Are there any soft tissue nodules outside the borders of the gastrointestinal tract? These may represent multiple neurofibromas.

Differential Diagnosis

The above imaging appearances are characteristic of a "target lesion."

Notes

As with any barium series, always ask to look at the rest of the images if they are not immediately available.

A "target" or "bull's eye" lesion corresponds to an *en face* view of an ulcer with a central depression filled with barium. Gastric erosions with surrounding raised mucosal oedema may give a similar appearance.

Multiple lesions are more suggestive of metastases, of which melanoma is the most common. Others include lung and breast metastases, as well as gastric lymphoma.

Bibliography
Levine MS, Rubesin SE, Herlinger H, Laufer I. Double-contrast upper gastrointestinal examination: technique and interpretation. Radiology 1988; 168(3):593–602

Robinson C, Punwani S, Taylor S. Imaging the gastrointestinal tract in 2008. Clin Med 2009; 9(6):609–612

2 Introduction to Chest Imaging

Joseph Jacob and Sujal Desai

It almost goes without saying that candidates appearing for any postgraduate radiology examination can expect to be tested on chest radiology. Despite major advances in CT, the increasing emphasis on positron emission tomography (PET)-CT, and the sophistication of ultrasound and MRI techniques, candidates are still more likely to be shown plain films. This is reflected in the chest cases shown in the following section: the overwhelming majority of cases begin with a test of observational and interpretative skills using plain chest X-rays. There is sometimes an irrational expectation among candidates that they will be shown complex, high-resolution CT cases—a fear that is almost always unfounded. Thus, the prospective examination candidate would do better to have a sounder grasp of standard plain chest radiology than attempting to master the finer points of the various (rare) diffuse interstitial lung diseases.

In the context of the examination, the chest cases shown will broadly fall into two groups: first, those cases which are "standards" and which candidates will be expected to deal with competently (e.g., lobar collapse, lung cancer, pneumothorax under tension, and air under the diaphragm), and second, those in which the diagnosis may not be immediately apparent. Regardless of the "category" of the film, a methodical approach is to be adopted. However, for cases in the first category—for instance, an examination showing a probable lung cancer or a right upper lobe collapse—the candidate must make sure that the "expected" signs (i.e., those which the examiner will almost certainly want to hear) are clearly stated. Thus, when describing the obvious right upper lobe cancer, it would be important to describe the size, outline, and differential densities (cavitation, calcification) that may or may not be visible. The examiner will also be waiting for the examinee to look for and comment on the presence or absence of important ancillary features (e.g., nodal enlargement, features indicating chronic airflow obstruction, pleural fluid, and/or bony lesions). For films such as these, it is then important to come to a swift and hopefully accurate conclusion (*"The chest X-ray appearances are highly suspicious for lung cancer with mediastinal lymph node enlargement in a patient who undoubtedly has a smoking history..."*).

It is clear that not all studies will be in the former category. However, for such examinations, it is important to commit to first principles, and the initial step must be to determine the dominant radiological sign or signs. When doing so, the candidate is strongly advised to use standard chest radiology terminology; loose descriptive terms such as "pleuroparenchymal change," "an interstitial pattern," and "air-space consolidation" are discouraged. Instead, the defined and widely accepted chest radiology terms must be used to describe the radiological pattern (e.g., a reticular pattern, consolidation, a nodule, or mass); the interested reader is referred to the most recent Fleischner Society glossary for both chest radiographs and CT.[1] An appreciation of the dominant sign(s) will allow the candidate to determine the likely anatomical compartment (i.e., air space, interstitial, and/or airway) in which the pathology is likely to be. Thus, in a patient with a pattern predominant consolidation, it is likely—barring a few (rare) examples—that the pathological process primarily affects the air spaces. Similarly, in the patient with a reticular pattern as the key finding, and particularly when this is associated with other signs of fibrosis (e.g., honeycombing or volume loss), it is reasonable to state that the process is likely to be an interstitial lung disease.

In the examination context (and also perhaps in daily practice), the clinical information should be asked for only after the description of predominant radiological signs and ancillary features. Finally, the candidate must realise that many radiological signs (on chest X-ray and CT) are wholly nonspecific. Thus, consolidation seen on chest radiographs or CT in a young patient with a history of cough and fever is most likely to reflect infection. While the same might be true in an elderly patient, the possibility that the same pattern might indicate sinister pathology (particularly when it is persistent despite treatment) must be borne in mind.

Reference

1. Hansell DM, Bankier AA, MacMahon H, McLoud TC, Müller NL, Remy J. Fleischner Society: glossary of terms for thoracic imaging. Radiology 2008;246(3): 697–722

2.1 Anterior Mediastinal Mass

Clinical History

*A young man presents with a cough (**Fig. 2.1.1**).*

Ideal Summary

This is an anteroposterior erect chest radiograph that shows a large left-sided mass that obscures the left heart, indicating that the mass is positioned anteriorly. There is a broad base to the mediastinum. There are no differential densities; specifically, there is no calcification and no foci of fat density. The left hilum is seen through the mass, indicating that the mass does not make contact with the hilum, and the lateral border of the descending aorta is also clearly visible through the mass.

No further abnormality is seen within the lung parenchyma. There are no pleural effusions.

The appearances are those of an anterior mediastinal mass, the common causes of which include lymph node enlargement, a thymic mass, and a germ cell tumour. A thyroid tumour seems less likely in this case as there is no obvious continuity with any mass in the superior mediastinum. I would take this further by recommending a contrast-enhanced CT scan of the chest.

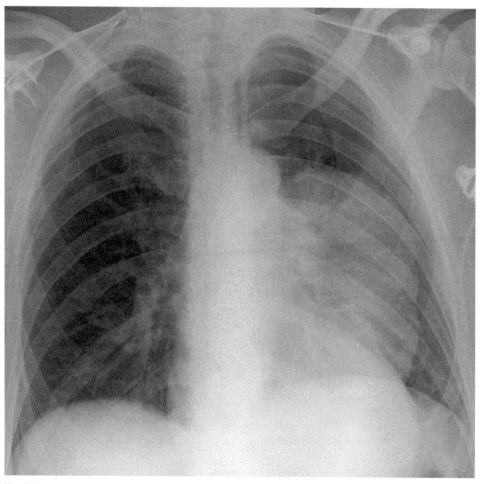

Fig. 2.1.1

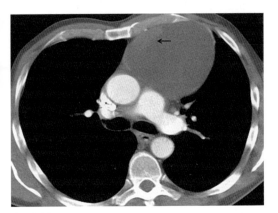

Fig. 2.1.2

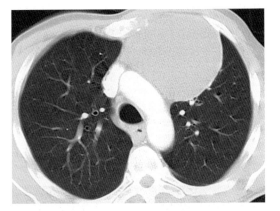

Fig. 2.1.3

*These are selected images from the thoracic CT examination of the same patient (**Figs. 2.1.2** and **2.1.3**).*

These are axial CT images slices on mediastinal and lung parenchymal windows that show a large lobulated mass in the anterior mediastinum. The mass is of predominantly fluid density, but there are solid components (**Fig. 2.1.2**, arrow). There are no foci of calcification or fatty components, as judged by the absence of low attenuation in this mass. The differential diagnoses for a predominantly cystic anterior mass include a mediastinal tumour such as a germ cell tumour undergoing cystic degeneration, a thymic cystic tumour, or a necrotic nodal mass (in a patient with lymphoma). Based on the signs shown, it is not possible to make a more specific CT diagnosis.

(Note: Biopsy in the above case confirmed the diagnosis of a teratoma.)

Examination Tips

If shown a large mediastinal mass on a chest X-ray or CT, look for and comment on:
- Features that confirm or suggest the mediastinal localisation: on chest X-ray, look for the broad base to the mediastinum, and the obtuse (as opposed to acute) angle with the mediastinum. The mediastinal origin of a mass is more easily confirmed on CT (so ask for axial images if no further information can be gleaned from the chest X-ray).
- The localisation in the mediastinum (e.g., superior mediastinum versus anterior mediastinum versus paracardiac).
- Differential densities (calcification or ossification, fat density, and fluid/fat–fluid levels) on CT.
- Ancillary features that might suggest aggressive "biological behaviour" (e.g., signs of invasion of the mediastinal structures, a mass effect, and pleural or pericardial effusions).

Differential Diagnosis

- Mediastinal germ cell tumour with cystic degeneration
- Thymic cyst
- Necrotic nodal mass (the most likely cause for isolated anterior mediastinal nodes would be a lymphoma)

Notes

- Teratomas are the most common tumours of germ cell origin to occur in the mediastinum, and "mature" teratomas account for up to 70% of cases.
- Other histopathological subtypes of germ cell tumours include seminomas, nonseminomatous tumours, and mixed types.
- The typical finding is of a well-defined mass that is either smooth or lobulated and, not infrequently, tends to be localised to one hemithorax. The mass may contain differential densities (soft tissue, fluid, fat, and occasionally calcification or ossification); a fat–fluid level is highly suggestive of the diagnosis but is not commonly present.

Bibliography

Ueno T, Tanaka YO, Nagata M, et al. Spectrum of germ cell tumours: from head to toe. Radiographics 2004;24(2): 387–404

2.2 Sickle Cell Disease

Clinical History

A young woman has a routine chest X-ray in the out-patient department (Fig. 2.2.1).

Ideal Summary

This is an anteroposterior radiograph of the chest in a young woman. The bones all appear generally sclerotic, with a loss of the normal corticomedullary differentiation. The humeral heads have a sclerotic margin, suggesting bilateral symmetric avascular necrosis. Additionally, there are H-shaped vertebrae seen behind the heart. Under the left hemidiaphragm, there are bowel loops that have a relatively lateral position, suggesting the absence of normal splenic tissue. There is no focal lung abnormality, and no pleural effusions can be seen.

The appearances indicate an underlying diagnosis of sickle cell disease with bone and pulmonary vascular changes. In addition, I suspect that there has been autosplenectomy. I would review previous chest radiographs and suggest a specialist review.

Examination Tips

This is a relatively straightforward chest case, but one in which the extrapulmonary findings (sclerotic bones, H-shaped vertebral bodies, and signs suggesting splenic infarction and atrophy) are perhaps the most important.

When shown a chest X-ray in which the bones are clearly the principal abnormality, the following key points should be remembered:
- Comment on the extent and severity of bone sclerosis (i.e., single versus multiple bones).
- Look for signs of bone destruction.
- In a female patient, check for breast soft tissue (has there been a previous mastectomy?). For male patients, ask about previous prostatic surgery or cancer *after* giving a full description of the bony abnormalities.

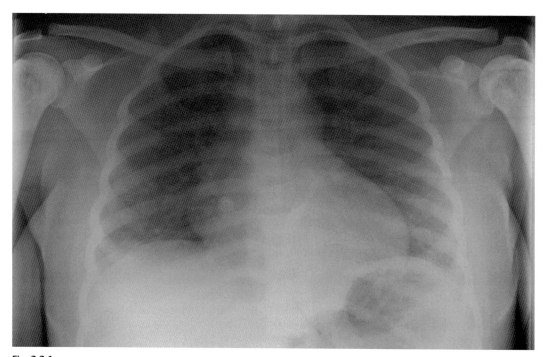

Fig. 2.2.1

- Look for features suggestive of avascular necrosis of the humeral heads.
- Look for signs suggestive of liver or spleen enlargement (myelofibrosis) or splenic atrophy (sickle cell disease).
- Closely inspect the mediastinal contours for posterior masses in patients with sickle cell disease (extramedullary haemopoiesis).

Differential Diagnosis

- Sickle cell disease
- Metastatic bone disease (e.g., prostatic carcinoma or breast cancer)
- Myelofibrosis
- Renal osteodystrophy
- Fluorosis

Notes

- In patients with sickle cell disease, marrow hyperplasia causes several skeletal abnormalities including biconcave vertebrae and narrowing of the bone cortices with coarsening of the trabecular pattern.
- Bone infarcts cause avascular necrosis of the humeral and femoral heads, but may be seen in the small tubular bones of the hands in children.
- The heart may be enlarged, and the central pulmonary vessels may appear prominent.
- In acute chest syndrome, focal areas of consolidation with or without pleural effusions can be seen. In chronic disease, there may be signs of fibrosis with volume loss.

Bibliography

Ejindu VC, Hine AL, Mashayekhi M, Shorvon PJ, Misra RR. Musculoskeletal manifestations of sickle cell disease. Radiographics 2007;27(4):1005–1021

Sylvester KP, Desai SR, Wells AU, et al. Computed tomography and pulmonary function abnormalities in sickle cell disease. Eur Respir J 2006;28(4):832–838

2.3 Cystic Fibrosis

Clinical History

A woman with a chronic condition presents with cough and fever (**Fig. 2.3.1**).

Ideal Summary

This is a frontal chest radiograph of an adult woman. There is a right-sided long line, which appears appropriately positioned, and no complication of line insertion is apparent. The lungs are of normal volume. Multiple ring and tramline opacities are seen, and these are most prominent in mid and upper zones. Both hila appear to be prominent, with no specific features to suggest lobulation. There are no focal areas of consolidation or pleural effusions. The findings indicate a diagnosis of bronchiectasis, and, given the mid and upper zone distribution, cystic fibrosis is the most likely diagnosis.

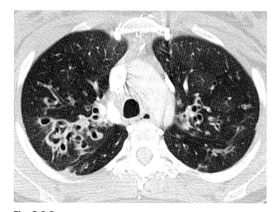

Fig. 2.3.2

This is an image from a thoracic CT examination of the same patient (**Fig. 2.3.2**).

This CT image at the level of the aortic arch demonstrates multiple dilated and thick-walled airways in

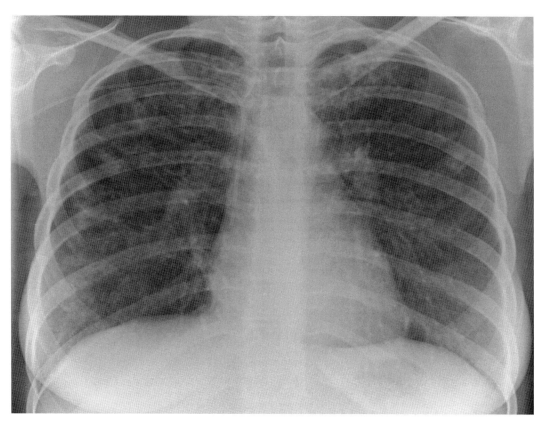

Fig. 2.3.1

both upper lobes. There is clear evidence of bronchial crowding, particularly in the right upper lobe. None of the airways appears plugged. A subtle but definite mosaic attenuation pattern is shown in both lungs. The findings on CT support the diagnosis of cystic fibrosis.

Examination Tips

In a patient in whom the predominant pattern comprises multiple ring and tramline opacities, look for and comment on the following.

Chest X-ray

- The predominant distribution (e.g., bilateral upper zone [typically cystic fibrosis], bilateral upper zone and central [allergic bronchopulmonary aspergillosis], and bilateral lower zone [idiopathic bronchiectasis])
- Lung volumes: airflow obstruction is the characteristic functional abnormality
- Large airway plugging (bronchocoeles): suggesting a diagnosis of allergic bronchopulmonary aspergillosis
- Air–fluid levels in dilated airways
- Hilar enlargement: usually bilateral; this may be due to nodal enlargement or vascular prominence caused by pulmonary hypertension
- The presence or absence of any complications: consolidation (relatively uncommon in cystic fibrosis), pneumothorax

CT

- Abnormal dilatation of the airways in comparison to the accompanying pulmonary arterial branch— best appreciated for airways that are perpendicular to the imaging plane (i.e., in the upper and lower lobes), giving the "signet-ring" sign

- Morphological type: cylindrical (tube-like), varicose ("nodular" outline), or cystic
- Crowding of the airways
- Volume loss
- Airway plugging: large ("finger-in-glove" appearance, bronchocoeles) or small (tree-in-bud pattern)
- Mosaic attenuation pattern: caused by obliterative bronchiolitis (found to a greater or lesser degree in all patients with bronchiectasis)
- Hilar or mediastinal lymph node enlargement
- Bronchial artery hypertrophy

Differential Diagnosis

Although there are many causes of bronchiectasis, the predominant upper zone distribution suggests two main possibilities:
- Cystic fibrosis
- Allergic bronchopulmonary aspergillosis

Notes

Bronchiectasis is the irreversible dilatation of bronchi that is typically caused by inflammation. Historically, infection (e.g., tuberculosis, pertussis) has been regarded as an important cause of bronchiectasis. While this is still probably true in developing nations, the same does not hold in Western countries, where the common aetiologies include cystic fibrosis and immunodeficiency states. In up to 50% of cases, a cause for bronchiectasis is not declared despite exhaustive investigations.

Bibliography
Hansell DM, Lynch DA, McAdams HP, Bankier AA (eds). Imaging of Diseases of the Chest. 5th ed. Philadelphia, PA: Mosby-Elsevier; 2010

2.4 Rib Destruction

Clinical History

*A middle-aged woman presents with right-sided chest pain (**Fig. 2.4.1**).*

Ideal Summary

This is an anteroposterior chest radiograph that demonstrates an abnormal soft tissue density in the right upper right lung field. This abnormal area is associated with destruction of the posterior aspect of the right fifth (**Fig. 2.4.1**, arrow). In addition, there is a pleurally based mass of soft tissue density in the left lower zone (**Fig. 2.4.1**, arrowhead). There is increased density at the left apex projected just over the anterior end of the first rib. There are no other focal lung masses, and there is no plain film sign of hilar or mediastinal lymph node enlargement. There are no pleural effusions.

The features are those of metastatic lung disease. The increased density at the anterior end of the left first rib is certainly suspicious, and if the patient is a

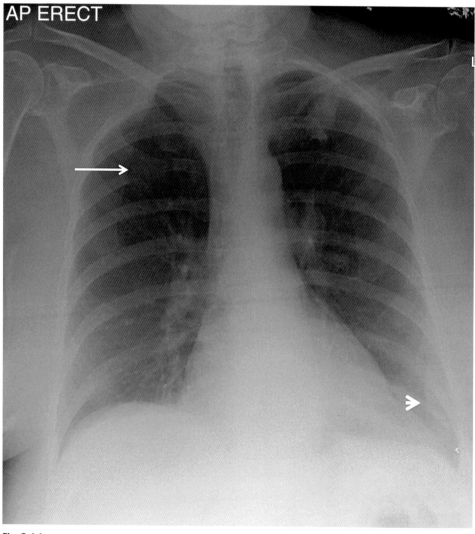

Fig. 2.4.1

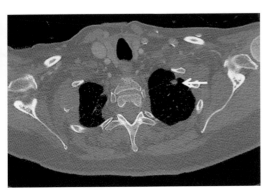

Fig. 2.4.2

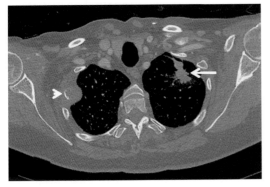

Fig. 2.4.3

smoker, the possibility of lung cancer must be considered. The patient should be referred to a lung cancer multidisciplinary team and a CT scan with intravenous contrast performed.

*These are images from the thoracic CT examination of the same patient (**Figs. 2.4.2** and **2.4.3**).*

The CT images on bone windows confirm the suspicion of a left apical mass (**Figs. 2.4.2** and **2.4.3**, long arrows). This has spiculate margins, is not calcified, and shows no evidence of cavitation. As on the chest radiograph, there is an expansile destructive rib lesion seen on the right (**Fig. 2.4.3**, arrowhead). Overall, the chest radiograph and CT appearances are those of lung cancer with bone metastases.

Examination Tips

This is a classic examination case that involves observation of the traditional "review areas." The following points are important:

- The practice of looking at the review areas and stating that "*I am looking at the bones,*" followed rapidly by the statement "*… and they are normal*" is all too common! A review of the all the bones shown on a chest X-ray takes some time and a cursory glance is to be avoided.
- Look for the obvious causes of rib metastases that might be shown on a chest X-ray (i.e., lung cancer [as in the case shown], breast cancer [is there evidence of a mastectomy and/or surgical clips in the axilla?], or renal tumour [are surgical clips seen at the "edge" of the film?]).

Differential Diagnosis

- Metastatic disease (e.g., lung or breast)
- Plasmacytoma
- Tuberculosis
- Rare fungal infections
- Brown tumour of hyperparathyroidism

Notes

- Metastatic disease is the most common cause of malignant involvement of the ribs.
- Metastases may be either lytic or sclerotic.
- Primary lung tumours may directly invade the chest wall and destroy the adjacent ribs.
- True primary neoplasms of the ribs are rare; chondroid lesions are the most common primary tumours and nearly always arise at or near the anterior end of the rib.
- Enchondromas cause focal expansion of the rib.

Bibliography

Guttentag AR, Salwen JK. Keep your eyes on the ribs: the spectrum of normal variants and diseases that involve the ribs. Radiographics 1999;19(5):1125–1142

2.5 Aspergilloma

Clinical History

A 53-year-old man presents with a chronic cough (**Fig. 2.5.1**).

Ideal Summary

This is an erect chest radiograph of an adult patient. There is homogeneous opacification at the left upper zone associated with apical pleural thickening. More importantly, at the left apex, there appears to be a cavity containing solid material (**Fig. 2.5.1**, long arrow). Around this there is a crescent of air lucency. No underlying rib abnormality is demonstrated. There are signs of volume loss as judged by the elevation of the left hilum and ipsilateral tracheal deviation. There is also possibly a thin-walled fibrocavity at the right apex with no obvious lateral pleural thickening (**Fig. 2.5.1**, short arrow). Multiple small calcified opacities that are likely to represent benign tuberculous granulomas are seen in the right lung. The findings at the left apex are those of a mycetoma in a patient who is likely to have had tuberculosis in the past. I would further investigate this case with CT examination.

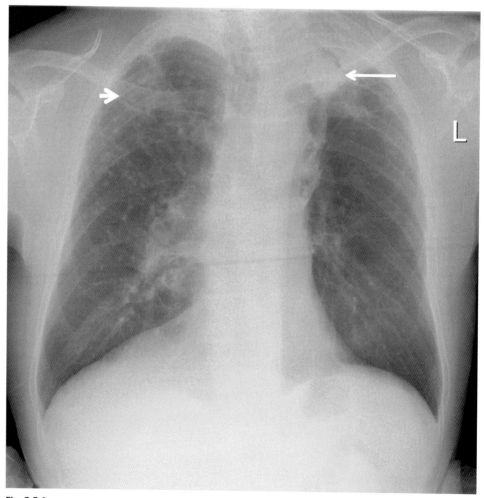

Fig. 2.5.1

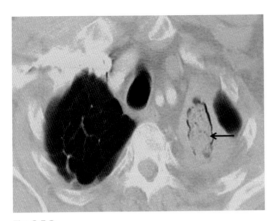

Fig. 2.5.2

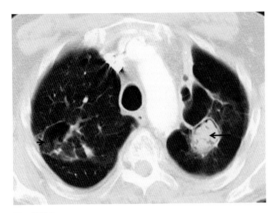

Fig. 2.5.3

These are the thoracic CT images of the same patient (**Figs. 2.5.2** and **2.5.3**).

The CT images support the suspicion on chest radiographs of fungal colonisation of the left apical fibrocavity (**Figs. 2.5.2** and **2.5.3**, long arrows), but additionally confirm the presence of another (noncolonised) cavity on the right. There is marked pleural thickening at the left apex (**Fig 2.5.3**, short arrow).

Examination Tips

When shown a chest X-ray with upper zone volume loss or fibrosis, look for and comment on:
- The presence or absence of intracavitary material.
- The presence or absence of air crescents.
- Thickening of the lateral pleura (particularly if shown serial chest X-rays—this may be the first sign that a mycetoma is forming in a pre-existing fibrocavity). This is a reactive phenomenon and may regress as the aspergilloma resolves.
- Look for and describe, where possible, the signs of an underlying cause of a "fibrocavity" in the upper zones (i.e., previous tuberculosis, sarcoidosis).
- Look for and attempt to exclude lung cancer as a possible cause (e.g., comment on rib destruction).

Differential Diagnosis

- Mycetoma (most commonly related to *Aspergillus fumigatus* infection)
- Lung cancer

Notes

- Fungal colonisation (also termed a "mycetoma" and most commonly caused by *Aspergillus fumigatus*) often occurs as a consequence of any fibrocavitary lung disease. The most common underlying causes of such fibrosis are tuberculosis and sarcoidosis.
- There is a characteristic appearance on chest X-ray and CT with intracavitary material—typically in the upper zones—surrounded by a crescent of air density (the "air crescent" sign).

Bibliography

Buckingham SJ, Hansell DM. *Aspergillus* in the lung: diverse and coincident forms. Eur Radiol 2003;13(8):1786–1800

Franquet T, Müller NL, Giménez A, Guembe P, de La Torre J, Bagué S. Spectrum of pulmonary aspergillosis: histologic, clinical, and radiologic findings. Radiographics 2001; 21(4):825–837

2.6 Carcinoid Tumour

Clinical History

*A young man, who is otherwise well, presents with a cough (**Fig. 2.6.1**).*

Ideal Summary

This is a chest radiograph of a young man. The lungs are clear, and the heart size is normal. The hila are also normal. Looking at the review areas confirms that the apices are normal. There are no abnormalities below the hemidiaphragms. The ribs, visible spine, and remaining bones are normal. Behind the heart and, specifically, in the left main bronchus, there is a well-defined smooth mass (**Fig. 2.6.1**, arrow). The mass is of soft tissue density, and there is no associated calcification. There is no evidence of distal atelectasis or consolidation. There are no pleural effusions.

The features indicate an endobronchial lesion. Possible causes include lung cancer, endobronchial metastases, and a carcinoid/neuroendocrine tumour. The patient should be referred to the lung cancer multidisciplinary team. Thoracic CT with intravenous contrast should also be requested.

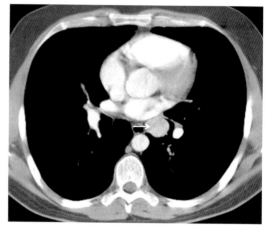

Fig. 2.6.2

*These are images from the thoracic CT examination of the same patient (**Figs. 2.6.2–2.6.4**)*

On these axial CT images on mediastinal and lung windows, there is evidence of a well-defined mass of soft tissue density protruding into the posterior aspect of the left main bronchus (**Fig. 2.6.2**, arrow). There is a definite extraluminal component. The mass is noncalcified. The lungs are clear, and there are no complicating features such as distal atelectasis or

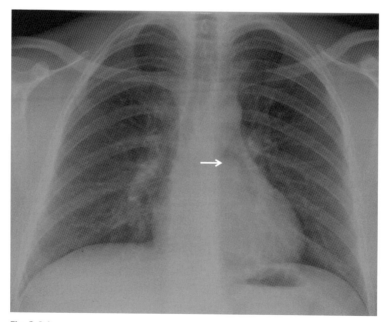

Fig. 2.6.1

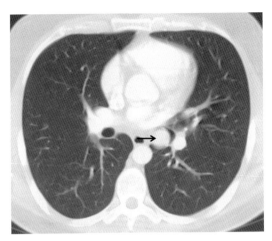

Fig. 2.6.3

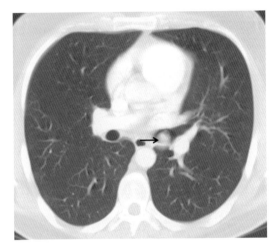

Fig. 2.6.4

consolidation. The findings on the chest radiograph and CT indicate an endobronchial mass. Although there is a possible differential diagnosis, the extraluminal component of this mass suggests the diagnosis of a carcinoid tumour. Biopsy confirmation will be required; a radionuclide (octreotide) scan would be of value.

Examination Tips

This case emphasises the importance of analysing the "review areas" when confronted with an apparently normal chest X-ray:

- Tell the examiner that you are looking at the apices, behind the heart, below the hemidiaphragms,

and at the central airways (trachea and main bronchi).

- When an abnormality has been spotted, as in this case, look for and comment on the shape, size, and density of any abnormality.
- Look for and comment on any ancillary features: consolidation, atelectasis/lobar or segmental collapse, or pleural effusions.

Differential Diagnosis

- Lung cancer
- Carcinoid tumour
- Endobronchial metastases (rare—typically from kidney, breast, or colon cancer)

Notes

- Bronchial carcinoids are rare tumours of neuro-endocrine origin that exhibit a range of biological behaviour; so-called "typical" carcinoids are the most common subtype (accounting for 85 to 90% of all cases) and are usually benign. Atypical carcinoids may demonstrate aggressive (malignant) features.
- Most carcinoid tumours are found in relation to the central airways.
- On chest X-ray, there may be indirect signs (e.g., segmental or lobar volume loss, or airway plugging) or a central mass may be seen.
- On CT, the relationship of the tumour to the airway is better shown: the tumour may be largely or wholly extraluminal—the appearance of the former being likened to an "iceberg." The tumour is generally well defined and of soft tissue attenuation, and may enhance markedly following intravenous contrast.

Bibliography

Jeung MY, Gasser B, Gangi A, et al. Bronchial carcinoid tumors of the thorax: spectrum of radiologic findings. Radiographics 2002;22(2):351–365

Ko JM, Jung JI, Park SH, et al. Benign tumors of the tracheobronchial tree: CT-pathologic correlation. AJR Am J Roentgenol 2006;186(5):1304–1313

Wilson RW, Kirejczyk W. Pathological and radiological correlation of endobronchial neoplasms: Part I, Benign tumors. Ann Diagn Pathol 1997;1(1):31–46

2.7 Tuberculosis

Clinical History

A young man presents with a cough, weight loss, and fever (**Fig. 2.7.1**).

Ideal Summary

This is an erect chest radiograph, which shows multiple small soft tissue density nodules throughout the lungs. There is no particular zonal predilection. There are no associated pleural effusions and the hila appear normal. Although there is a differential diagnosis for this appearance, the most important diagnosis to consider is that of miliary tuberculosis. If that diagnosis has been excluded, the alternative possibilities to consider would be miliary metastases, fungal infection, lung disease caused by exposure to a variety of organic or inorganic dusts, and rarely sarcoidosis. I would like to ask if there is a history of any infection and recent travel history, and to discuss the case with the respiratory team. Further imaging with a CT of the thorax would be helpful.

These are CT images of the thorax in the same patient (**Figs. 2.7.2** and **2.7.3**).

The CT study shows widespread small nodules. The lesions are noncalcified and randomly distributed throughout the lungs. There are no other ancillary findings. The CT findings indicate that disseminated tuberculosis is the most likely diagnosis.

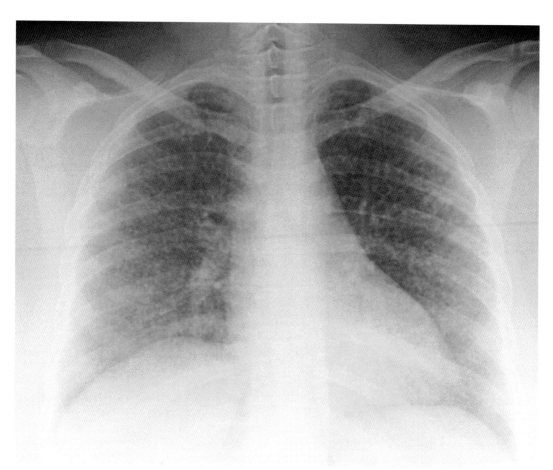

Fig. 2.7.1

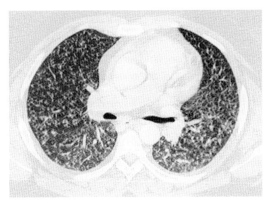

Fig. 2.7.2

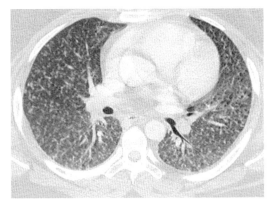

Fig. 2.7.3

Examination Tips

This is a classical examination case that should be "dispatched" quickly. The following points should be noted:

- Discuss the key pattern and mention the word "miliary" in the description.
- Comment on the distribution (random versus upper zone versus lower zone).

- Look for and comment on any ancillary features:
  - Nodal enlargement (with or without calcification): could this be a pneumoconiosis?
  - Pleural effusions
  - (Destructive) bone lesions: is the lung appearance part of a disseminated cancer?
- Ask about a history of travel (e.g., visits to areas with endemic fungal infection) and occupation (could this be pneumoconiosis?).

Differential Diagnosis

- Disseminated tuberculosis
- Metastases (e.g., thyroid cancer)
- Fungal infection (e.g., histoplasmosis, blastomycosis, or coccidioidomycosis)
- Pneumoconioses
- Sarcoidosis (rare)

Notes

- The term "miliary" refers to a radiological pattern that is recognisable on chest X-ray and CT. When this pattern is seen in the context of tuberculosis, it indicates haematogenous dissemination.
- The pattern is not pathognomonic of tuberculosis and may be seen in patients with pneumoconiosis, fungal infections (blastomycosis or coccidioidomycosis), and haematogenous spread of cancer.
- Miliary tuberculosis can occur when there is mild immunocompromise.

Bibliography
Hansell DM, Lynch DA, McAdams HP, Bankier AA, eds. Imaging of Diseases of the Chest. 5th ed. Philadelphia, PA: Mosby-Elsevier; 2010

2.8 Lung Metastases and Mastectomy

Clinical History

A 34-year-old woman presents with back pain (**Fig. 2.8.1**).

Ideal Summary

This is a chest radiograph of an adult woman that shows asymmetry of the breast outlines, with the left appearing smaller. The other dominant abnormality is in the lungs, where there are numerous large rounded masses of soft tissue density. The masses are predominantly in a central location but with at least one seen more peripherally. No pleural effusions are seen. There are no obvious destructive bone lesions.

There are many possible causes of multiple pulmonary nodules, but in a patient whom I suspect has had a mastectomy, the most likely diagnosis is that of multiple metastases. I would suggest further imaging with a CT examination, both to evaluate the chest findings and also to assess the vertebral bodies given the clinical history of back pain.

These are some selected images from a CT series (**Figs. 2.8.2** and **2.8.3**).

This is a CT scan of the chest on mediastinal and lung parenchymal windows. There is evidence of a breast prosthesis on the left, the inner membrane of which appears to have ruptured. There are numerous masses within the lungs in keeping with the findings on

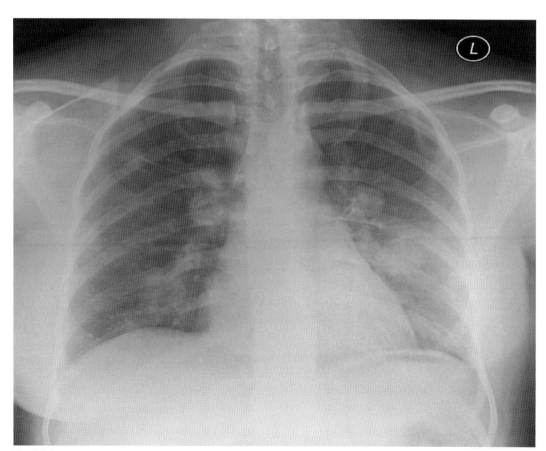

Fig. 2.8.1

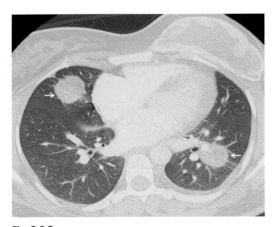

Fig. 2.8.2

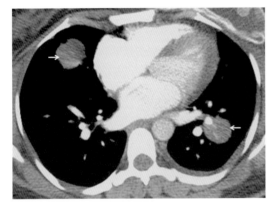

Fig. 2.8.3

the chest radiograph and likely to indicate metastases from a breast cancer (**Figs. 2.8.2** and **2.8.3**, arrows). There is also a small left pleural effusion not well shown on the initial chest radiograph. In addition to assessment of the CT on bone windows settings, a bone scan would be necessary to evaluate the extent of dissemination of cancer.

Examination Tips

When shown a chest radiograph and/or CT with multiple rounded nodules, look for and comment on:

- The approximate size (use descriptive terms such as *miliary*, *small*, *large*, and *varying in size*) and profusion of nodules

- Density characteristics (soft tissue, calcification [think about metastases from an osteosarcoma or chondrosarcoma], and cavitation [metastases from a squamous primary cancer, septic emboli, or Wegener's granulomatosis])
- Ancillary features: mastectomy, lymph node enlargement, and destructive or expansile bony lesions. (Remember: there are 24 ribs, 12 vertebral bodies, 2 clavicles, 2 scapulae, and the proximal end of 2 humeri – if you tell the examiner that you are "*looking at the bones*," make sure you look at *all* of the bones!)
- In the examination, you may need to think about some of the more "exotic" causes of multiple lung nodules (e.g., Carney's triad or benign metastasising leiomyomas)

Differential Diagnosis

- Multiple metastases
- Infection or multiple abscesses (in the appropriate clinical context)
- Immunological (e.g., Wegener's granulomatosis or rheumatoid arthritis)
- Vascular (multiple arteriovenous malformations)

Notes

- The lung is a common site for metastases.
- With extrathoracic malignancies, pulmonary metastases occur in 20 to 54% of patients.
- The breast, colon, kidneys, uterus, and head and neck are the most common primary site.
- Choriocarcinoma, osteosarcoma, testicular tumour, melanoma, Ewing's tumour, and thyroid carcinoma frequently metastasise to the lung.
- Typical radiological findings of a pulmonary metastasis include multiple located, round, variably sized nodules and diffuse thickening of the interstitium.

Bibliography

Seo JB, Im JG, Goo JM, Chung MJ, Kim MY. Atypical pulmonary metastases: spectrum of radiologic findings. Radiographics 2001;21(2):403–417

2.9 Pleural Fibroma

Clinical History

*A young woman presents to her general practitioner with a cough (**Fig. 2.9.1**).*

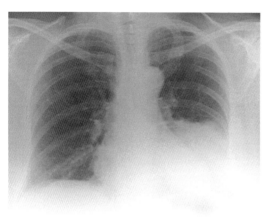

Fig. 2.9.1

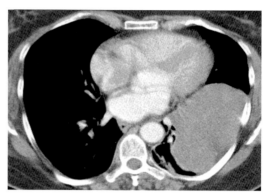

Fig. 2.9.2

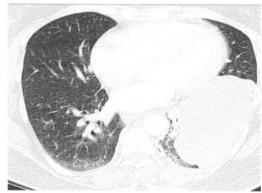

Fig. 2.9.3

Ideal Summary

This is an erect chest radiograph of an adult woman with an ill-defined rounded mass in the left lower zone that has a relatively well-defined upper margin. The mass appears to make contact with the pleural surface, but there are no obvious signs to suggest rib destruction or chest wall invasion. The mass seems to form an acute angle with the pleural surface suggesting, at least on the chest X-ray, that the mass is primarily intrapulmonary. There is no calcification or cavitation. The left heart border and hemidiaphragm are well visualised, indicating that the lesion is posterior. The hilar points are in their normal position, indicating no associated volume loss. The right lung and pleural space are clear. No pleural effusions are seen.

The appearance on chest X-ray suggests a large lung mass. In a smoker, the first diagnosis to consider would be that of lung cancer. In the first instance, after considering the history, it would be reasonable to recommend contrast-enhanced thoracic CT scan to better evaluate this lesion.

*These are two images from the chest CT examination of the same patient (**Figs. 2.9.2** and **2.9.3**).*

On these axial lung and mediastinal window images of the chest CT, there is a large lobulated mass of homogeneous density in the left hemithorax. There are no differential densities—specifically, there is no calcification or fat. There is broad contact with the lateral pleural margin, but there are acute angles where the mass makes apparent contact, and there are no CT signs suggesting invasion. A plane of fat density is also visible adjacent to the cardiac border. No pleural effusions are seen.

Discerning the exact anatomical origin of this mass is difficult—the acute angles formed where the mass makes contact with the pleural surface or chest wall suggest that this is intrapulmonary. That being the case, the first diagnosis to consider and exclude for this large mass would be lung cancer, and it would be important to know the smoking history. The absence of any aggressive radiological features raises the possibility that this might be a benign lung lesion such as a hamartoma (even though there are no calcific densities). If this is not a lung lesion, an alternative diagnosis is that of a benign pleural tumour such as a localised fibrous tumour of the pleura. CT in the prone position might help because around 50% of these tumours are pedunculated and can change shape when the patient's position is changed.

Examination Tips

Making a confident diagnosis of a solitary intrathoracic mass based on imaging findings is not straightforward. This is true for the examination and is certainly true in daily practice! Nevertheless, the candidate would be expected to offer a practical and sensible list of differential diagnoses. The following teaching points should be noted:

- As with other nodules or masses, look for and discuss the size, site, and shape and outline of the lesion. Comment on any differential densities (e.g., calcification, fat, or air).
- Try to judge the likely anatomical origin of the lesion (i.e., lung versus pleural or mediastinal). This is not always easy, particularly for large lesions. The apparent angle of contact with the pleural or mediastinal surface may help: acute angles suggest that the lesion is likely to be pulmonary, whereas obtuse (broad-based) angles suggest that the mass may be of pleural or mediastinal origin.
- Ancillary features of likely "biological behaviour"—the presence of rib destruction, or chest wall or vascular invasion—indicate an aggressive mass. Also look for pleural effusion and lymph node enlargement.

Differential Diagnosis

The list of differential diagnoses for an intrathoracic mass or nodule, even a large mass as in the case shown, is long. A confident (and, more importantly, correct) diagnosis is often not made solely on the basis of chest X-ray and CT findings. The histopathological diagnosis in the case presented was a localised fibrous tumour of the pleura. However, the important diagnoses to consider for a (large) mass of the type shown would be as follows.

Pulmonary

- Lung cancer
- Other tumours: hamartoma, carcinoid, solitary metastasis, and rare lung tumours (e.g., lymphoma, pulmonary blastoma, and haemangiopericytoma)
- Infectious causes: abscess, hydatid disease, or "round" pneumonia
- Inflammatory or vascular causes: rheumatoid nodule, Wegener's granulomatosis, organising pneumonia, sarcoidosis, mucoid impaction, or haematoma

Pleural

- Fibroma
- Fluid loculated in a fissure

Notes

- A localised fibrous tumour of the pleura (synonymous with pleura fibroma, localised pleural mesothelioma, benign mesothelioma, and solitary fibrous tumour) is a rare intrathoracic tumour that most often presents in the fifth to seventh decades.
- There is no association with previous asbestos exposure (compare with malignant pleural mesothelioma).
- Most tumours are benign, but there is a spectrum, and up to one-third of localised fibrous tumours are malignant.
- The common presenting symptoms are breathlessness and chest pain, but around half of tumours are discovered incidentally on imaging tests.
- Localised fibrous tumours tend to be large at presentation.
- On CT, lesions tend to be soft tissue density, show homogenous enhancement, and are mobile.
- Larger tumours there may contain areas of low attenuation because of necrosis.

Bibliography

Cardillo G, Carbone L, Carleo F, et al. Solitary fibrous tumors of the pleura: an analysis of 110 patients treated in a single institution. Ann Thorac Surg 2009;88(5): 1632–1637

Qureshi NR, Gleeson FV. Imaging of pleural disease. Clin Chest Med 2006;27(2):193–213

2.10 Malignant Pleural Mesothelioma

Clinical History

*A 59-year-old woman presents with chest pain and shortness of breath (**Fig. 2.10.1**).*

Ideal Summary

This is an erect chest radiograph. There is lobulated pleural thickening in the left hemithorax that is associated with a moderate-volume pleural effusion.

There is no contralateral mediastinal shift, and the right lung is clear. There are no obvious signs of pleural calcification on this chest radiograph. The appearances on the chest radiograph suggest malignant pleural thickening, and the two principal differential diagnoses are malignant pleural mesothelioma and (metastatic) adenocarcinoma to the pleura. The latter is usually secondary to lung cancer. Other tumours that can spread to or involve the pleura include thymoma and lymphoma. To take this case forward, I would recommend a CT scan of the chest with intravenous contrast.

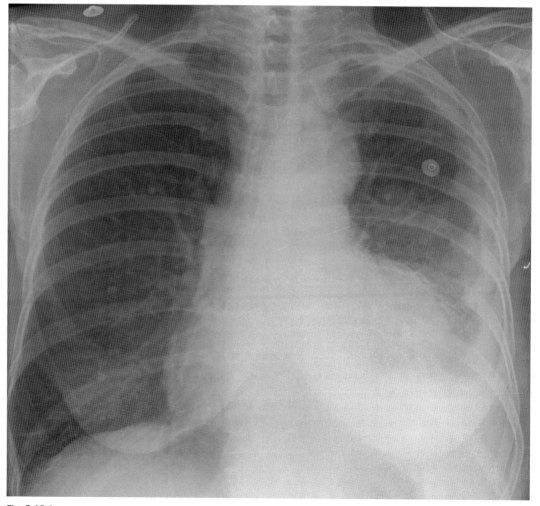

Fig. 2.10.1

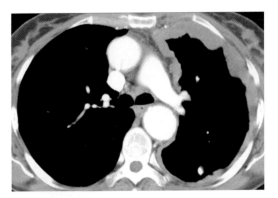

Fig. 2.10.2

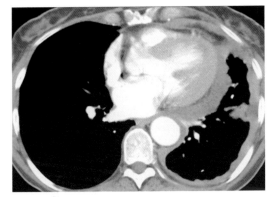

Fig. 2.10.3

*These are two images from the CT chest for the same patient (**Figs. 2.10.2** and **2.10.3**).*

The axial CT images show almost circumferential and nodular pleural thickening. In places the pleura is thicker than 1 cm, and this thickening involves the mediastinal pleura. The pleura on the right is normal. In these images, no obvious lung mass is seen, and there are no pleural plaques.

The CT features are those of malignant pleural thickening, the two main diagnoses being malignant pleural mesothelioma and adenocarcinoma of the pleura. There are no imaging features on chest X-ray or CT that will distinguish between these two possibilities.

Examination Tips

If shown a case of pleural thickening, look for and comment on the following:

- Nodularity, thickening of the pleural exceeding 1 cm, involvement of the mediastinal pleura, and/or circumferential thickening: any one of

these features is strongly suggestive of malignant pleural disease. Note that chest X-ray and CT cannot differentiate between malignant pleural mesothelioma and pleural adenocarcinoma (or, for that matter, any other cause of diffuse malignant pleural disease)

- Volume loss on the side of pleural thickening (even with apparently limited disease) or the absence of significant contralateral mediastinal displacement in the presence of a large pleural effusion; a lack of ipsilateral lung collapse is, however, suggestive of malignant pleural mesothelioma
- Pleural plaques (calcified or noncalcified)
- Additional features: obvious signs of chest wall invasion (malignant mesothelioma can "track" along a biopsy site), diaphragmatic invasion (ask for coronal or sagittal CT reconstructions, if available), lymph node enlargement, and extrathoracic metastatic disease

Differential Diagnosis

- Malignant pleural mesothelioma
- Pleural adenocarcinoma
- Others - metastatic thymoma, lymphoma

Notes

- Malignant pleural mesothelioma, which accounts for < 1% of all thoracic tumours, is a relentlessly aggressive neoplasm caused by exposure to asbestos.
- There is an estimated 30-fold increased risk of developing malignant pleural mesothelioma in patients exposed to asbestos.
- The diagnosis is not infrequently delayed, and the outlook for patients is bleak.
- Chest X-ray and CT may suggest the diagnosis of malignant pleural thickening, but the distinction between malignant pleural mesothelioma and metastatic adenocarcinoma of the pleura is often impossible.
- In practice, histopathological and immunohistochemical examinations are required to confirm the diagnosis.

Bibliography

Desai SR, Hansell DM. Pleural tumours. In: Husband JE, Reznek RH, eds. Husband & Reznek's Imaging in Oncology. 3rd ed. London, UK: Informa Healthcare; 2010

Ismail-Khan R, Robinson LA, Williams CC Jr, Garrett CR, Bepler G, Simon GR. Malignant pleural mesothelioma: a comprehensive review. Cancer Contr 2006;13(4): 255–263

2.11 Septic Emboli

Clinical History

*A young man presents with fever (**Fig. 2.11.1**).*

Ideal Summary

This is an erect chest radiograph of an adult patient. There is a right-sided internal jugular line that is appropriately positioned. This finding suggests that the patient may be acutely unwell. There are several small cavitating lesions in the left upper and right mid-zone (**Fig. 2.11.1**, arrows). There is no obvious hilar or paratracheal lymph node enlargement, but there is a right-sided pleural effusion.

There is a relatively wide differential diagnosis for multiple lung cavities but, in a young patient, who is likely to be acutely unwell, the most likely underlying cause is infection. Typical infective causes include *Staphylococcus aureus* (e.g., in an intravenous drug abuser) or *Klebsiella* and other gram-negative pneumonias. In an immunocompromised or neutropenic patient, these appearances may be caused by angioinvasive aspergillosis during the phase of neutrophil recovery. Wegener's granulomatosis is another possible cause. Metastases from a primary squamous cancer may lead to this appearance, but in a young man, this diagnosis is less likely. I would confirm these appearances with a chest CT examination, and inform the clinical team of the appearances.

*These are two CT images of the same patient (**Figs. 2.11.2** and **2.11.3**).*

The axial CT images demonstrate multiple thin-walled cavities of roughly similar size (**Figs. 2.11.2** and **2.11.3**, arrows). There is no particular zonal predilection. A moderate pleural effusion is seen on the

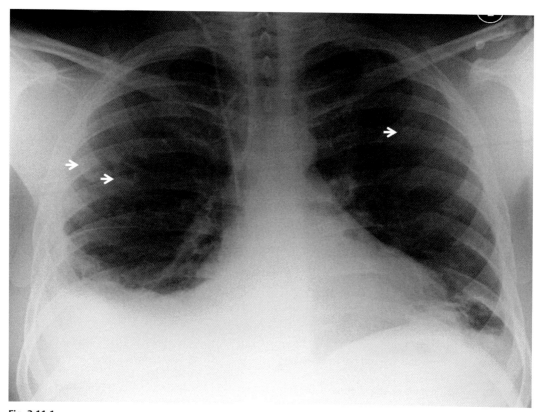

Fig. 2.11.1

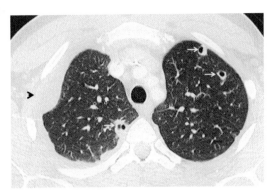

Fig. 2.11.2

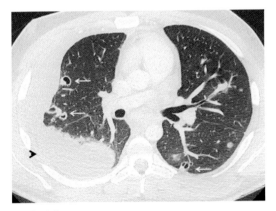

Fig. 2.11.3

right (**Figs. 2.11.2** and **2.11.3**, arrowhead). The differential diagnosis for these CT findings is identical to that for the chest radiographs. Infection again seems to be the most likely diagnosis.

Examination Tips

When shown a chest X-ray or CT with multiple cavities, look for and comment on the following:
- The distribution of cavitating lesions (a predominantly upper zone distribution may be seen in tuberculosis; peripheral cavities may suggest that the lesions are infarcts), and sparing of the tips of the middle and/or lingula lobe and the extreme lung bases (Langerhans' cell histiocytosis).

- Ancillary features. Look for: destructive bone (i.e., vertebral/rib) lesions, which may suggest that the cavities are metastatic; indwelling catheters (septic emboli); associated nodules (Langerhans' cell histiocytosis); enlarged intrathoracic nodes lymph nodes; and "vegetations" on the heart valves (septic emboli).

Differential Diagnosis

Multiple lung cavities may be seen in the following clinical scenarios:
- Infection: *Staphylococcus aureus, Klebsiella pneumoniae*, fungal, and mycobacterial
- Metastases: squamous carcinoma or sarcoma
- Inflammatory: Wegener's granulomatosis, rheumatoid nodules, or Langerhans' cell histiocytosis
- Vascular: infarcts (septic or otherwise)
- Miscellaneous: "cystic" bronchiectasis, sequestered segment

Notes

- The multiple cavities in this patient were caused by septic emboli secondary to infective endocarditis, a well-recognised pulmonary complication of intravenous drug abuse.
- Thromboembolic material may originate from deep venous thrombosis, indwelling catheters, or septic vegetations on the tricuspid valve.
- Peripheral cavities may rupture into the pleural space and cause empyema or a pyopneumothorax.
- Staphylococcal infection is the most common.

Bibliography

Gotway MB, Marder SR, Hanks DK, et al. Thoracic complications of illicit drug use: an organ system approach. Radiographics 2002;22(Spec No):S119–S135

Hagan IG, Burney K. Radiology of recreational drug abuse. Radiographics 2007;27(4):919–940

Vourtsi A, Gouliamos A, Moulopoulos L, et al. CT appearance of solitary and multiple cystic and cavitary lung lesions. Eur Radiol 2001;11(4):612–622

2.12 Sarcoidosis

Clinical History

A young man presents with a persistent dry cough (**Fig. 2.12.1**).

This chest radiograph of an adult man shows right paratracheal and bilateral symmetrical hilar lymph node enlargement. Additionally, there is filling-in of the aortopulmonary window. The azygoesophageal line is not well shown on this examination, but there is no obvious splaying of the carina. There are no obvious signs of parenchymal infiltration on this study.

The findings on this chest radiograph are highly characteristic of sarcoidosis. Tuberculosis generally does not cause symmetrical hilar nodal enlargement, and lymphoma is usually associated with asymmetrical nodal disease. However, if there are continuing clinical suspicions, biopsy confirmation may be warranted.

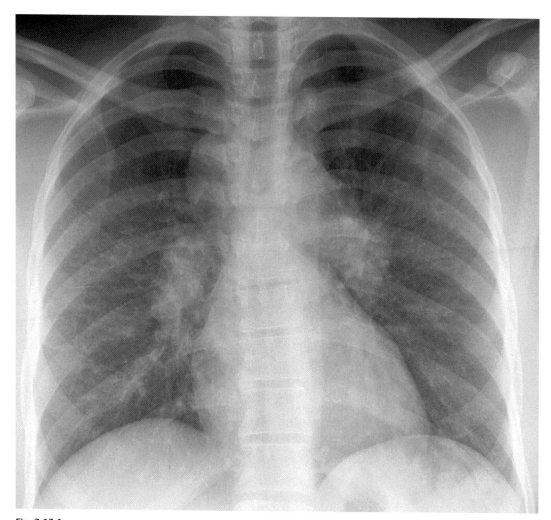

Fig. 2.12.1

Examination Tips

This case shows the classical distribution of lymph node enlargement in sarcoidosis. If shown such a case, comment on the symmetrical nature of the hilar nodal enlargement—a typical finding in sarcoidosis (in contrast to lymphoma [asymmetric] and tuberculosis [unilateral]). Remember to look for and comment on the following:

- Calcification in the lymph nodes. On CT, calcification of the nodes in sarcoidosis tends to have a "softer" quality (likened to icing sugar), in contrast to what is seen in tuberculosis. Moreover, in sarcoidosis, nodal calcification tends to be more focal within the nodes, unlike tuberculosis in which calcification involves the whole node. Calcification of lymphomatous nodes is very uncommon (< 1% of cases) except as a posttreatment finding.
- The presence or absence of lung abnormality. Bronchocentric reticulation in the upper zone, which is roughly symmetrical, is a typical finding in sarcoidosis. Parenchymal calcification is most often indicative of tuberculosis rather than sarcoidosis. The presence of cavities should also prompt the diagnosis of tuberculosis rather than sarcoidosis.
- The presence or absence of pleural effusions or thickening. Pleural disease is uncommon in sarcoidosis.

Differential Diagnosis

- Sarcoidosis
- Lymphoma
- Tuberculosis

Notes

- The majority of patients with sarcoidosis have an abnormal chest X-ray at some time during the course of the disease.
- Nodal enlargement is a feature in up to 80% cases.
- The most common pattern of nodal enlargement is as shown in the case above, namely symmetrical bilateral hilar and right paratracheal.
- Unilateral hilar nodal enlargement is uncommon, as is isolated anterior or posterior mediastinal enlargement.
- The natural history is for nodal enlargement to resolve over a period of up to 2 years, the general rule being that nodes will not enlarge again; the corollary is that an increase in size of the nodes after resolution must raise the suspicion of alternative diagnoses (e.g., lung cancer, lymphoma, or tuberculosis).

Bibliography

Brauner MW, Grenier P, Mompoint D, Lenoir S, de Crémoux H. Pulmonary sarcoidosis: evaluation with high-resolution CT. Radiology 1989;172(2):467–471

Bein ME, Putman CE, McLoud TC, Mink JH. A reevaluation of intrathoracic lymphadenopathy in sarcoidosis. AJR Am J Roentgenol 1978;131(3):409–415

Hamper UM, Fishman EK, Khouri NF, Johns CJ, Wang KP, Siegelman SS. Typical and atypical CT manifestations of pulmonary sarcoidosis. J Comput Assist Tomogr 1986;10(6):928–936

2.13 Posterior Mediastinal Mass

Clinical History

*A young man presents with a persistent cough, but is otherwise well (**Fig. 2.13.1**).*

Ideal Summary

This is an erect chest radiograph. There is increased density behind the left heart that is obscuring the medial half of the left hemidiaphragm. The density has a curved lateral border, and there is a broad base to the mediastinum. No differential densities are shown. The left hilum is seen, as is the inferior aspect of the left heart border. However, the descending aorta is not seen as being separate from the mass. There is no splaying of ribs on this side, and the vertebral bodies, which are visible, appear normal. Air in the gastric fundus is subdiaphragmatic. The lungs are clear, and no pleural effusions can be seen. The findings suggest a posterior mediastinal mass. The possible causes of a mass in the posterior mediastinum include a neurogenic tumour, lymph node enlargement, and, less commonly, extramedullary haemopoiesis. An aneurysm of the descending thoracic aorta is another possibility.

I would normally recommend a thoracic CT with contrast to confirm the posterior mediastinal location and better evaluate the anatomical relationship.

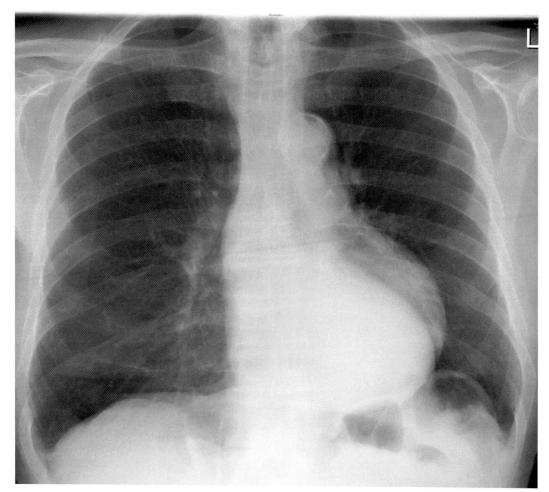

Fig. 2.13.1

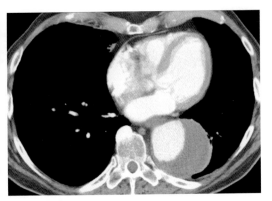

Fig. 2.13.2

*This is a CT image from the same patient (**Fig. 2.13.2**).*

The contrast-enhanced CT image through the chest on mediastinal settings demonstrates an aneurysmal dilatation of the descending thoracic aorta. There is considerable eccentric thrombus in the aortic lumen. On the image provided, there is no sign of a dissection flap or penetrating ulcer. The aneurysmal dilatation corresponds to the findings seen on the chest radiograph. The diagnosis is of an aneurysm of the descending aorta.

Examination Tips

If you are shown a mass that you believe to be mediastinal in origin, demonstrate to the examiner that you are aware of the signs suggesting that the mass is truly mediastinal. Ask yourself these questions and tailor your description accordingly:

- Does the mass have a broad base to the mediastinum and a convex lateral margin?
- Is there an obtuse angle where the mass "makes contact" with the mediastinum?
- Does the mass obscure any normal mediastinal structures (e.g., heart border, aorta, hemidiaphragm)?
- Which location or anatomical "compartment" (e.g., superior, posterior, or anterior) is it in?

- Is there any displacement or absence of the paraspinal lines?

Also look for and comment on:
- Any differential densities: look specifically for fat and calcification
- Rib anomalies or destruction

Differential Diagnosis

- Neurogenic tumours
- Hiatus hernia
- Lymphoma
- (Descending) aortic aneurysm
- (Oesophageal) duplication cyst

Notes

- The boundaries of the posterior mediastinum are as follows:
  - Anteriorly, the posterior trachea and pericardium
  - Anteroinferiorly, the diaphragm
  - Posteroinferiorly, the vertebral column
  - Superiorly, the thoracic inlet.
- The true anatomical posterior boundary is the vertebral column.
- With mediastinal disease, masses in the paraspinal regions are included in the posterior mediastinum.
- The contents of the posterior mediastinum are:
  - Oesphagus
  - Descending aorta
  - Azygous and hemiazygous veins
  - Thoracic duct
  - Vagus and splanchnic nerves
  - Lymph nodes
  - Fat

Bibliography

Whitten CR, Khan S, Munneke GJ, Grubnic S. A diagnostic approach to mediastinal abnormalities. Radiographics 2007;27(3):657–671

2.14 Langerhans' Cell Histiocytosis

Clinical History

*A young man presents with a persistent cough and breathlessness of recent onset (**Fig. 2.14.1**).*

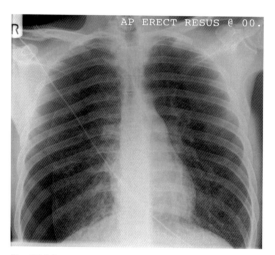

Fig. 2.14.1

Ideal Summary

This is an erect chest radiograph of an adult man. There is a right-sided pneumothorax and, perhaps more importantly, there are subtle but definite signs of mediastinal shift as judged by displacement of the right heart border to the left. This suggests a degree of tension, and having seen this radiograph, I would immediately inform the medical team in charge.

The background lung parenchyma is also diffusely abnormal with widespread reticulation and suggestive of multiple thin-walled cysts. No large pleural effusions can be seen, but the costophrenic recesses are not seen on this study. Despite the widespread reticulation, the lung volumes are preserved and, if anything, increased. No obvious skin nodules are seen, and there is no convincing evidence of hilar or mediastinal nodal enlargement.

In a young man with such extensive disease, Langerhans' cell histiocytosis, complicated by a right-sided pneumothorax (possibly under tension) is the most likely diagnosis. A high-resolution CT scan would be of value to evaluate this further.

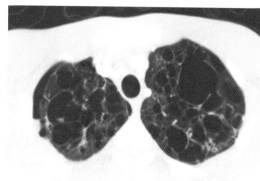

Fig. 2.14.2

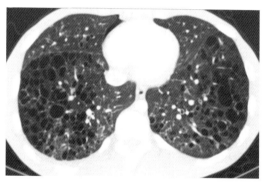

Fig. 2.14.3

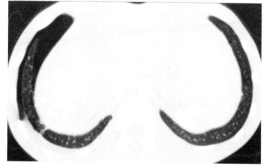

Fig. 2.14.4

*These are some selected images from the CT series in the same patient (**Figs. 2.14.2−2.14.4**).*

On these axial CT images, there is evidence of a right-sided pneumothorax associated with a small ipsilateral pleural effusion at the base. Additionally, there are multiple thin-walled cysts of varying size. Many cysts have bizarre shapes, for example, at the left apex and in the left lower lobe. There is sparing of the tips of the middle lobe and lingula. Furthermore, there are no cysts in the costophrenic recesses. As on the chest radiograph, there are no obvious cutaneous nodules, and no posterior mediastinal masses are shown. The CT appearances are those of Langerhans' cell histiocytosis, complicated by a right-sided pneumothorax.

Examination Tips

If you are shown a chest X-ray with a diffuse reticular or reticulonodular pattern and a preservation (or even sometimes an increase) of lung volumes, the following diagnoses should be considered:
- Langerhans' cell histiocytosis
- Lymphangioleiomyomatosis
- Tuberose sclerosis
- Neurofibromatosis

On CT, it is important to identify the predominant pattern. In the case shown, the dominant abnormality is the presence of multifocal low-attenuation lesions throughout the lungs. Importantly, in contrast to emphysema, the low-density foci all seem to have a definable wall, indicating that these are cysts. Once the predominant pattern(s) has been identified, the following should be looked for or ascertained:
- Distribution of the cysts. In "classical" Langerhans' cell histiocytosis, there is sparing of the tips of the middle lobe, the lingula, and the extreme lung bases. In lymphangioleiomyomatosis and tuberose sclerosis complex, the distribution of cysts is generally uniform with no particular zonal predilection. In some patients with Birt–Hogg–Dubé's disease, a lower zone predominance of cysts and/or paracardiac cysts may be seen.
- Shape of the cysts. Langerhans' cell histiocytosis is classically associated with bizarre cysts of variable sizes.
- Nodules. These are seen in Langerhans' cell histiocytosis (with or without cavitation) and in some patients with tuberose sclerosis complex.
- Pneumothoraces.

- Gender and smoking history. Tuberose sclerosis complex (almost always occurring in women) and lymphangioleiomyomatosis (exclusively in women) have a striking gender predisposition. Pulmonary Langerhans' cell histiocytosis (but *not* Langerhans' cell histiocytosis in other organs) is very strikingly associated with smoking.

Differential Diagnosis

- Langerhans' cell histiocytosis
- Postinfective pneumatocoeles
- Lymphoid interstitial pneumonia
- Neurofibromatosis
- Tuberous sclerosis complex
- Birt–Hogg–Dubé disease

Notes

- Pulmonary Langerhans' cell histiocytosis is strongly associated with smoking and usually occurs in the absence of other organ involvement.
- The radiological findings will depend on the "stage" at which imaging is done:
  - In early disease, the dominant finding is that of multiple nodules in the mid and upper zones, sometimes with a peribronchovascular distribution; large nodules are uncommon.
  - With progression, nodules will be seen to cavitate, and in the late phase, there will be cysts.
- Some cysts have an odd outline (thought to be a result of the coalescence of multiple cysts).
- There is a recognisable zonal predilection with sparing of the extreme lung bases and the tips of the middle lobe and lingula.

Bibliography
Brauner MW, Grenier P, Tijani K, Battesti JP, Valeyre D. Pulmonary Langerhans cell histiocytosis: evolution of lesions on CT scans. Radiology 1997;204(2):497–502

Lacronique J, Roth C, Battesti JP, Basset F, Chretien J. Chest radiological features of pulmonary histiocytosis X: a report based on 50 adult cases. Thorax 1982;37(2): 104–109

2.15 *Pneumocystis jirovecii* Pneumonia

Clinical History

A man presents with recent onset of shortness of breath (**Fig. 2.15.1**).

Ideal Summary

This is an anteroposterior erect chest radiograph. There is a Hickman line projected over the right hemithorax, and this appears to be correctly positioned and without complication. There is diffuse ground-glass opacification in both lungs. The heart size is normal, and there are no pleural effusions. I can see no obvious septal lines. The presence of the Hickman line suggests that this patient may be undergoing chemotherapy and hence may be immunosuppressed. Given this, the diagnosis that needs to be considered first is *Pneumocystis jirovecii* pneumonia (PCP).

I would recommend referral to the chest physicians with a view to performing induced sputum analysis and/or diagnostic bronchoscopy with lavage. A CT scan may be of value to evaluate the extent of lung abnormality and to identify complications.

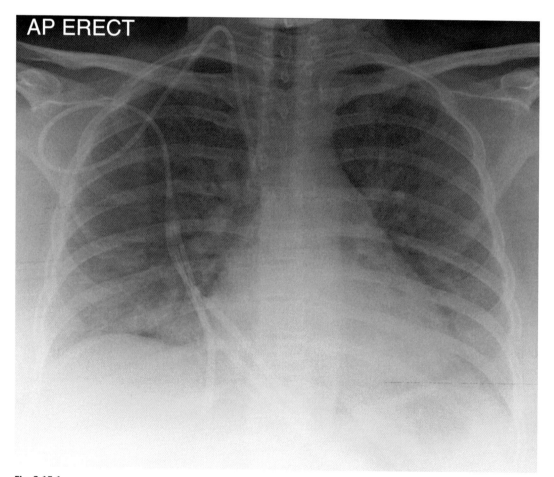

Fig. 2.15.1

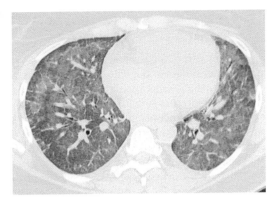

Fig. 2.15.2

This is a single CT image obtained soon after the chest X-ray examination (**Fig. 2.15.2**).

This is an axial slice from a CT scan of the chest on lung parenchymal windows. There is diffuse ground-glass opacification involving all lobes. There is perhaps some sparing of the lung periphery. There is no thickening of the interlobular septa, and no pleural effusions are seen.

Although pulmonary oedema would be the most common cause of widespread ground-glass opacities, the normal heart size, absence of septal lines, and pleural effusion make this a little less likely. The likely history of immunosuppression is important, and the diagnosis of PCP certainly needs to be considered. An alternative diagnosis would be diffuse pulmonary haemorrhage (even in the absence of an obvious history of haemoptysis).

Examination Tips

- PCP typically affects immunocompromised patients including those with:
  - Congenital immune deficiency
  - HIV infection with AIDS
  - Organ transplantation
  - On long-term steroids or chemotherapy.
- The infection is classically central in distribution, sparing the peripheries of the lung.
- Pleural effusions and hilar lymph node enlargement are uncommon.
- Patients with AIDS receiving aerosolised pentamidine prophylaxis show an atypical distribution, with a ground-glass pattern predominantly affecting the upper lobes.

Differential Diagnosis

- PCP
- Pulmonary oedema
- Diffuse pulmonary haemorrhage

Notes

In equivocal cases, the patient may be treated for pulmonary oedema with diuresis and monitored for a radiological and symptomatic response to treatment. If no response is shown, either induced sputum sampling or bronchoalveolar lavage is required to obtain histopathological confirmation.

Bibliography

Baughman RP, Dohn MN, Shipley R, Buchsbaum JA, Frame PT. Increased *Pneumocystis carinii* recovery from the upper lobes in *Pneumocystis pneumonia*. The effect of aerosol pentamidine prophylaxis. Chest 1993;103(2):426–432

Turner D, Schwarz Y, Yust I. Induced sputum for diagnosing *Pneumocystis carinii* pneumonia in HIV patients: new data, new issues. Eur Respir J 2003;21(2):204–208

2.16 Lobar Collapse

Clinical History

*A middle-aged woman presents with shortness of breath (**Fig. 2.16.1**).*

Ideal Summary

This is an erect radiograph of a woman. There is increased density with a well-defined upper border seen in the right mid and lower zones. This is obscuring the right heart border and right hemidiaphragm. There is mediastinal shift to the right as judged by the deviation of the trachea to this side. The right hilum is depressed and not visible on this radiograph. The left lung and pleural space are clear with no effusion seen on the side of the abnormality. Some flattening of the left hemidiaphragm is noted, suggesting that there might be a history of smoking. The findings are those of combined middle and right lower lobe collapse, indicating an obstructing lesion in the bronchus intermedius. In smokers, the features must be considered suspicious for lung cancer, and appropriate urgent referral (for CT and bronchoscopy) is warranted.

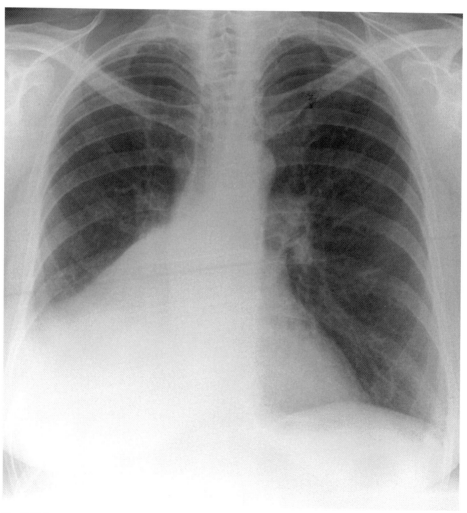

Fig. 2.16.1

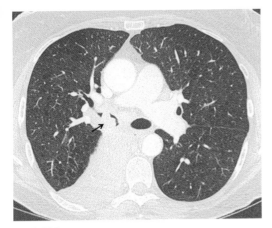

Fig. 2.16.2

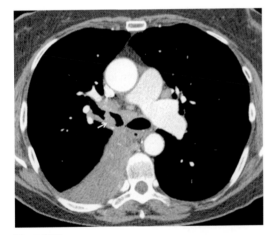

Fig. 2.16.3

*These are some images from a CT examination in the same patient (**Figs. 2.16.2** and **2.16.3**).*

The axial CT images confirm complete collapse of the middle and right lower lobes. This is associated with an irregular endobronchial mass (**Figs. 2.16.2** and **2.16.3**, arrow), and again, in a smoker, the most likely diagnosis is that of lung cancer.

Examination Tips

It is imperative that candidates revise and recognise the signs of all forms of lobar collapse. Remember

also that the film may not show all the recognised features of a particular type of collapse; for instance, there may be negligible volume loss (tracheal or mediastinal shift, or diaphragmatic elevation) in some patients.

Differential Diagnosis

- Lung cancer
- Carcinoid tumour
- Mucous plugging
- Endobronchial metastases (e.g., breast, colon, or renal cancer and malignant melanoma)

Notes

Remember and comment on the following in patients with lobar collapse:
- The silhouette sign: look for and comment on the loss of normally visible borders on a chest X-ray (e.g., the left or right heart borders [lingula or middle lobe, respectively], hemidiaphragms [lower lobes], and aortic arch [left upper lobe]).
- In infants, remember that an aspirated foreign body may be the cause of the collapse (note that with a "check-valve" effect, there may be air-trapping and hyperexpansion of the distal lung as opposed to collapse).
- In older children and young adults, think of mucous plugging (particularly if there is a history of asthma).
- In adults, lung cancer (or other neoplasm) must be the first diagnosis to consider. Look for ancillary features (e.g., flattening of the hemidiaphragms [indicating chronic obstructive pulmonary disease], hilar/mediastinal lymph node enlargement, and pleural effusions), which may point to the most likely diagnosis.

Bibliography

Hansell DM, Lynch DA, McAdams HP, Bankier AA, eds. Imaging of Diseases of the Chest. 5th ed. Philadelphia, PA: Mosby-Elsevier; 2010

2.17 Lung Cancer

Clinical History

*A middle-aged man presents with a new and persistent cough (**Fig. 2.17.1**).*

Ideal Summary

This is an erect radiograph of the chest showing an area of increased density seen at the right apex (**Fig. 2.17.1**, arrow). This has an irregular lateral border. No differential densities are seen. Specifically, there is no obvious calcification or cavitation. Both hemidiaphragms are flattened, suggesting that there is underlying chronic airflow limitation and that the patient is a smoker. There are no other focal opacities, and no pleural effusions can be seen. There is no plain film evidence of hilar or mediastinal lymph node enlargement. In a smoker, the opacity at the

right apex must, in the first instance, be considered suspicious for lung cancer. A CT scan of the chest and abdomen is recommended, and the patient should be referred to the local lung cancer multidisciplinary team meeting.

*These are some CT images of the same patient (**Figs. 2.17.2** and **2.17.3**).*

These are axial slice CT images taken on lung windows and showing a spiculated mass at the right apex that abuts the pleura posteromedially. There are no obvious signs of chest wall or rib invasion on these images, but a review of the soft tissue and bone windows would be needed. There are focal lucencies in the mass, but these are likely to be caused by the background emphysema rather than cavitation. On the given images, there are no other focal lesions. Similarly, the soft tissue window settings are not

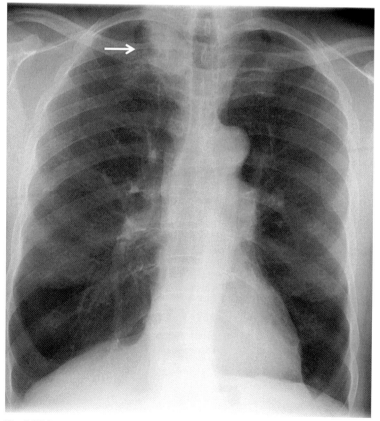

Fig. 2.17.1

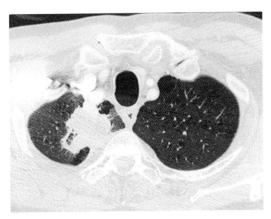

Fig. 2.17.2

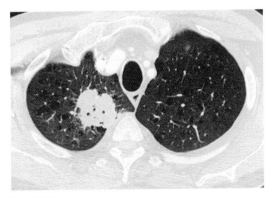

Fig. 2.17.3

seen—these would be required for evaluation of the hila and mediastinum. The visible features are highly suspicious for lung cancer.

Examination Tips

- This is a classical examination case that should pose little difficulty. The case involves a right apical opacity in a patient whose chest X-ray appearances indicate chronic obstructive airways disease. The first (and perhaps the only) diagnosis to consider must be lung cancer.
- You should look for and comment on:
  - Site (upper versus mid versus lower zones), size, shape, and margins (lobulated, smooth, or spiculated).
  - Presence/absence of calcification or cavitation.

- Always check for features that may have staging significance:
  - Enlarged ipsilateral hilar/bronchopulmonary (N1), ipsilateral mediastinal (N2), or contralateral mediastinal, hilar, or supraclavicular (N3) lymph nodes
  - Pleural or pericardial effusions (M1a)
  - Other lung nodules (T3, T4, or M1a)
  - Destroyed ribs adjacent to a peripheral tumour (T3), or remote destructive bone lesions or other signs of distant metastasis (M1b).

Differential Diagnosis

- Lung cancer
- Infection (in the apical region, tuberculosis should probably be considered)

Notes

- Lung cancer is the most common cause of death caused by malignancy, accounting for at least 40,000 deaths in the United Kingdom.
- The overwhelming majority of patients have a history of smoking.
- The diagnosis of lung cancer is often first suspected on the basis of chest X-ray findings, but CT is almost always then required.
- There is a growing reliance on positron emission tomography (PET)-CT imaging in the management of patients with lung cancer.

Bibliography

Goldstraw P, Crowley J, Chansky K, et al; International Association for the Study of Lung Cancer International Staging Committee; Participating Institutions. The IASLC Lung Cancer Staging Project: proposals for the revision of the TNM stage groupings in the forthcoming (seventh) edition of the TNM Classification of malignant tumours. J Thorac Oncol 2007;2(8):706–714

Hansell DM, Lynch DA, McAdams HP, Bankier AA. Imaging of Diseases of the Chest. 5th ed. Philadelphia, PA: Mosby-Elsevier; 2010

Nair A, Klusmann MJ, Jogeesvaran KH, Grubnic S, Green SJ, Vlahos I. Revisions to the TNM staging of non-small cell lung cancer: rationale, clinicoradiologic implications, and persistent limitations. Radiographics 2011;31(1):215–238

2.18 Lung Collapse Caused by a Saccular Aneurysm

Clinical History

*A young man presents acutely short of breath with no history of trauma (**Fig. 2.18.1**).*

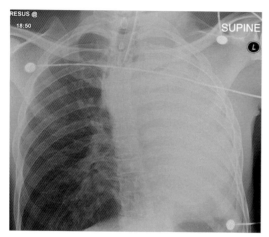

Fig. 2.18.1

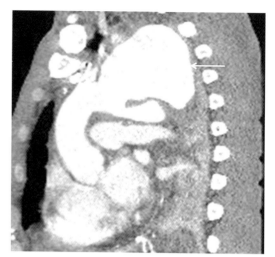

Fig. 2.18.2

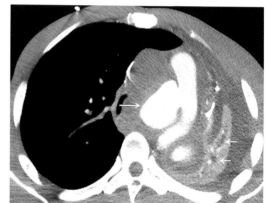

Fig. 2.18.3

Ideal Summary

This is a supine radiograph in a patient who has been intubated. The endotracheal tube is correctly positioned. There is a "white-out" of the left hemithorax. The right heart border is shifted to the left, indicating marked volume loss. There is no sign of aerated lung on this side. The right lung and pleural space are clear, although the costophrenic recess is not seen. The findings indicate total left lung collapse caused by central obstruction. In a young patient, lung cancer is not a likely diagnosis. In the absence of any further history from the patient, the possibility of an aspirated foreign body may need to be considered. A central carcinoid tumour or a mediastinal mass are two other possibilities. The patient should be referred for contrast-enhanced CT.

*These are some selected images from the CT examination (**Figs. 2.18.2–2.18.4**).*

The sagittal and axial CT images confirm complete collapse of the left lung. Some fluid-filled airways ("fluid bronchograms," **Fig. 2.18.3**, short arrows) are

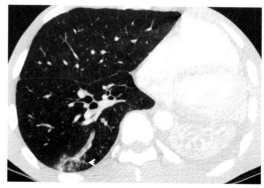

Fig. 2.18.4

seen in the collapsed lung, and there is an ipsilateral pleural effusion. The aortic arch is abnormal, with a saccular aneurysm communicating with its medial wall via an apparently narrow neck (**Fig. 2.18.2**, arrow). No obvious aortic calcifications or gaseous lucencies are seen. The aneurysm is surrounded by homogeneous soft tissue density that is displacing and compressing the trachea. This would account for the collapse of the left lung in this young patient. The appearances are those of contained contrast extravasation from this large aneurysm. On lung windows, there is a "tree-in-bud" pattern at the right lung base (**Fig. 2.18.4**, arrowhead), indicating inflammatory or infective exudate in the peripheral airways.

Examination Tips

- This case highlights the importance of identifying the signs of complete lung collapse and, in the absence of a known congenital anomaly, deducing that there must be central obstruction.
- When shown such a case, the candidate must demonstrate that he or she is able to distinguish, as far as is reasonably possible, between the causes of a total "white-out" (i.e., total lung collapse versus a large pleural effusion).

Look for and comment on the following:
- Marked ipsilateral mediastinal shift, which favours complete lung collapse as opposed to a large effusion (note that with large effusions, there may be remarkably little contralateral shift if there is significant underlying [passive] lung collapse or if there is relative "fixation" of the mediastinum [e.g., malignant mesothelioma])
- The presence or absence of aerated lung on the side of interest
- Central radiopaque (foreign) bodies, especially in children

- Mediastinal calcification or fat density—germ cell tumours or vascular lesions

Differential Diagnosis

- Central tumours:
  - Lung cancer (in patients aged over 40 years)
  - Carcinoid tumour
  - Mediastinal masses
- Aspirated foreign body
- Congenital
  - Lung agenesis or aplasia

Notes

The diagnosis in this young patient was a mycotic aneurysm.
- Aortic mycotic aneurysms most commonly occur in predisposed patients.
- There is often a history of intravenous drug abuse or immune compromise.
- Congenital heart disease, previous surgery, and adjacent infections are also recognised factors.
- Most mycotic aneurysms tend to be saccular and progress relatively rapidly, in contrast to atherosclerotic aneurysms.
- This is a surgical emergency with a poor prognosis; endovascular repair may be the only option for the patient.

Bibliography

Agarwal PP, Chughtai A, Matzinger FRK, Kazerooni EA. Multidetector CT of thoracic aortic aneurysms. Radiographics 2009;29(2):537–552

Razavi MK, Razavi MD. Stent-graft treatment of mycotic aneurysms: a review of the current literature. J Vasc Interv Radiol 2008; 19(6, Suppl)S51–S56

2.19 Anomalous Right Coronary Artery

Clinical History

A 43-year-old patient presents with arrhythmia and intermittent chest pain on exercise. There is no family history of ischaemic heart disease (**Figs. 2.19.1—2.19.4**).

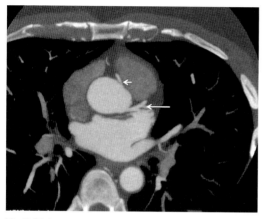

Fig. 2.19.1

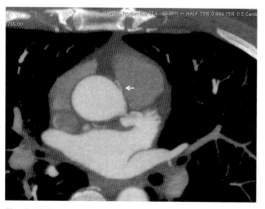

Fig. 2.19.2

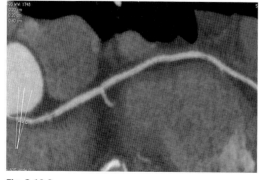

Fig. 2.19.3

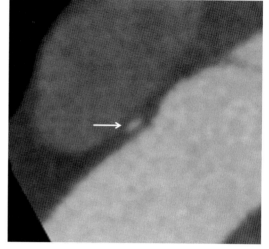

Fig. 2.19.4

Ideal Summary

These maximum-intensity projection reconstructions from a coronary CT angiogram demonstrate that the left coronary artery arises from the posterior aspect of the left sinus of Valsalva (**Fig. 2.19.1**, long arrow). The right coronary artery has an anomalous origin; the image shows a very narrow-calibre right coronary artery with a slit-like orifice arising from the anterior aspect of the left sinus (**Figs. 2.19.1 and 2.19.2**, short arrow). The curved multiplanar reconstruction and the orthogonal image through this confirm the slit-like orifice of the right coronary artery and the narrowed proximal course of the right coronary artery. This is optimally seen in **Fig. 2.19.4** (arrow), where the right coronary artery is visible between the well-opacified aorta and the nonopacified pulmonary artery. The diagnosis is that of an anomalous right coronary artery origin with a potentially "malignant" interarterial course between the aorta and pulmonary artery.

Examination Tips

Cardiac and, specifically, coronary CT examinations are being requested with increasing frequency by cardiologists and other clinicians. Therefore, over time, it is likely that examination candidates will be shown coronary CT studies.

Before looking for disease, it is important for the candidate to be mindful of normal coronary anatomy

- The origin and course of the left and right coronary arteries and the "dominance" (the artery that gives rise to the posterior descending artery) should be noted.
- In the majority of subjects, the left coronary artery arises from the left and the right coronary artery from the right sinus of Valsalva.
- The left main stem divides to give rise to two main branches: the left anterior descending artery (with its diagonal branches and septal perforators) and the circumflex arteries (which give off the obtuse marginal divisions).
- The right coronary gives rise to acute marginal branches and usually terminates as the posterior descending artery (running in the inferior interventricular groove) and a posterolateral branch.

Differential Diagnosis

The causes of chest pain are lengthy and clinically based.

Notes

- In the majority of patients, CT coronary angiography is requested for the evaluation of atherosclerotic disease. The key advantages of CT coronary angiography are that the examination is minimally invasive (in contrast to conventional catheter angiography) and that a normal study has a high negative predictive value.
- Anomalies of coronary artery origin are rare but potentially important congenital abnormalities.
- Overall, coronary anomalies are detected incidentally in around 1% of the population who are otherwise healthy.
- The real importance of an anomalous origin is whether or not the subsequent course of the artery is deemed "malignant" (i.e., it passes between two [high-pressure] arterial structures).
- An anomalous right coronary artery originating from the left coronary sinus and passing between the aorta and pulmonary artery is a possibly life-threatening abnormality; this is a rare anomaly with an estimated prevalence of < 0.5%.

Bibliography

Bastarrika G, Lee YS, Huda W, Ruzsics B, Costello P, Schoepf UJ. CT of coronary artery disease. Radiology 2009;253(2):317–338

Kim SY, SeoJB, Do KH, et al. Coronary artery anomalies: classification and ECG-gated multi-detector row CT findings with angiographic correlation. Radiographics 2006;26(2):317–333, discussion 333–334

2.20 Cannonball Secondaries from Adrenal Carcinoma

Clinical History

*A middle-aged man presents with cough and abdominal discomfort (**Fig. 2.20.1**).*

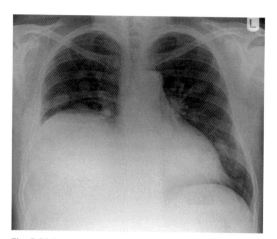

Fig. 2.20.1

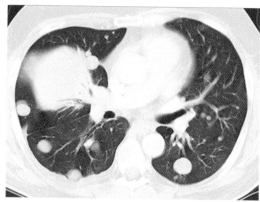

Fig. 2.20.2

Ideal Summary

This is an erect chest radiograph of an adult man. There are numerous well-defined rounded masses throughout both lungs. There is elevation of the right hemidiaphragm. There is slight blunting of the right costophrenic angle caused by pleural fluid. No effusion is seen on the left. No abnormality is seen in the bones. There are many possible causes of multiple rounded nodules in the lungs, but the most likely diagnosis is that of "cannonball" metastases. Typical causes of large metastases of this type in an adult man include renal or colon cancer and melanoma. Other possible causes of multiple rounded nodules include Wegener's granulomatosis and rheumatoid arthritis. A CT scan of the chest, abdomen, and pelvis would be of value to investigate this further.

*These are selected images of the CT you have requested (**Figs. 2.20.2–2.20.5**).*

These axial CT images confirm that there are numerous large bilateral lung nodules with a small right-sided pleural effusion seen. In the abdomen, there is a large heterogeneous mass. The epicentre of the mass seems to be superomedial to the right

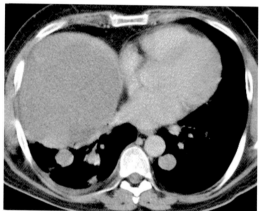

Fig. 2.20.3

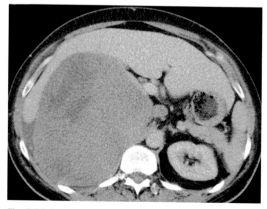

Fig. 2.20.4

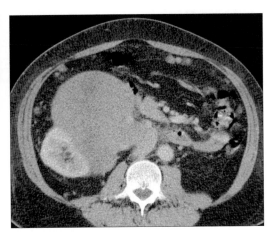

Fig. 2.20.5

kidney, which itself appears to be displaced inferiorly. The liver is displaced anteriorly and superiorly, accounting for the elevated right hemidiaphragm. There are numerous discrete nodules, of soft tissue density, in the peritoneum, which are likely to represent peritoneal tumour deposits. The most likely diagnosis in this patient is that of disseminated adrenal carcinoma. A review of all the abdominal CT imaging on soft tissue and bone windows would be needed to stage the patient, and further investigations would include nuclear medicine radioisotope imaging with either an octreotide or MIBG scan to direct chemotherapeutic intervention.

Examination Tips

The examiner will not give you a simple X-ray of lung secondaries; look for evidence of the primary tumour:

- Absent breast following surgery for a primary breast tumour
- Trachea displacement by a thyroid tumour
- An absent "long bone" with primary bone tumour
- Intra-abdominal abnormality, for example, elevation of the hemidiaphragm
- Calcification in an abdominal tumour

Differential Diagnosis

- Calcified metastases (rare):
  - Mucinous adenocarcinomas
  - Osteosarcomas or synovial sarcomas
  - Thyroid carcinomas (papillary and medullary)
  - Malignant germ cell tumours
- Miliary metastases (from vascular tumours):
  - Breast
  - Thyroid
  - Kidney
  - Prostate
  - Soft tissue and bone sarcomas
  - Choriocarcinomas
- Cavitating metastases:
  - Squamous cell carcinoma from head and neck and cervix
  - Osteosarcoma
- Haemorrhagic metastases (typically ill-defined):
  - Choriocarcinoma
  - Kaposi's sarcoma

Notes

- "Cannonball" metastases of the type shown in the case presented here are most common in patients with renal or colon cancers and melanomas. Rarer causes include choriocarcinoma and adrenal carcinoma.
- Metastases from sarcomatous primary tumours may be cystic and peripheral, predisposing patients to pneumothoraces; in a patient with an amputation and a pneumothorax, think about the possibility of metastatic osteosarcoma.
- The candidate should revise a working list of the different types and origins that can be shown by examiners.

Bibliography

Flavin R, Finn S, McErlean A, et al. Cannonball metastases with favourable prognosis. Ir J Med Sci 2005;174(1): 61–64

2.21 Atherosclerotic Coronary Artery Disease

Clinical History

*A 49-year-old patient presents with atypical chest pain, raised cholesterol levels, and a family history of premature coronary artery disease (**Figs. 2.21.1–21.3**).*

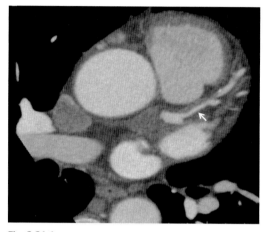

Fig. 2.21.1

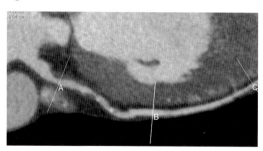

Fig. 2.21.2

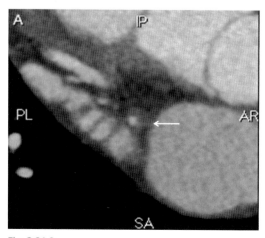

Fig. 2.21.3

Ideal Summary

The reconstructed axial image demonstrates soft plaque at the ostium of the left anterior descending coronary artery (LAD), which extends into the proximal LAD down to the approximate level where the first diagonal originates (**Fig. 2.21.1**, arrow). The curved multiplanar reconstruction demonstrates the overall extent of disease, and the orthogonal section at the level where the first section (labelled A on **Fig. 2.21.2**) dissects the artery shows that the severity of narrowing is greater than 70% (**Fig. 2.21.3**, arrow) and is likely to be significant. These are appearances of atherosclerotic coronary artery disease, and referral for invasive angiography is warranted.

Examination Tips

- Interpretation of coronary artery disease requires a systematic approach in which all arterial segments are evaluated.
- In addition to the basic review on the axial images, the candidate should be in the habit of looking at the arterial segments in multiple planes: two orthogonal planes (at 90° to each other) are particularly useful when determining the severity of stenosis.
- When reporting the severity of stenosis, most experienced observers use relatively broad categories (< 30%, 30 to 50%, 50 to 70%, and > 70%) to describe the severity of luminal narrowing.
- In simple terms, narrowing of less than < 50% is not likely to be flow-limiting.
- Disease that causes greater than 70% narrowing is likely to be significant and probably warrants invasive angiography, particularly if the patient is symptomatic.
- Disease in the 50 to 70% category is of uncertain physiological significance, and a confirmatory functional test (e.g., stress echocardiography) may be needed before proceeding to more invasive tests.

Bibliography

Bastarrika G, Lee YS, Huda W, Ruzsics B, Costello P, Schoepf UJ. CT of coronary artery disease. Radiology 2009;253(2):317–338

3   Introduction to Musculoskeletal Imaging

Ounali S. Jaffer, Imran Khan, and David A. Elias

Musculoskeletal imaging cases are among the most commonly presented in any radiology examination. This is obviously a reflection of general radiological clinical practice, but, additionally, the fact that all imaging modalities may contribute uniquely to the diagnosis and staging of many musculoskeletal pathologies means that such cases lend themselves to a discussion by the examiner and the candidate. Some general principles should be borne in mind in the approach to a musculoskeletal case:

❶ Anatomy is usually critical to making an accurate diagnosis. When faced with a lesion, always ask yourself where the "epicentre" of the process is likely to be (i.e., where do you think the process started?). This will form the basis of your differential diagnostic list. Consider whether the epicentre of a lesion is:

   i. Within a bone or in a joint (e.g., avascular necrosis of the hip has its epicentre in the femoral head, whereas an arthritis of the hip has its epicentre in the joint itself).

   ii. Within a bone or soft tissue (e.g., osteosarcoma has its epicentre in the bone with an adjacent soft tissue mass, while a soft tissue tumour will have an epicentre in the soft tissue but may erode adjacent bone).

   iii. If within a bone, is the epicentre medullary or cortical? Is it epiphyseal, metaphyseal, or diaphyseal? Each of these will have separate differential diagnostic possibilities.

   iv. If within a soft tissue, is the epicentre within muscle, tendon, ligament, enthesis (i.e., the organ that attaches a ligament or tendon onto bone), fascia, nerve, vessel, or fat?

❷ Only provide differential diagnoses that are relevant to the patient's age group.

- Always check if the age is printed somewhere on the film.
- If no age clues are present and the age group is critical to your differential list, just before listing the differential diagnoses you should say to the examiner something like, "Assuming the patient is 20 to 30 years of age…." If you have seen enough films, you should in most cases be able to make a reasonable attempt at estimating the age, and this approach avoids asking the examiner direct questions, which can be uncomfortable!

- With bone tumours, many lesions are relatively age-specific. In general, always consider metastases and myeloma in patients above the age of 40 years. Do not include metastases and myeloma for much younger patients (except if you think there may be a particular malignancy such as neuroblastoma, which occurs in childhood).
- Paediatric hip disease is another classic example in which the differential diagnosis is age-dependent:

   i. Developmental dysplasia (in newborns, but missed cases may present at any age)

   ii. Septic arthritis (may occur at any age but most commonly at 0 to 6 years)

   iii. Transient synovitis (age 2 to 10 years)

   iv. Perthes' disease (typically 5 to 8 years)

   v. Slipped upper femoral epiphysis (during the adolescent growth spurt—mean age 12 years in girls and 13.5 years in boys)

   vi. Juvenile chronic arthritis (may be at any age).

❸ The presence of a single lesion versus multiple lesions often critically alters the differential diagnosis. This applies to joint disease (i.e., monoarthropathy versus polyarthropathy) as well as focal bone lesions. If you see only one lesion and you want to use a differential diagnostic list for a single lesion (which usually is shorter than the list for multiple lesions), you may say something like, "Assuming this is a solitary lesion…." Again, this avoids a direct question to the examiner and allows the examiner to redirect you comfortably if they want to lead you down another route.

❹ Try to be ordered in your presentation:

- List findings, including pertinent negatives. While doing this, you should be thinking (but not saying):

   i. What are the diagnostic possibilities and what are the other findings that each possibility may show on this film? That way you will actively look for all the possible relevant findings and mention pertinent negatives.

   ii. If you think you know the diagnosis, resist the temptation to come up with it and bring your presentation to a close. Continue listing relevant positive and negative findings and think of the "3 Cs"—Causes, Consequences, and Concomitant findings. Good radiology examination cases may have all of these on the film, allowing you to score highly. See Case 3.14 (Transient Lateral Patellar Dislocation) for an example of this.

- Summarise. This is not essential to do but can be useful if your description was long, and it provides you with a bit of extra thinking time. However, the summary should not be a repetition of all your findings. Rather, it should be a single sentence with the key findings that are going to form the heading of your differential diagnostic list. Therefore, you will include findings that lead to a short differential list (or if possible a single diagnosis) and ignore findings that are nonspecific.
- Differential diagnosis. If you can confidently give a single diagnosis, do so. If you need to list differential diagnoses, aim to include no more than three. It is crucial that they must all be relevant to the case. Try to avoid listing diagnoses and then explaining why you think they are unlikely (a surprisingly common temptation).
- Emergency management. If there are any issues requiring emergency management, remember to say what you would do.
- Further investigation. Remember to be specific (i.e., do not just say "I would arrange an MRI," say "I would arrange an MRI *of the knee to identify....*").

⑤ Do not forget to ask for old films where relevant. They often sort out a diagnostic dilemma in real life as well as in the examination, and are cheaper than carrying out an MRI.

Descriptive Approach to Joint Disease in the Hands

- Distribution:
  - Which joints are involved?
  - Is it a monoarthropathy or polyarthropathy?
  - If a polyarthropathy, is it unilateral or bilateral?
  - If bilateral, is the process symmetrical or asymmetrical?
- Periarticular soft tissues:
  - Swelling
  - Calcification
- Periarticular bone mineral density:
  - Periarticular osteopaenia/subchondral sclerosis?
- Joint space:
  - Widened/narrowed/ankylosed/normal?
  - Dislocation/subluxation?

- Erosions:
  - Location: central/marginal/juxta-articular?
  - Character:
    - Ill-defined/well-defined?
    - If well-defined, are the erosions proliferative (i.e., is there new bone formation at the margin)?
    - Are there overhanging margins?
- Osteophytes
- Periosteal reaction
- Tuft resorption

Descriptive Approach to a Focal Bone Lesion

The following approach describes three key features of location, and then describes all the potential features of a lesion from inside out:

- Location (where is the epicentre?):
  - Which bone?
  - Diaphysis/metaphysis/epiphysis?
  - Central medullary/eccentric medullary/cortical/extraosseous (soft tissue)?
- Matrix:
  - Lytic
  - Sclerotic
  - "Ground glass"
  - Chondroid ("rings and arcs")
- Margin:
  - Well-defined/ill-defined (a narrow or wide zone of transition)
  - If well-defined, is the border sclerotic?
- Supplementary features:
  - Expansile/nonexpansile
  - Endosteal scalloping
  - Cortical breach
  - Pathological fracture
  - Periosteal reaction
  - Soft tissue mass

Acknowledgements

In passing on these tips, I must acknowledge their source, and thank my many pre-examination teachers at the Royal London and St. Bartholomew's Hospital, London, United Kingdom. In particular, much of the above advice comes from Dr. Otto Chan's many tutorials. A first-rate radiologist, and teacher with unlimited enthusiasm, he continues to inspire radiologists and clinicians alike.

-David A. Elias

3.1 Ankylosing Spondylitis

Clinical History

A 50-year-old man presents with acute back pain following trauma (**Fig. 3.1.1**).

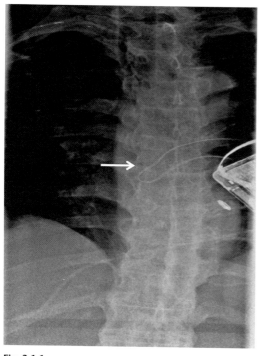

Fig. 3.1.1

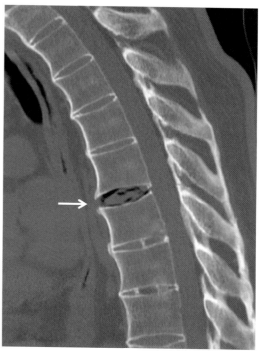

Fig. 3.1.2

Ideal Summary

This is an anteroposterior radiograph of the thoracic spine. A pacemaker can be seen. There are fused syndesmophytes across multiple lower thoracic vertebral bodies. There is a horizontal linear lucency across a midthoracic disk (**Fig. 3.1.1**, arrow), with no displacement seen on this single view. This likely represents a diskal insufficiency fracture (Andersson lesion) in a patient with inflammatory spondyloarthropathy. I would advise spinal immobilisation and CT for further evaluation. MRI is contraindicated in this case due to the pacemaker.

This is a further image of the abnormality in the same patient (**Fig. 3.1.2**).

This is a sagittal reformatted image from a CT scan of the thoracic spine. This confirms bridging syndesmophytes at the anterior and posterior vertebral body margins, as well as bridging ossification of the interspinous ligament. This is consistent with a chronic inflammatory spondyloarthropathy, likely ankylosing spondylitis. The diskal fracture is also confirmed, with widening of a midthoracic disk space with a vacuum phenomenon, and fracture of the anterior and posterior bridging syndesmophytes and the ossified ligamentum flavum posteriorly (**Fig. 3.1.2**, arrow). The appearances are those of an unstable thoracic diskal insufficiency fracture (Andersson lesion) in a patient with chronic inflammatory spondyloarthropathy. Spinal immobilisation and neurosurgical referral are advised.

Examination Tips

- Seronegative spondyloarthritis may affect the vertebra, intervertebral disks, facet and costovertebral joints, and tendon and ligament attachments (entheses). It is therefore important to review all of these areas.

Syndesmophytes, which represent ossification in the annulus fibrosus of the disk, run vertically from the margin of the vertebral body. These can be distinguished from osteophytes, which run horizontally from the margin of the vertebral body, even if only for a short distance, before turning vertically.

Diskal lesions occurring in ankylosing spondylitis are termed Andersson lesions.

- Inflammatory involvement of the intervertebral disks, known as spondylodiscitis or an "inflammatory Andersson lesion," is a noninfective lesion of the central disk.
  - Radiography demonstrates erosions at the centre of end plates and disk height loss.
  - On MRI, there is signal change (hyperintense on short T1 inversion recovery [STIR] and hypointense on T1-weighted images) within the central disk and adjacent end plates, with central end plate erosions.

Spinal insufficiency fractures are also common, especially in the presence of osteoporosis.

- This may occur spontaneously or following minor trauma.
- Fractures are typically horizontally oriented and may occur through the mid portion of a vertebral body or (as in this case) through the disk.
- Diskal fractures are termed "non-inflammatory Andersson lesions."

Differential Diagnosis

The radiographic features in this case are characteristic of an Andersson fracture in a chronic inflammatory spondyloarthropathy, and no differential diagnosis needs to be provided. Differentiation between spondyloarthritides can be difficult on the basis of imaging alone. Usually, a detailed history should help differentiate them (skin changes in psoriasis, bowel symptoms for inflammatory bowel disease, and urethritis/cervicitis in reactive arthritis).

Ankylosing spondylitis:

- This predominately affects the axial as opposed to the appendicular skeleton and is most common in young males.
- Sacroiliitis is typically symmetrical.

Psoriasis:

- This produces parasyndesmophytes (ossification of the paravertebral connective tissue), as opposed to syndesmophytes (ossification of the annulus fibrosus).

- Sacroiliitis is typically bilateral, but asymmetrical.
- Absence of sacroiliitis is more frequently encountered than in ankylosing spondylitis.

Reactive arthritis:

- Absence of severe cervical involvement is more typical.
- Sacroiliitis is typically bilateral, but asymmetrical.
- Absence of concomitant sacroiliitis is more frequently encountered than in ankylosing spondylitis.

Inflammatory bowel disease:

- Appearances typically are similar to those of ankylosing spondylitis, with a symmetrical sacroiliitis.

Notes

Ankylosing spondylitis typically presents between the ages of 30 and 55 years, and is much more prevalent in males (4–10:1).

The aetiology is not completely understood; however, a strong genetic predisposition exists. A direct relationship with the *HLA-B27* gene has been determined.

Usually, patients will initially report a transient ache within the lower back indicative of sacroiliac disease. Progression of the disease is usually segmental, with subsequent involvement of the lumbar and then thoracic and cervical segments.

Sacroiliitis is identified radiographically as loss of definition of the subchondral bone plate at the inferior sacroiliac joint. This is followed by erosions, sclerosis (on both sides of the joint), and eventual ankylosis.

Romanus lesions, which manifest as irregularities and erosions involving the anterior and posterior margins of the vertebral end plates, are the earliest changes of spondylitis seen on radiographs. Disease progression leads to sclerotic changes ("shiny corners") of the vertebral end plates.

Bibliography

Hermann KG, Althoff CE, Schneider U, et al. Spinal changes in patients with spondyloarthritis: comparison of MR imaging and radiographic appearances. Radiographics 2005;25(3):559–569, discussion 569–570

Levine DS, Forbat SM, Saifuddin A. MRI of the axial skeletal manifestations of ankylosing spondylitis. Clin Radiol 2004;59(5):400–413

3.2 Avascular Necrosis

Clinical History

A 25-year-old woman presents complaining of left hip pain (**Fig. 3.2.1**).

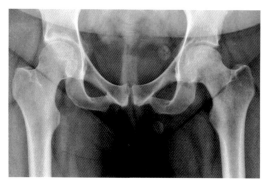

Fig. 3.2.1

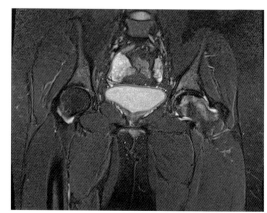

Fig. 3.2.2

Ideal Summary

This is an anteroposterior radiograph of the hips in an adult woman. There is patchy sclerosis and lucency of the left femoral head associated with mild flattening of the superior femoral head. No subchondral fracture line is evident on the plain radiograph. The joint space is preserved, and there is no abnormality on the acetabular side of the joint. The rest of the visualised bones and joints are unremarkable. In particular, the right hip is normal. The appearances are of avascular necrosis (AVN) of the left hip. I do not see evidence of an underlying cause on this radiograph. Orthopaedic review would be advised.

These are some further images of the same patient (**Figs. 3.2.2–3.2.4**).

These are coronal short T1 inversion recovery and coronal and sagittal T1-weighted MR images of the hips. There is serpiginous subchondral signal change in the left femoral head with areas of low signal on all sequences consistent with sclerosis. There is marrow oedema within the femoral head and neck, and a joint effusion is present. There is slight flattening of the femoral head, consistent with early collapse, and there are early ring osteophytes around the femoral head consistent with early secondary degenerative changes. The acetabular side of the joint appears normal, and there is no abnormality of the right hip.

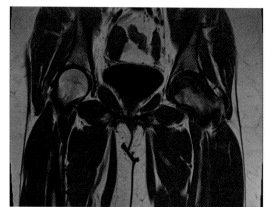

Fig. 3.2.3

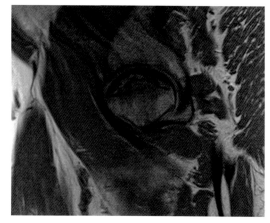

Fig. 3.2.4

This confirms the diagnosis of AVN seen on the plain radiograph. Further management by the orthopaedic team is indicated.

Examination Tips

- The radiographic diagnosis of AVN relies on identifying that the epicentre of the abnormality lies within the femoral head itself and not within the joint. Even when there is secondary degenerative change such that there are changes on the acetabular side of the joint and joint space loss, the changes are typically asymmetrically distributed across the joint, with much more advanced changes on the femoral side, such that the epicentre of the process appears to remain within the femoral head.
- Causes of AVN that may be identifiable on the pelvic radiograph should be sought. Examples include:
  - An underlying fracture of the femoral neck
  - Sacroiliitis or pubic symphysitis, which may indicate inflammatory spondyloarthropathy and steroid treatment
  - Chronic renal failure, which may be indicated by heavy vascular calcification or the soft tissue of a renal transplant in the pelvis
  - Sickle cell disease, which may be shown by bone sclerosis and "H-shaped" vertebral bodies
  - A massive spleen may occasionally extend into the left hemipelvis and indicate myelofibrosis
  - Gaucher's disease, commonly associated with AVN of the femoral heads; there may be generalised osteopaenia, cortical thinning with endosteal scalloping, broadened distal femoral metaphyses (Erlenmeyer's flask deformity), focal lucencies, and bone infarcts.
- The contralateral hip has an elevated risk of AVN and its normality (or otherwise) should be commented upon.

Differential Diagnosis

- In view of the pathognomonic imaging findings, there is no other differential diagnosis.
- Osteoarthritis can cause sclerosis of the femoral head and some contour deformity, but it is associated with osteophyte formation and loss of joint space, and changes should equally affect the acetabular side of the joint.

Notes

- Avascular necrosis is a result of interrupted blood supply resulting in bone infarction.
- It can occur in a host of conditions, including trauma. However, a significant proportion of patients have no predisposing factors.
- Radiographs are not sensitive in the early stages. Radiographic staging is as follows:
  - Stage I—normal appearances
  - Stage II—patchy sclerosis and lucency as a result of bone hyperemia and an osteoblastic response
  - Stage IIIA—subchondral crescent sign, indicating subchondral fracture
  - Stage IIIB—collapse of the femoral head
  - Stage IV—secondary osteoarthritis
- MRI is sensitive in preradiographic AVN:
  - On T1-weighted images, there is typically a low signal intensity serpiginous band in the early stages surrounding a normal fat signal intensity. On T2-weighted images, there may be a "double-line sign" visible, with a low-signal band in keeping with osteoblastic activity and a high-signal inner band in keeping with granulation tissue.
  - MRI can also demonstrate any associated femoral neck marrow oedema and joint effusion, and these features may correlate with pain.
  - MRI can also determine the volume of the involvement of the femoral head. The risk of femoral head collapse increases where over 25% of the weight-bearing portion of the femoral head is involved.
- Bone scans are also more sensitive than radiographs in diagnosing AVN, although less sensitive than MRI:
  - In the early stages, there may be a photopaenic defect. In later stages, there is increased activity due to the hyperemic response and osteoblastic activity, or due to secondary degenerative changes.
- Treatment of AVN consists of core decompression, vascularised bone grafts, or arthroplasty for late-stage disease.

Bibliography

Saini A, Saifuddin A. MRI of osteonecrosis. Clin Radiol 2004;59(12):1079–1093

Manaster BJ. From the RSNA Refresher Courses. Radiological Society of North America. Adult chronic hip pain: radiographic evaluation. Radiographics 2000;20(Spec No: S3–S25)

3.3 Bucket Handle Tear of the Medial Meniscus

Clinical History

A 25-year-old man presents with pain in right knee following an injury (**Figs. 3.3.1** and **3.3.2**).

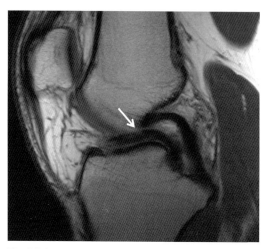

Fig. 3.3.1

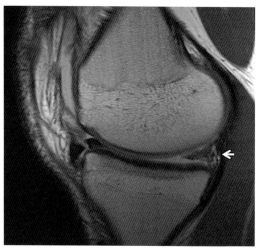

Fig. 3.3.2

Ideal Summary

These are selected sagittal MR proton density images of the intercondylar region and medial compartment of the knee. An intact posterior cruciate ligament (PCL) is demonstrated on the intercondylar image, with a structure anteroinferior to it consistent with a "double PCL sign" (**Fig. 3.3.1**, arrow); this represents a displaced meniscal fragment. The medial compartment demonstrates a "ghost" (absent; **Fig. 3.3.2**, arrow) posterior horn of the medial meniscus, with an additional structure adjacent to the anterior horn consistent with a displaced meniscal fragment. A joint effusion is also seen on the medial compartment image. The appearances are consistent with a bucket handle tear of the medial meniscus. It would be my normal practice to review the remainder or the MR examination to identify associated ligamentous and cartilage injuries. Urgent orthopaedic referral is advised, particularly if the knee is locked.

Examination Tips

- It is useful to be able to locate a sagittal MRI of the knee to the medial or lateral compartment or the intercondylar region:
  - In the intercondylar region, the anterior and/or PCLs will be identified, and the obliquely sloping roof of the intercondylar notch (Blumensaat's line) is seen (**Fig. 3.3.1**).
  - In the medial compartment, the tibia has the shape of a golf tee.
  - In the lateral compartment, the tibia has the shape of the butt of a gun (or on some slices the fibula may be identifiable).
- On either the medial or lateral meniscus, the posterior horn should never normally be smaller than the anterior horn. If the posterior horn is smaller, there is either a meniscal tear with a displaced fragment, or there has been a partial meniscectomy.
- A displaced meniscal fragment lying adjacent to the anterior meniscus (**Fig. 3.3.2**) is sometimes called a "fast-forward sign."
- The patellar tendon is only partially in the plane of the section in **Fig. 3.3.1**, and examination of this image alone may result in the erroneous conclusion that it is torn. Before making that diagnosis, you would need to ask to see the adjacent images.

Differential Diagnosis

Differential diagnosis of the double PCL sign:
- Anterior cruciate ligament (ACL) tear:
  - The normal ACL should run parallel to the roof of the intercondylar notch (Blumensaat's line).

- In a complete proximal tear of the ACL, its torn fibers may lie horizontally in the intercondylar notch, potentially mimicking a "double PCL sign."
- An ACL tear is distinguished from a meniscal bucket handle tear by reviewing full image series and identifying whether a normal ACL is seen separately or whether the meniscus is deficient in volume. Additionally, the ACL will be seen to insert onto the tibial footplate even when torn from its proximal origin.
- Prominent intact meniscofemoral ligament:
  - The meniscofemoral ligaments extend from the posterior horn of the lateral meniscus to the lateral aspect of the medial femoral condyle.
  - The meniscofemoral ligament of Humphrey runs anterior to the PCL, while the ligament of Wrisberg runs posterior to the PCL.
  - When a normal meniscofemoral ligament is prominent, it can mimic a "double PCL sign."
  - A meniscofemoral ligament may be distinguished from a displaced meniscal fragment by identifying the expected attachments of the ligament on successive MR images and identifying whether a meniscus is deficient in volume.

Notes

- Medial meniscal tears may be asymptomatic or present with joint line tenderness or grinding, and there may be a positive McMurray's test on clinical examination.
- Torn menisci with displaced fragments may present with locking and require urgent arthroscopic repair or partial meniscectomy.
- Meniscal tears may be described by their orientation relative to the normally c-shaped meniscus:
  - Horizontal tears cleave the meniscus into superior and inferior fragments.

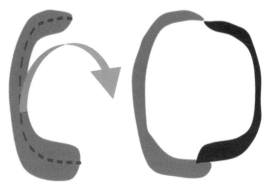

Fig. 3.3.3

- Vertical tears may be radial (directed like the spokes in a bicycle wheel) or longitudinal (directed along the curve of the c-shape, separating an inner portion of the c-shape from an outer portion of the c-shape).
- Oblique tears are intermediate between vertical and horizontal tears.
- Complex tears contain a mixture of tear morphologies.
- Where a longitudinal tear extends to involve the entire meniscus, the inner fragment may separate from the outer fragment and flip centrally into the intercondylar notch. This is known as a bucket handle tear (**Fig. 3.3.3**).

Bibliography

Saifuddin A. The Knee in Musculoskeletal MRI: A Rapid Reference Guide. Oxford University Press. Oxford, UK: Oxford University Press; 2008

Venkatanarasimha N, Kamath A, Mukherjee K, Kamath S. Potential pitfalls of a double PCL sign. Skeletal Radiol. 2009;38:735-9.

3.4 Diaphyseal Aclasis

Clinical History

*A 23-year-old man presents with a long-standing mass in his left leg. He feels that the mass is increasing in size, causing more pain (**Figs. 3.4.1** and **3.4.2**).*

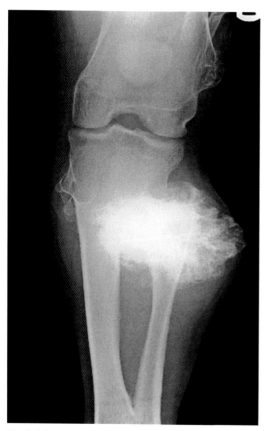

Fig. 3.4.1

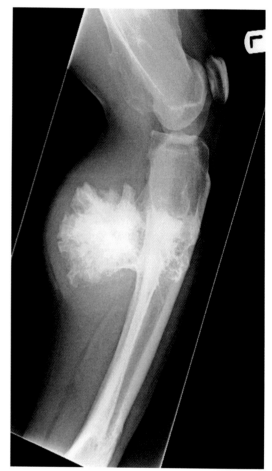

Fig. 3.4.2

Ideal Summary

These are frontal and lateral radiographs of the left lower limb of a young adult with fused epiphyses. There is a large sclerotic bony lesion arising from the proximal fibula that extends posterolaterally and anteriorly. There is continuation of the bony cortex of the lesion with the fibula on the lateral image. Further bony lesions are present at the medial and lateral aspects of the distal femur, and also at the proximal tibia, and at the distal tibia and fibula within the metaphyseal regions. These also demonstrate contiguity of the cortex and medulla of the lesions with the underlying bone. The distal femur and proximal tibia show associated metaphyseal widening, and there is some varus bowing of the tibia. There is no knee joint involvement and no effusion.

The appearances are in keeping with multiple osteochondromas consistent with diaphyseal aclasis. Comparison with available previous radiographs would be important to assess for any change in the largest lesion, which might indicate malignant change. Given the large size of this lesion, clinical assessment should be made for evidence of mechanical impingement. In particular, peroneal neurovascular symptoms may be expected. Given the clinical history of enlargement, MRI should be performed to assess for a cartilage cap. Orthopaedic review is suggested.

Examination Tips

- The radiological diagnosis of an osteochondroma relies on the presence of contiguity between the cortex of the lesion and the cortex of the host bone, and contiguity between the medulla of the lesion and the medulla of the host bone.
- Solitary lesions generally arise from the metaphyseal regions and grow away from the adjacent joint. However, lesions in diaphyseal aclasis may not conform to this pattern.
- It is important to comment on fusion of the epiphysis, as osteochondromas can grow with the growth of the underlying bone in an immature skeleton.
- Evidence for potential complications of an osteochondroma should be sought:
  - Overlying bursa
  - Extrinsic compression (which may be due to the lesion or due to an overlying bursa) causing impingement upon:
    - Joint
    - Muscle
    - Neurovascular structures
  - Fracture
  - Malignant transformation (see below)
  - Bony deformity

Differential Diagnosis

The findings are characteristic, and no differential diagnosis should be provided.

Notes

- Osteochondromas are common benign bone tumours, composed of cortical and medullary bone with an overlying cartilage cap.
- Osteochondromas can be solitary or multiple, as encountered in diaphyseal aclasis (hereditary multiple exostoses), which is an autosomal dominant condition.
- When multiple, they are usually encountered around the knee or in the humerus. However, they are also commonly identified around the ribs, scapula, and hips.
- Malignant transformation may occur in 1 to 2% of solitary osteochondromas and 3 to 5% of patients with diaphyseal aclasis. Approximately 90% of cases of malignant transformation are to chondrosarcoma, and this is usually of low grade.
- Clinical features suspicious for malignant degeneration include new otherwise unexplained pain or continued growth after skeletal maturity.
- Radiographic features of malignant change, particularly if these are seen to be new, include:
  - Scattered calcifications in the soft tissue part of a lesion (i.e., within the cartilage cap)
  - An irregular or ill-defined osteochondral surface of a lesion
  - A soft tissue mass (which may be due to a bursa rather than malignant degeneration)
  - Focal lucencies developing within a lesion
  - Destruction or scalloping of the host bone.
- MRI demonstrates the overlying cartilage cap. A cap of more than 1.5 cm in thickness after skeletal maturity is considered suspicious for malignant change, and MRI can help direct biopsy to the thickest region.
- Osteochondromas may require resection for cosmetic reasons or symptomatic relief. In patients with diaphyseal aclasis, surgery is also performed to correct deformities.
- Patients with diaphyseal aclasis require surveillance to evaluate for possible malignant complication. Malignant transformation is treated with wide surgical excision.

Bibliography

Lee KC, Davies AM, Cassar-Pullicino VN. Imaging the complications of osteochondromas. Clin Radiol 2002;57(1):18–28

Murphey MD, Choi JJ, Kransdorf MJ, Flemming DJ, Gannon FH. Imaging of osteochondroma: variants and complications with radiologic-pathologic correlation. Radiographics 2000;20(5):1407–1434

3.5 Enchondroma

Clinical History

A 30-year-old woman presents to the emergency department complaining of pain in her left thigh following a fall (**Figs. 3.5.1** and **3.5.2**).

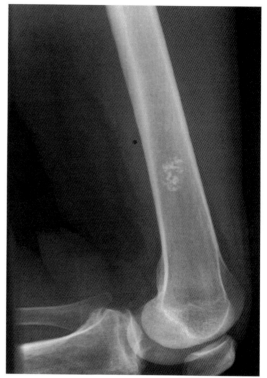

Fig. 3.5.2

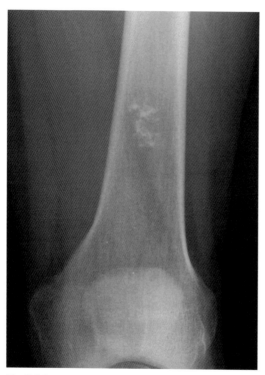

Fig. 3.5.1

Ideal Summary

These are anteroposterior and lateral radiographs of the distal femur of an adult patient. There is a calcified lesion within the medulla of the distal diaphysis of the femur. The lesion is nonexpansile and appears well defined. The calcification has the morphology of "arcs and rings" consistent with chondroid matrix. I cannot see evidence of any fractures, cortical involvement, periosteal reaction, or soft tissue masses. No other lesions are present on the available radiographs. The appearances are typical for a well-differentiated chondroid lesion, likely an

enchondroma, although a well-differentiated chondrosarcoma may have similar appearances and may need to be excluded, especially if the lesion has become painful. The differential diagnosis would be of a medullary infarct, although the calcification in an infarct is typically more peripheral and serpiginous, unlike the more central "arcs and rings" seen in this case. It would be helpful to review any previous imaging, if available, to identify any change in appearances. In the absence of previous imaging, further assessment with MRI or CT is advised.

This is another image from the same patient (**Fig. 3.5.3**).

On this single sagittal CT reformatted image, the lesion is confined within the medulla without involvement of the cortex. The pattern of calcification appears consistent with chondroid matrix, with a "ring and arc" pattern evident. There is no significant

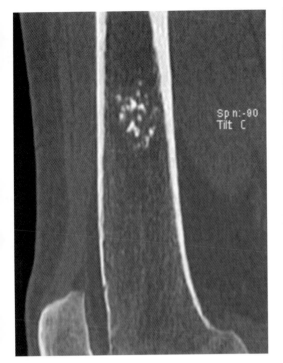

Fig. 3.5.3

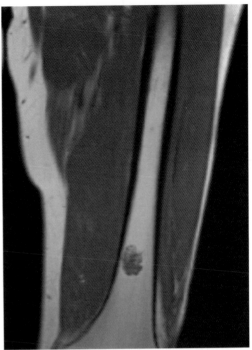

Fig. 3.5.4

endosteal scalloping, cortical breach, periosteal reaction, or soft tissue mass.

These are the MR images from the same patient (**Figs. 3.5.4** and **3.5.5**).

These are coronal T1-weighted and T2 fat-saturated images of the left femur. On T1-weighted imaging, there is a predominant low-to-intermediate signal intensity lesion, with high signal foci superiorly. The lesion has a lobulated contour. On the T2 fat-saturated image, there are more clearly defined clusters of numerous high signal intensity locules. The foci of low signal present are likely to represent the calcification already observed on the other imaging modalities. There are no associated features to suggest an aggressive pathology.

This is the nuclear medicine study (**Fig. 3.5.6**).

This whole-body bone scan demonstrates moderate uptake within the left femoral lesion, with a degree of uptake less than that seen within the anterior iliac crest. There are no other lesions identified elsewhere within the skeleton. The given features of all the imaging modalities are in keeping with

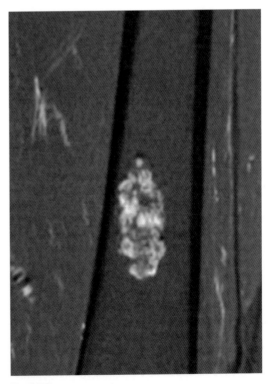

Fig. 3.5.5

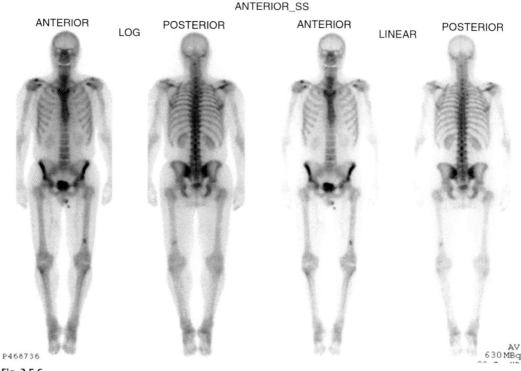

Fig. 3.5.6

a well-differentiated chondroid lesion and would make enchondroma the most likely diagnosis. I would suggest follow-up at 6 months with conventional radiographs.

Examination Tips

The main differential diagnoses of such a lesion within the long bones are chondrosarcoma and bone infarct.

- The presence of pain should always alert the observer to the possibility of a malignant tumour as most patients with chondrosarcomas (81 to 95%) will complain of this symptom. Enchondromas (34%) may also present with pain, but do so less frequently. Usually, pain associated with enchondromas can be attributed to an associated fracture or a concurrent intra-articular disorder (e.g., meniscal tear or osteoarthritis). Patients with bone infarcts often present with pain but may also be asymptomatic. In practical terms, if the patient complains of pain, further imaging is usually warranted.
- The typical appearance of chondroid matrix mineralisation may not always be obvious on plain

films, especially in the long bones. In such cases, it is reasonable to request a CT study to differentiate the dystrophic ossification of bone infarcts from the "ring and arcs" pattern of chondroid calcification.

- Always ask for any old films for comparison. If the degree of calcification within the lesion has decreased, this may be an indicator of malignant transformation.
- Lobulated borders on MRI are suggestive of chondroid pathology, but this does not distinguish enchondromas from an infarction or a chondrosarcoma. Typical MRI features of enchondromas include multiple thin septa, a low-to-intermediate T1-weighted and high T2-weighted signal, and a "ring and arcs" pattern on contrast enhancement. Calcification is usually seen as signal voids on all sequences.
- A useful discriminator on bone scintigraphy is the degree of uptake within the lesion. If the uptake is less than that observed within the anterior iliac crest (which is normally an active site), the lesion is more likely to be an enchondroma. Conversely, if lesion uptake is greater than that seen within the anterior iliac crest, a chondrosarcoma is the more likely diagnosis.

Radionuclide scanning is not reliable in differentiating an enchondroma from an ossified marrow infarct.

Differential Diagnosis

- Bone infarct:
  - This shows dystrophic ossification as opposed to "ring and arc" calcification.
  - A serpiginous rind of sclerosis encapsulating the lesion is strongly suggestive of a bone infarct. On MRI, this will be of low signal intensity on both T1- and T2-weighted imaging.
- Chondrosarcoma:
  - The following features are strong indicators of chondrosarcoma and should trigger referral to a bone tumour unit for potential biopsy and excision:
    - Pathological fracture occurring with minimal trauma
    - Multilayered or spiculate periosteal reaction
    - Permeative or moth-eaten osteolysis
    - Cortical destruction
    - A soft tissue mass
  - The following features are weaker potential indicators of chondrosarcoma, and the lesion may require biopsy and excision (at a bone tumour unit):
    - Endosteal scalloping of over two-thirds of the cortical thickness in depth
    - Endosteal scalloping along over two-thirds of the length of the lesion
    - Cortical thickening or hyperostosis
    - Activity greater than that of the anterior iliac crest on delayed-phase bone scintigraphy
    - Early and exponential enhancement on dynamic gadolinium-enhanced MRI
    - Pain not otherwise explained

Notes

- Solitary enchondromas are usually discovered between the second and fourth decades.
- Polyostotic forms of the disease (Ollier's disease and Maffucci's syndrome) carry a greater risk for malignant transformation than for solitary lesions (< 1%).
- Enchondromas are most commonly located within the hands and feet, with chondrosarcomas a rare occurrence in this location. Pathological fracture, expansion, and scalloping in this location are common features and not generally indicators of malignant transformation.
- In the axial skeleton, enchondromas are unusual and chondrosarcomas more common; lesions within the axial skeleton should evoke a high degree of suspicion for malignancy.
- Biopsy should only be performed if there are defined features of an aggressive lesion suggestive of chondrosarcoma or imaging ambiguity. In most cases, the imaging features should be sufficient to achieve a confident diagnosis of enchondroma. Biopsies should ideally be undertaken in specialist units.
- If imaging confirms a benign enchondroma, follow-up with periodic radiographs (after 3 to 6 months initially and then annually is sufficient).

Bibliography

Murphey MD, Flemming DJ, Boyea SR, Bojescul JA, Sweet DE, Temple HT. Enchondroma versus chondrosarcoma in the appendicular skeleton: differentiating features. Radiographics 1998;18(5):1213–1237, quiz 1244–1245

Parlier-Cuau C, Bousson V, Ogilvie CM, Lackman RD, Laredo JD. When should we biopsy a solitary central cartilaginous tumor of long bones? Literature review and management proposal. Eur J Radiol 2011;77(1):6–12

3.6 Primary Hyperparathyroidism

Clinical History

*A 35-year-old man presents with leg pain (**Fig. 3.6.1**).*

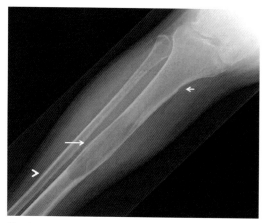

Fig. 3.6.1

Ideal Summary

This is an anteroposterior radiograph of the right tibia. A large lytic lesion is located in the central medulla of the mid-tibial diaphysis, with some thin trabeculae within the lesion but no matrix. The lesion is well defined. It is mildly expansile and there is cortical thinning. Laterally, there is a small area of cortical breach with adjacent periosteal elevation (**Fig. 3.6.1**, long arrow). There is no soft tissue mass. The bones appear generally osteopaenic. There is a subperiosteal erosion at the medial aspect of the proximal tibial metaphysis (**Fig. 3.6.1**, short arrow). There is a thin unilaminar periosteal reaction at the lateral mid-fibular diaphysis (**Fig. 3.6.1**, arrowhead). A small focus of ossification is seen at the site of the interosseous membrane between the lower tibial and fibular shafts. No vascular calcification is present.

The appearances are most likely consistent with hyperparathyroidism, most likely primary, with a brown tumour of the tibia. I would like to review the lateral view and any old films, and recommend blood tests for renal function and calcium and parathyroid hormone levels. Radiographs of the hands or a bone scan would help confirm the diagnosis. Orthopaedic referral is advised for review of the tibial lesion, as the focal cortical irregularity may indicate the presence of a pathological fracture, and the degree of cortical thinning is concerning for risk of further fracture.

*These are the magnified hand radiographs (**Fig. 3.6.2**).*

This is a radiograph of portions of the index and middle fingers. Subperiosteal resorption can be seen at the radial aspects of most of the visualised phalanges, most marked for the middle phalanges (**Fig. 3.6.2**, long arrow). There is early acro-osteolysis at the terminal tuft of the left index finger, and small marginal erosions are present at the proximal interphalangeal joint of the same finger (**Fig. 3.6.2**, short arrow). No soft tissue calcification is seen. Appearances are in keeping with bony manifestations of hyperparathyroidism.

Examination Tips

- Identification of subperiosteal bone resorption reduces the wide potential differential diagnosis of a lytic bone lesion to a single diagnosis.
- In general, a brown tumour would not be included in the differential diagnosis of a lytic bone lesion without the presence of other features of hyperparathyroidism.
- Be sure to identify possible pathological fractures in bone lesions, which may be a cause of presentation. Additionally, large lesions with cortical thinning or breach may need orthopaedic management due to the potential fracture risk.
- Primary is more likely than secondary hyperparathyroidism here as brown tumours are more common in the primary form. In contrast, secondary hyperparathyroidism, most commonly due to renal osteodystrophy, is characterised by vascular and other soft tissue calcifications and osteosclerosis, which are absent in this case.

Differential Diagnosis

In the absence of subperiosteal bone resorption, the differential diagnosis of this lytic tibial lesion might include:
- Fibrous dysplasia:
  - Typically, this shows a ground-glass matrix.

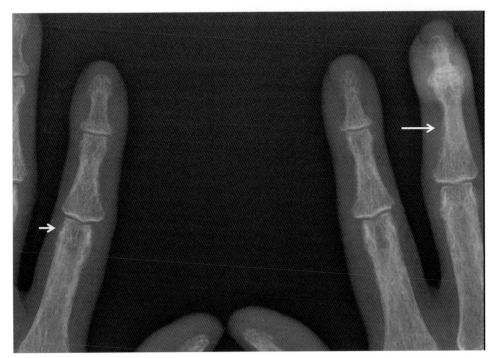

Fig. 3.6.2

- Osteoblastoma:
  - These usually occur in the second or third decade, but can occur later.
  - In tubular bones, lesions are commonly diaphyseal.
  - The radiographic characteristics are variable and may not allow a specific diagnosis to be made.
- Plasmacytoma:
  - Typically, these occur in an older age group, but they may be seen in the thirties age group.
  - They commonly cause endosteal scalloping.

Notes

- Hyperparathyroidism is due to excessive parathyroid hormone production and is characterised by decreased bone mass due to increased numbers of osteoclasts.
- Primary hyperparathyroidism is usually due to a single parathyroid adenoma. Less commonly, parathyroid hyperplasia or carcinoma may be the cause.
- Radiographic features include:
  - Bone resorption, which may be:
    - Subperiosteal
    - Subchondral (i.e., intra-articular), producing joint erosions
    - Intracortical, producing cortical tunnelling
    - Endosteal, producing cortical thinning
    - Subligamentous, producing erosions at the ligament and tendon attachments
    - Trabecular.
  - Brown tumour:
    - Typically appears as a well-defined, expansile, lytic lesion with endosteal scalloping.
  - Bone softening:
    - Vertebral collapses and bowing of the long bones.
  - Periosteal new bone formation
  - Features more common in secondary than primary hyperparathyroidism include:
    - Soft tissue calcification (including vascular calcification)
    - Osteosclerosis (e.g., a "rugger jersey" spine).

Bibliography

McDonald DK, Parman L, Speights VO Jr. Best cases from the AFIP: primary hyperparathyroidism due to parathyroid adenoma. Radiographics 2005;25(3):829–834

Stacy GS, Kapur A. Mimics of bone and soft tissue neoplasms. Radiol Clin North Am 2011;49(6): 1261–1286, vii

3.7 Avulsion of the Lesser Trochanter

Clinical History

A 64-year-old man presents with left groin pain (**Fig. 3.7.1**).

Ideal Summary

There is an irregular focus of ossification projected over the left groin, and the left lesser trochanter is absent. This is consistent with a lesser trochanteric avulsion (**Fig. 3.7.1**, arrow). At the site of the defect, there is a small focal lucency, but no destructive femoral lesion is seen. There are no other focal bony lesions. Vascular calcification can be noted. The finding of a lesser trochanteric avulsion in an adult is considered to indicate the presence of an underlying malignant bone tumour until proven otherwise. Given the age of the patient, this would most likely be a bone metastasis or myeloma. A lateral radiograph of the hip may be useful in identifying any underlying lesion. MRI or CT of the hip would identify the presence of a femoral bone lesion.

This is another image from the same patient (**Fig. 3.7.2**).

This is a coronal reformatted image from a CT scan of the pelvis. CT confirms the presence of a lytic lesion at the site of lesser trochanteric avulsion, consistent with a pathological avulsion fracture (**Fig. 3.7.2**, arrow). There is no matrix. The lesion is well defined laterally with a sclerotic margin, but there is cortical loss medially. There is no periosteal reaction or soft tissue mass identifiable on this image. Given the age of the patient, metastatic disease or myeloma is the most likely diagnosis. A bone scan, CT of the chest, abdomen, and pelvis, and a myeloma screen are advised.

This is an image from the chest CT examination (**Fig. 3.7.3**).

This is an image from CT of the chest that demonstrates a mass in the right upper lobe with a spiculate margin consistent with a primary lung carcinoma. This confirms the primary tumour responsible for the lytic abnormality of the left lesser trochanter and the avulsion fracture.

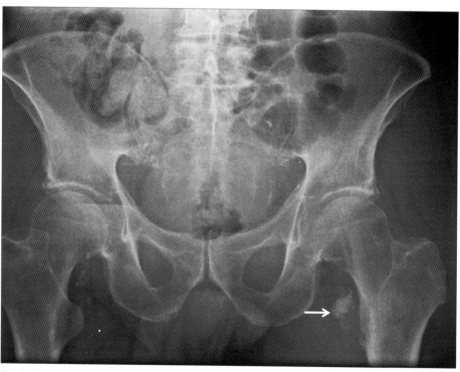

Fig. 3.7.1

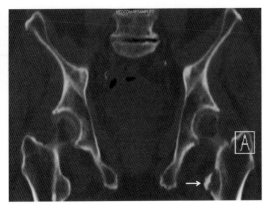

Fig. 3.7.2

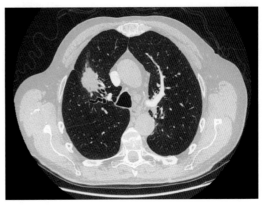

Fig. 3.7.3

Examination Tips

- It is sometimes critical to identify what is *absent* on an image—in this case, the lesser trochanter.
- The pull of the iliopsoas displaces the avulsed lesser trochanter cranially.
- In adults, atraumatic avulsions are considered virtually pathognomonic for the presence of an underlying bone lesion.
- A lytic bone lesion identified in the over 40-year age group is most commonly due to metastatic disease or myeloma. Investigations usually include:
  - Bone scan to identify other lesions
  - CT of the chest, abdomen, and pelvis—to identify a primary
  - Myeloma screen

Differential Diagnosis

The combination of an ossific mass with an absent lesser trochanter is diagnostic of lesser trochanteric avulsion. Causes of an ossific mass in the groin can be classified by structure of origin and could include:
- Hip joint:
  - Intra-articular body
- Bony avulsions:
  - For example, by rectus femoris (avulsion of the anterior inferior iliac spine) or adductor avulsions from the inferior pubic body

- Muscles
  - Myositis ossificans
  - Sarcoma
- Scrotal
  - Scrotal pearl
  - Testicular tumour or infarct
- Lymph node

Notes

- The iliopsoas attaches to the lesser trochanter, and if the femur is relatively weakened at this site, the lesser trochanter may be avulsed by this relatively powerful muscle.
- In a child or adolescent, lesser trochanteric avulsions occur following acute trauma in the absence of an underlying bone lesion, as the unfused apophysis is a site of relative weakness.
- In adults with atraumatic avulsion, metastatic disease or myeloma is the usual underlying cause, but a variety of malignant primary bone tumours have also been described.

Bibliography
James SL, Davies AM. Atraumatic avulsion of the lesser trochanter as an indicator of tumour infiltration. Eur Radiol 2006;16(2):512–514

3.8 Osteoid Osteoma

Clinical History

*A 19-year-old man presents with left leg pain that is worse at night (**Fig. 3.8.1**).*

Ideal Summary

The lateral radiograph of the left tibia demonstrates cortical thickening and sclerosis on the anterior aspect of the mid-diaphysis of the tibia (**Fig. 3.8.1**, arrow). There is no evidence of a central radiolucency within the sclerotic region, and no linear cortical lucency is identified. The lesion appears solitary on the radiograph provided. The differential diagnosis would include osteoid osteoma and tibial stress fracture. Given the provided history, the former is more likely. I would recommend further investigation of the lesion to identify a central nidus or a fracture line. An anteroposterior radiograph would normally be first assessed for these features. If that were negative, CT or MRI could be performed.

*This is another image from the same patient (**Fig. 3.8.2**).*

This is an axial CT image of the left leg. There is marked cortical thickening at the anterolateral aspect of the tibial shaft. Within the thickened cortex, there is a small rounded lucent nidus with mineralisation within it (**Fig. 3.8.2**, arrow). These findings are typical of cortical osteoid osteoma of the tibia. I would advise orthopaedic referral for further management. If clinically appropriate, this lesion may be treated with CT-guided radiofrequency ablation.

Examination Tips

- Osteoid osteoma typically appears as an area of dense sclerosis with a central rounded lucency, known as a nidus, which is less than 2 cm in diameter. The lucent nidus may show central mineralisation within it.
- CT is generally thought to demonstrate the nidus more clearly than MRI, but with improving MRI resolution this may no longer apply.

Differential Diagnosis

- Stress fracture:
  - The usual differential diagnosis is of a stress fracture. Distinction between osteoid osteoma and stress fracture relies on the identification

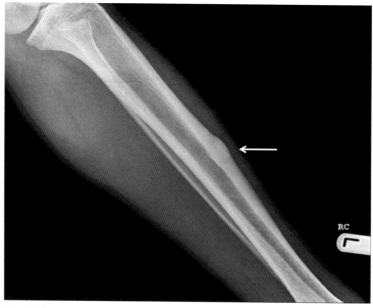

Fig. 3.8.1

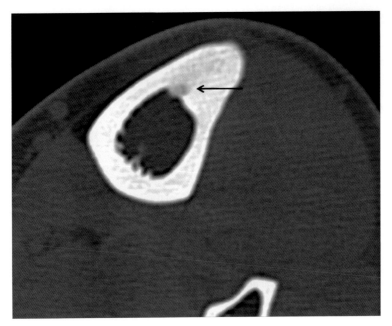

Fig. 3.8.2

of a rounded lucent nidus in osteoid osteoma versus a linear lucent fracture perpendicular to the long axis of the bone in a stress fracture.

- CT or MRI is often required to identify these features.
- Intracortical abscess:
  - The presence of a sequestrum within an intracortical abscess can make differentiation from osteoid osteoma difficult on plain radiographs.
  - CT imaging in an abscess may show that the inner margin of the cavity is irregular and sequestrum is present eccentrically.
  - MRI can also differentiate between the two lesions, as the unmineralised nidus in osteoid osteoma will enhance with gadolinium, whereas the abscess will demonstrate only peripheral enhancement and lack central enhancement.

Notes

- Osteoid osteoma is a benign bony tumour predominantly seen in males between the ages of 7 and 25 years.
- Osteoid osteoma is generally classified by location into cortical, medullary, and subperiosteal (in descending order of frequency of occurrence).
- The majority of the lesions are extra-articular, with 50% of lesions occurring in the tibia and femur. Approximately 30% occur in the spine, hands, and feet.
- Extra-articular lesions usually present with pain, which is typically worse at night and is relieved by aspirin.
- In the spine, osteoid osteoma typically occurs in the neural arch and causes radicular pain and painful scoliosis (the lesion being present on the concave side). Lesions are most frequent within the lumbar spine, followed by the cervical spine.
- Technetium 99m bone scintigraphy demonstrates a "double-density sign" with intense focal activity in the nidus superimposed on a larger area of moderate activity as a result of reactive changes.
- Intra-articular osteoid osteoma, which occurs within or near a joint, is distinct from the extra articular form and has a nonspecific clinical presentation. Pain is not typically worse at night. The hip is the most common joint affected. There is minimal reactive cortical thickening but there may be a joint effusion.
- Treatment consists of radiofrequency ablation or en bloc excision.

Bibliography

Chai JW, Hong SH, Choi JY, et al. Radiologic diagnosis of osteoid osteoma: from simple to challenging findings. Radiographics 2010;30(3):737–749

Kransdorf MJ, Stull MA, Gilkey FW, Moser RP Jr. Osteoid osteoma. Radiographics 1991;11(4):671–696

3.9 Osteopathia Striata/Osteopoikilosis

Clinical History

*A 70-year-old man has suspected multiple myeloma. This is an image from the skeletal survey (**Fig. 3.9.1**).*

Ideal Summary

This is an anteroposterior radiograph of the pelvis in an adult. There are dense linear medullary striations within both femora, centred on the metaphysis, with extension into the diaphysis. Similar striations are seen within the acetabulum, extending to the iliac and ischial bones. The distribution of findings is symmetrical in nature. Present in the same areas are small, more rounded sclerotic deposits. There is no cortical abnormality and no bony expansion. The findings are in keeping with a diagnosis of osteopathia striata, but the more rounded sclerotic foci suggest osteopoikilosis. This is likely to be an overlap syndrome of the two conditions. Comparison with any old films would confirm that appearances have not changed.

*The patient has a known history of breast cancer. This is a bone scan of the same patient (**Fig. 3.9.2**).*

This is a whole-body bone scan. No abnormal increased uptake is demonstrated to suggest the presence of bony metastatic disease from the known breast cancer. This confirms the diagnosis of a sclerosing bone dysplasia.

Examination Tips

- Osteopathia striata is a hereditary sclerosing bone dysplasia that should not be confused with metastatic or metabolic causes of bone sclerosis.
- There are typical dense linear striations in the diaphysis and metaphysis of the tubular bones. In the iliac bones, these can produce a "fan-shaped" appearance.
- Overlap syndromes with a combination of sclerosing bone dysplasias coexisting within the same patient are well recognised: the combination of osteopathia striata, osteopoikilosis (multiple rounded or ovoid sclerotic deposits in the meta-epiphyseal regions of the long bones and pelvis), and melorheostosis (a typical "dripping candle wax" appearance of dense sclerosis along a bony cortex) is well described.
- Both osteopoikilosis and osteopathia striata are characterised by their symmetrical distribution.
- Both entities are benign, so aggressive features such as a periosteal reaction and osseous destruction are not found. If encountered, an alternate diagnosis should be sought.

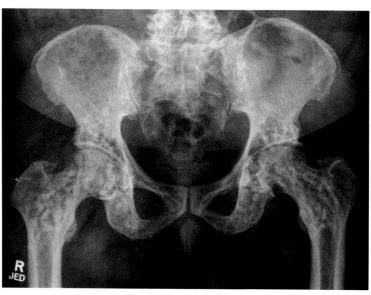

Fig. 3.9.1

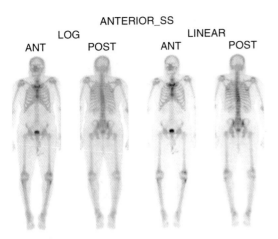

ANTERIOR_SS

LOG   LINEAR
ANT   POST   ANT   POST

Fig. 3.9.2

- The conditions will manifest in childhood; therefore, always ask for the old films for comparison. Stability of appearances enhances the certainty of diagnosis.
- If uncertain, a bone scan should be ordered. A normal bone scan is helpful in confirming the benign diagnosis.

Differential Diagnosis

The case here has characteristic appearances, and no differential diagnosis is required. Osteopathia striata should not generally be confused with other entities. Although the linear striations in osteopathia striata may resemble the coarsened trabeculae of Paget's disease, there is no expansion or cortical thickening. The multiple small rounded sclerotic foci in osteopoikilosis tend to be symmetrical and of uniform size (2–10 mm) and shape, and have a predilection for ends of tubular bones, extending along the trabeculae. These features should distinguish osteopoikilosis from all of the following causes of multiple sclerotic focal bone lesions:

- Osteoblastic metastases:
  - Breast and prostate cancer.
  - They have a predilection for the axial skeleton.
  - There are positive scintigraphic findings.
- Multiple myeloma:
  - Lesions are sclerotic in 1 to 3% of cases.
  - Lesions may become sclerotic after therapy.
  - Sclerotic myeloma lesions are typically associated with POEMS syndrome (polyneuropathy, organomegaly, endocrinopathy, monoclonal protein, and skin changes).

- Tuberous sclerosis:
  - Sclerotic deposits may occur in tuberous sclerosis.
  - Sclerotic deposits are irregular in shape.
  - Typically, cystic bony lesions occur.
  - Extraskeletal manifestations are generally clinically apparent.
- Mastocytosis:
  - Focal sclerotic deposits may occur in mastocystosis.
  - There is usually osteoporosis and areas of bony rarefaction.
  - Extraskeletal manifestations are generally clinically apparent.

Notes

- Both osteopathia striata and osteopoikilosis are dysplasias of secondary spongiosa (mature bone). They are characterised by failure of bone remodeling, resulting in the persistence of mature bony trabeculae and being manifest as focal densities and/or striations.
- Osteopoikilosis is inherited as an autosomal dominant trait and is frequently associated with dermatofibrosis lenticularis disseminata (papular fibromas over the back, arms, and thighs). The finding of small, symmetrically scattered opacities at the articular ends of long, tarsal, and carpal bones is characteristic. Lesions may also be found around the acetabulum and glenoid fossa, with the skull, spine, and ribs less common but recognised sites of involvement.
- Osteopathia striata primarily affects the long bones. Striations normally run parallel to the long axis of the bone and are found within the metaphysis, with extension into the diaphysis. Involvement of the epiphysis is rare but a recognised feature. Inheritance was initially thought to be autosomal dominant but, more recently, an X-linked inheritance pattern has been suggested. In some patients, sclerosis of the skull may occur, which can lead to cranial nerve palsies.

Bibliography

Greenspan A. Sclerosing bone dysplasias—a target-site approach. Skeletal Radiol 1991;20(8):561–583

Ihde LL, Forrester DM, Gottsegen CJ, et al. Sclerosing bone dysplasias: review and differentiation from other causes of osteosclerosis. Radiographics 2011;31(7): 1865–1882

3.10 Chronic Osteomyelitis

Clinical History

*A 38-year-old man presents with chronic lower limb pain (**Fig. 3.10.1**).*

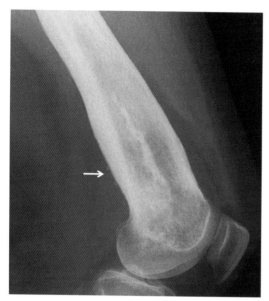

Fig. 3.10.1

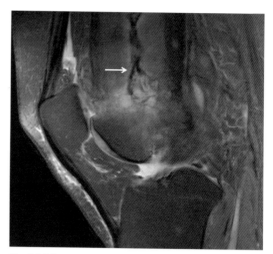

Fig. 3.10.2

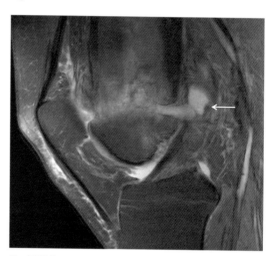

Fig. 3.10.3

Ideal Summary

This is a lateral radiograph of the lower femur. There is distal metaphyseal medullary expansile lesion with an ill-defined lucency inferiorly and ill-defined sclerosis superiorly. Additionally, there is an elongated area of central medullary sclerosis. There is diffuse metaphyseal cortical thickening seen tracking into the diaphysis above the field of view of the radiograph. There is no cortical breach. Posteriorly, there are irregular foci of periosteal reaction (**Fig. 3.10.1**, arrow). There is no soft tissue mass present, and no knee joint effusion is seen. The appearances are most typical for a chronic osteomyelitis, with the central medullary sclerosis representing a sequestrum. It would be my normal practice to review the frontal radiograph and radiographs of the remainder of the femur. Comparison with old radiographs would be helpful to assess for any progression. Further imaging with MRI may then be helpful to determine the extent of bony involvement, particularly if surgery is contemplated.

*These are two MR images from the same patient (**Figs. 3.10.2** and **3.10.3**).*

These are proton density fat-saturated sagittal MR images of the knee. These confirm the presence of the central sequestrum in the distal femoral metaphysis with surrounding marrow oedema (**Fig. 3.10.2**, arrow). There is cortical thickening but, at the posterior distal femoral metaphyseal region, there is an area of cortical breach with high-signal lobulated tissue extending through it into the adjacent soft tissues of the popliteal fossa (**Fig. 3.10.3**, arrow). There is a small knee joint effusion. The appearances confirm the diagnosis of chronic osteomyelitis with a sequestrum centrally, a thickened cortex representing the involucrum, with a defect within it consistent with a cloaca.

Examination Tips

- Chronic osteomyelitis is characterised by:
  - Sequestrum—a central area of sclerotic dead bone
  - Involucrum—a peripheral rim of new bone formation
  - Cloaca—a defect through the involucrum through which pus extrudes into the soft tissue. If this reaches the skin, it forms a sinus.
- Chronic osteomyelitis has a waxing and waning chronic course, and this is reflected in the pattern of periosteal new bone formation. Classically, there are areas of thick, benign-appearing periosteal reaction, with other areas of broken or laminar, more aggressive-appearing periosteal reaction. This may help distinguish chronic osteomyelitis from bone tumours in which the periosteal reaction, whether benign or aggressive, tends to be more uniform.

Differential Diagnosis

The radiographic features are characteristic in this case, and no differential diagnosis should be provided. Several other bone lesions show the presence of a sequestrum as a recognised finding but would generally have other distinguishing features:

- Eosinophilic granuloma (typically a button sequestrum in a skull lesion).
- Metastatic carcinoma (likely to be multiple focal lesions that may show prominent cortical destruction).
- Primary lymphoma of bone (usually permeative bone destruction with an aggressive periosteal reaction).
- Malignant fibrous tumours (ill-defined lesions with cortical destruction and an aggressive periosteal reaction).
- Radiation necrosis (a button sequestrum described in the skull).

- Other primary bone tumours produce central calcification or ossification that may appear as a sequestrum radiographically.
  - These include bone-forming tumours (e.g., osteoid osteoma or osteoblastoma), cartilage-forming tumours (enchondroma and chondroblastoma), and lipoma of bone.
  - All these lesions have characteristics that would not be confused with those of the given case.

Notes

- Osteomyelitis usually develops via haematogenous spread of infection. Local infection can occur in the presence of a soft tissue wound or local surgery.
- About 80 to 90% of cases are due to *Staphylococcus aureus* infection.
- Osteomyelitis can be divided into:
  - Acute:
    - Typically in children or in adults over 50 years of age with clinical evidence of sepsis
    - Radiographs may be negative for the first 10 to 21 days
    - Osteopaenia and variable lucency, cortical destruction, laminated periosteal reaction, and soft tissue mass are seen
  - Subacute:
    - Typically appears as a Brodie's abscess.
    - Focal bony lucency with surrounding sclerosis and sometimes a periosteal reaction.
  - Chronic:
    - Sequestrum, involucrum, and cloaca formation with chronic draining sinuses
    - Lucency, sclerosis, cortical thickening, and periosteal reaction of differing types.
  - MRI is valuable to confirm the diagnosis of chronic osteomyelitis and also to delineate the extent of bone involvement for surgical planning.

Bibliography

Bohndorf K. Infection of the appendicular skeleton. Eur Radiol 2004;14(Suppl 3):E53–E63

Jennin F, Bousson V, Parlier C, Jomaah N, Khanine V, Laredo JD. Bony sequestrum: a radiologic review. Skeletal Radiol 2011;40(8):963–975

Wenaden AE, Szyszko TA, Saifuddin A. Imaging of periosteal reactions associated with focal lesions of bone. Clin Radiol 2005;60(4):439–456

3.11 Calcium Pyrophosphate Dihydrate Deposition Disease and Haemochromatosis

Clinical History

A 68-year-old man presents with pain in the hands (**Fig. 3.11.1**).

Ideal Summary

This is a dorsopalmar radiograph of the hand. There is joint space loss at all of the metacarpophalangeal joints and the interphalangeal joint of the thumb, but the joint space loss particularly affects the thumb and index and middle fingers. Periarticular bone mineral density is preserved at all these joints. There are osteophytes at the thumb metacarpophalangeal

and interphalangeal joints. At the index and middle metacarpophalangeal joints, there are prominent hook-shaped osteophytes at the radial margin of the metacarpal heads.

In the carpus, there is radioscaphoid, scaphoid/trapezoid/trapezium (STT), and thumb carpometacarpal joint space loss. Periarticular bone mineral density is preserved. There are subchondral cysts at the distal radius and ulna and throughout the carpal bones. There are no erosions. Chondrocalcinosis can be seen at the triangular fibrocartilage complex, in the lunotriquetral ligament, at the radial margin of the wrist, and within the index and middle metacarpophalangeal joints. The radiographic appearances

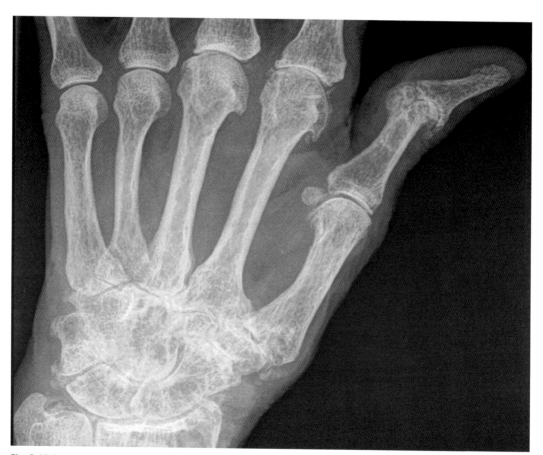

Fig. 3.11.1

are consistent with either calcium pyrophosphate dihydrate deposition (CPDD) disease or haemochromatosis. The changes in the joints of the thumb may indicate additional osteoarthritis.

Radiographs of the remainder of both hands should be performed. A chest radiograph may be helpful to identify cardiomegaly in haemochromatosis. Ferritin or transferrin blood tests are advised.

Examination Tips

- This arthritis is characterised by osteophyte formation with an absence of erosions. This is therefore a variant or mimic of osteoarthritis rather than an inflammatory erosive arthropathy.
- Haemochromatosis and CPDD disease have similar (and often indistinguishable) features in the hands:
  - Particularly affect the wrist and index and middle metacarpophalangeal joints
  - Subchondral cysts
  - Hook osteophytes
  - Chondrocalcinosis.
- Radiographic features more likely in keeping with haemochromatosis include:
  - Joint space narrowing affecting the ring and little finger metacarpophalangeal joints (as well as the index and middle finger metacarpophalangeal joints, which are affected in both conditions)
  - Hook osteophytes at the index and middle metacarpal heads.
- Radiographic features more likely in keeping with CPDD disease than haemochromatosis include:
  - Scapholunate dissociation.
- Osteoarthritis is so common that it may frequently be present in addition to another arthropathy, and in this case it may be responsible for the changes in the thumb ray (STT, carpometacarpal, MCP and IP joints).
- The distribution of osteoarthritis in the hands is different from that of haemochromatosis and CPDD disease:
  - The thumb ray (STT, carpometacarpal, metacarpophalangeal, and interphalangeal joints of the thumb)
  - Distal and proximal interphalangeal joints

- The second to fifth metacarpophalangeal and radiocarpal joints are typically relatively much less affected.
- Osteoarthritis should not cause hook osteophytes and heavy chondrocalcinosis.

Differential Diagnosis

There is no differential diagnosis to offer the examiner.

Notes

- CPDD disease:
  - CPDD may cause calcification in cartilage, synovium, ligaments, and tendons.
  - Acute synovitis may occur and is termed *pseudogout*.
  - Pyrophosphate arthropathy refers to chronic arthritis with osteoarthritis-like changes in an atypical distribution.
  - CPDD most commonly affects the knee (especially the patellofemoral joint), and subchondral cysts are often large and dominant
- Haemochromatosis:
  - Haemochromatosis is due to excessive iron deposition in the tissues.
  - Primary haemochromatosis is most commonly autosomal recessive in inheritance.
  - Secondary haemochromatosis is due to haemolytic anaemias, multiple blood transfusion, or dietary excess of iron.
  - Clinical findings include fatigue, bronzing of the skin, cirrhosis, cardiomyopathy, diabetes mellitus, and hypogonadism.
  - Arthropathy in haemochromatosis most commonly affects the hands, knees, and hips.

Bibliography

Adamson TC III, Resnik CS, Guerra J Jr, Vint VC, Weisman MH, Resnick D. Hand and wrist arthropathies of hemochromatosis and calcium pyrophosphate deposition disease: distinct radiographic features. Radiology 1983;147(2): 377–381

Jacobson JA, Girish G, Jiang Y, Sabb BJ. Radiographic evaluation of arthritis: degenerative joint disease and variations. Radiology 2008;248(3):737–747

3.12 Geode

Clinical History

A 32-year-old man presents with elbow pain (**Figs. 3.12.1** and **3.12.2**).

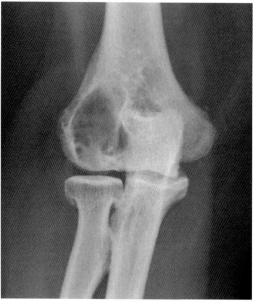

Fig. 3.12.1

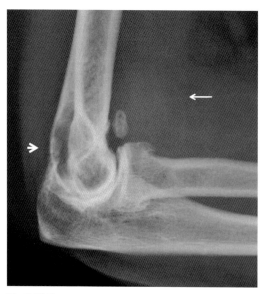

Fig. 3.12.2

Ideal Summary

These are anteroposterior and lateral radiographs of the elbow. There is a lucent lesion seen in the lateral humeral condyle extending to the articular surface of the capitellum and up into the distal humeral metaphysis. The lesion shows some internal trabeculation but no matrix. The lesion is well defined with, at least in part, a thin sclerotic rim. The lesion is not expansile. There is some cortical thinning on the lateral view but no cortical breach. No periosteal reaction or soft tissue mass is seen. There is a joint effusion as evidenced by marked elevation of the anterior fat pad (**Fig. 3.12.2**, long arrow) and visualisation of the posterior fat pad (**Fig. 3.12.2**, short arrow). There is osteophyte formation surrounding the radial head and, on the lateral view, at the capitellum and the tip of the olecranon. There is subchondral sclerosis. The joint space appears relatively well preserved on these views. There is a large intra-articular osseous body in the anterior joint. The appearances are of osteoarthritis of the elbow with a joint effusion and intra-articular body. In view of these findings, the humeral condylar lesion is likely to represent a large geode. A giant cell tumour is possible but less likely. I would like to review any available old images.

Examination Tips

- An elbow joint effusion elevates the anterior and posterior fat pads. A positive anterior fat pad sign appears as *elevation* of the normally visible anterior fat pad ("sail sign"). A positive posterior fat pad sign is seen as *visualisation* of the normally invisible posterior fat pad (which is obscured within the olecranon fossa on a normal lateral elbow view).
- Focusing on the features that give the narrowest differential diagnosis is key here:
  - A lytic lesion in the humerus has a wide differential diagnosis.
  - A lytic lesion centred in the subarticular region has a relatively narrow differential diagnosis.
  - A lytic lesion in the subarticular region associated with osteoarthritis of the joint has the narrowest differential of all. Clearly, the osteoarthritis could be incidental, but osteoarthritis is relatively uncommon in the elbow,

and the arthritic changes are prominent here. For this reason, you should not dismiss the arthritis as incidental.

Differential Diagnosis

The general differential diagnosis of a lytic lesion in a subarticular location is as follows:

- Geode
- Giant cell tumour:
  - 80% of lesions occur between ages 20 and 50 years
  - Lytic lesion centred in the metaphyseal region but extending to the subarticular bone
- Chondroblastoma:
  - Occurs between ages 5 and 20 years (i.e., *not* applicable in this case)
  - Arises before epiphyseal fusion
  - Internal calcification in 60%
- Clear cell chondrosarcoma:
  - Rare tumour (0.2% of biopsied primary bone tumours)
  - Third to fifth decades
  - Internal calcification in 30%
- Metastases or myeloma:
  - Can occur in a subarticular location but would be quite unusual in the absence of other lesions in the axial skeleton or metaphyseal regions

Notes

Geode (subchondral cyst)
- Forms in association with osteoarthritis either due to the ingress of synovial fluid into subarticular bone or due to bone necrosis in an area of subarticular marrow contusion.
- May be seen in virtually any arthritis, including:
  - Osteoarthritis
  - Rheumatoid arthritis
  - Seronegative inflammatory arthritis
  - Gout
  - Calcium pyrophosphate dihydrate deposition disease
  - Synovial proliferative disorders (pigmented villonodular synovitis or synovial osteochondromatosis)
  - Subchondral cysts are often particularly prominent in CPDD disease.

Bibliography

Jacobson JA, Girish G, Jiang Y, Sabb BJ. Radiographic evaluation of arthritis: degenerative joint disease and variations. Radiology 2008;248(3):737–747

Resnick D, Niwayama G, Coutts RD. Subchondral cysts (geodes) in arthritic disorders: pathologic and radiographic appearance of the hip joint. AJR Am J Roentgenol 1977;128(5):799–806

3.13 Paget's Disease

Clinical History

A 72-year-old man presents with pain in his right leg (**Figs. 3.13.1–3.13.3**).

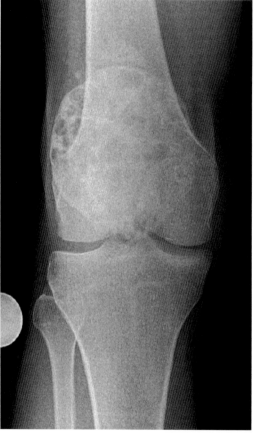

Fig. 3.13.1

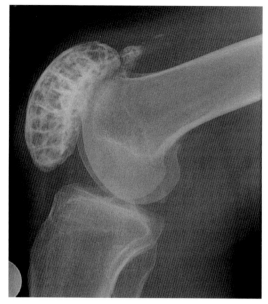

Fig. 3.13.2

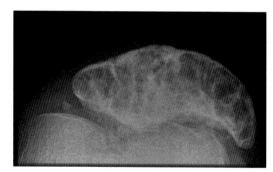

Fig. 3.13.3

Ideal Summary

These are anteroposterior, lateral, and skyline radiographs of the right knee. There is gross bony enlargement of right patella with marked cortical thickening, as well as thickening and sclerosis of the trabeculae giving a coarsened appearance. There is an osseous fragment within the suprapatellar pouch consistent with an intra-articular body, which may have fragmented from the patella. There is no associated joint effusion, cortical destruction, periosteal reaction, or soft tissue mass. The findings are in keeping with "mega-patella" secondary to Paget's disease. I would review other bone radiographs to ascertain the presence of Paget's disease elsewhere.

Examination Tips

- The findings of bony enlargement, coarsening of the trabeculae, and thickening of the cortex without any accompanying aggressive features are virtually diagnostic of Paget's disease.
- This is an example of a common pathology with classical features but occurring in an unusual location. Careful analysis of the radiographic signs allows the correct diagnosis to be made.

Differential Diagnosis

Given the classic radiographic signs, no differential diagnoses should be offered in this case. Monostotic Paget's disease of the knee could, however, pose a diagnostic conundrum in the following scenarios:

- Sclerosing lymphoma/osteoblastic metastasis could appear similar to the osteoblastic phase of Paget's disease, but should not cause uniform bony expansion. Features of cortical destruction, periosteal reaction, and a soft tissue mass would point to a malignant process.
- Haemangioma can uncommonly occur in the patella, and may show a web-like trabecular pattern that may mimic the coarse trabecular pattern in Paget's disease, demonstrating mild bony expansion, but not cortical thickening.
- Chronic osteomyelitis. This may be sclerotic with patchy areas of osteopaenia. Cortical destruction, periosteal reaction, soft tissue mass, and appropriate clinical history would indicate osteomyelitis rather than Paget's disease.

Other less likely but potential causes of an expanded patella (in different age groups) could include:

- Giant cell tumour (age 20 to 40 years)
- Aneurysmal bone cyst (age 10 to 30 years)
- Expansile metastasis (age over 40 years; highly unlikely in the absence of known metastatic disease)

These entities would not be expected to cause the cortical thickening and coarsened trabeculation as seen in this case.

Notes

- Paget's disease is a common disorder affecting 1 to 4% of people over the age of 40 years.
- The disease is usually polyostotic, with monostotoic disease accounting for 10 to 35% of cases. The most commonly involved sites are the pelvis, spine, skull, and proximal long bones (especially the femur). Involvement of the knee is rare.
- There are three distinct pathological phases:
  - An osteolytic phase, where osteoclasts predominate. In the long bones, the typical initial manifestation is of subchondral lucency, with progression of osteolysis resulting in a sharp margin described as a "blade of grass" or "flame-shaped."
  - Mixed-phase manifestations are consequent of osteoblastic repair, with radiographic findings

of coarsening and thickening of the trabecular pattern and cortex. This is the phase most often encountered by radiologists, the features are almost pathognomonic of the disease entity.

- The osteoblastic phase is commonly associated with bony enlargement. Areas of sclerosis may develop and can obliterate areas of previous trabecular thickening.
- Imaging features on other modalities:
  - Bone scintigraphy. Increased radionuclide uptake is demonstrable in all three phases of Paget's disease, and activity is usually marked on early and delayed phases in the active phase of the disease.
  - CT imaging is not normally required, but Paget's disease can often be encountered as an incidental finding.
  - MRI findings can vary according to the pathological phase of disease, from heterogeneous T1 and T2 signal in mixed-phase disease (usually predominately reduced T1 and increased T2 signal) to low-signal marrow intensity in osteoblastic disease.
- Biochemical testing: a raised serum alkaline phosphatase can help with the diagnosis.
- Local complications of Paget's disease should be sought on imaging and may include:
  - Insufficiency fractures. These are common in the long bones or the spine. Classically, a Pagetic insufficiency fracture occurs as a horizontal lucency in the subtrochanteric region at the convex (lateral) cortex of the femur ("banana fractures"), distinguishing them from Looser's zones in osteomalacia, which classically occur at the concave (medial) femoral cortex.
  - Neoplasm. Malignancy is suggested to occur in approximately 1% of cases and includes sarcomatous degeneration, myeloma, and metastatic disease from other primary sites. A lytic lesion and soft tissue mass in Pagetic bone should suggest possible malignancy.
  - Degenerative disease. This is commonly reported adjacent to sites of involvement in Paget's disease, particularly at the hip.

Bibliography

Cortis K, Micallef K, Mizzi A. Imaging Paget's disease of bone—from head to toe. Clin Radiol 2011;66(7):662–672

Ihde LL, Forrester DM, Gottsegen CJ, et al. Sclerosing bone dysplasias: review and differentiation from other causes of osteosclerosis. Radiographics 2011;31(7):1865–1882

3.14 Transient Lateral Patellar Dislocation

Clinical History

*A 25-year-old woman presents following an acute episode of "giving way" of the knee (**Fig. 3.14.1**).*

Ideal Summary

This is an axial fat-saturated proton density MR image of the left knee. The patella is laterally subluxed. There is a large osteochondral defect at the medial margin of the patellar with extensive marrow contusion at its base. There is further marrow contusion at the anterolateral margin of the lateral femoral condyle. There is a joint effusion, and within the lateral recess of the joint there is an elongated low signal body consistent with a displaced osteochondral fragment (**Fig. 3.14.1**, arrow). The medial patellar retinaculum is avulsed from its femoral attachment. The trochlear articular surface appears relatively flattened, consistent with trochlear dysplasia. The appearances are consistent with prior transient lateral patellar dislocation. Orthopaedic referral is advised for consideration of arthroscopy, particularly in view of the large intra-articular body.

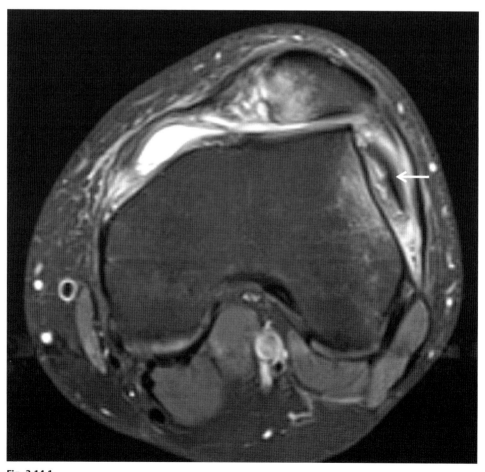

Fig. 3.14.1

Examination Tips

- In the absence of side markers, it is important to be able to identify which side is medial and which is lateral. The clues in this image are:
  - The anterior margin of the lateral femoral condyle is wider and projects more anteriorly than the corresponding anterior margin of the medial femoral condyle.
  - The anterior cruciate ligament origin can be seen in this image within the intercondylar notch. It lies on the medial aspect of the lateral femoral condyle.
  - The soft tissues are thicker on the medial side of the thigh (not visible in this case but often the easiest clue).
- Contusions give a clue to the mechanism of injury. In this case, these are "kissing" contusions, meaning that the medial margin of the patella impacted with the anterolateral margin of the lateral femoral condyle at the time of injury.
  - Anterior cruciate ligament injury may also lead to marrow contusion at the lateral femoral condyle, but this occurs more posteromedially, at the notch of the lateral femoral condyle seen on the sagittal image. There will usually be a corresponding "kissing contusion" at the posterior margin of the lateral tibial plateau, and obviously the medial patellar contusion will be absent.
- This is an image on which there are a surprisingly large number of findings related to the pathology. You may make the diagnosis quickly on the basis of the most obvious findings (in this case, the characteristic marrow contusion pattern and the patellar osteochondral defect). It is highly tempting to then stop looking at the case and draw your conclusions. As with many examination cases, to score well you need to remember to look for the "3Cs":
  - Causes. In this case, the flattened (dysplastic) trochlea groove predisposes to patellar instability.

- Complications. If you do not actively look for the separated intra-articular body, you will almost certainly miss it.
- Concomitant findings. If you know something about patellar dislocation, you may be aware that there is often associated tearing of the medial patellar retinaculum. Again this is a sign you can easily miss if you do not actively look for it.

Differential Diagnosis

The marrow contusion pattern in this case is pathognomonic.

Notes

- Lateral patellar dislocation is a common cause of an acute traumatic haemarthrosis in young patients.
- There is usually a history of giving way and knee swelling, but patellar dislocation is usually transient and has almost always relocated by the time of clinical presentation.
- Lateral patellar dislocation is therefore commonly clinically unexpected, and the diagnosis is often made on imaging findings.
- Radiographs will typically show a joint effusion. The patellar may be laterally subluxed but is rarely dislocated. There may be patellar alta (which is associated with patellar instability). A "sliver sign" may be identified—a small curvilinear osteochondral fragment lying in the joint.
- MRI is often required to make the diagnosis.

Bibliography

Elias DA, White LM. Imaging of patellofemoral disorders. Clin Radiol 2004;59(7):543–557

Saifuddin A. The Knee in Musculoskeletal MRI. Oxford, UK: Oxford University Press; 2008

3.15 Polyostotic Fibrous Dysplasia

Clinical History

*A 21-year-old man presents with pain in his left hip after a fall (**Fig. 3.15.1**).*

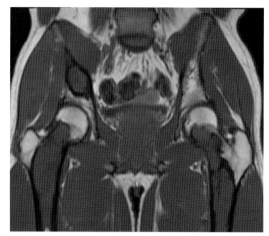

Fig. 3.15.2

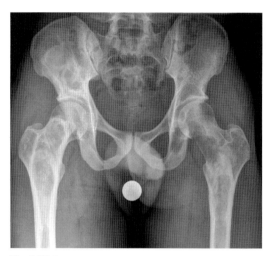

Fig. 3.15.1

Ideal Summary

This is an anteroposterior radiograph of the hips. There are lytic lesions within both proximal femora extending from the femoral necks down into the shafts. A further similar lesion lies in the right iliac wing. A smaller lesion is also present in the left ischium. The left femoral neck lesion shows no matrix, but the remaining lesions show a ground-glass appearance in some areas and thickened trabeculation in others. The lesions are well defined, with a thin rim in some areas and a thick sclerotic rim in others. The femoral neck lesions appear expansile, and there is endosteal scalloping in the femoral shafts. None of the lesions shows any definite cortical breach, although the left medial femoral neck is thin, which may be concerning for a fracture risk. There is no periosteal reaction or soft tissue mass. There is no evidence of an associated bowing deformity. The given findings would be typical for polyostotic fibrous dysplasia. MRI may be helpful to further assess the left femoral lesion to exclude an acute pathological fracture or potential malignant degeneration.

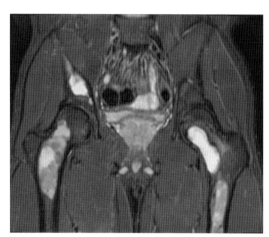

Fig. 3.15.3

*These are two MR images from the same patient (**Figs. 3.15.2** and **3.15.3**).*

These are coronal T1- and T2-weighted short T1 inversion recovery (STIR) images. On T1-weighted imaging, the three lesions all have low-to-intermediate signal intensity. On the STIR image, the lesions have a variable predominately intermediate-to-high signal. The left medial femoral neck cortex is quite thin, but there is no definite fracture line or soft tissue oedema to suggest acute fracture and no soft tissue mass. The MRI findings support a diagnosis of fibrous dysplasia.

Examination Tips

- Around 70 to 80% of fibrous dysplasia is monostotic; 20 to 30% is polyostotic.
- Fibrous dysplasia can have variable appearances on plain radiographs. Lesions typically:
  - Are diaphyseal or metadiaphyseal with the epicentre within the medulla
  - Are expansile, with endosteal scalloping
  - Have a "ground-glass" matrix
  - May have a sclerotic rim.
- Involvement of the epiphysis before closure of the growth plate and isolated epiphyseal lesions are rare.
- An MRI examination can help delineate the extent of the lesion and assess for a soft tissue component.
- Malignant sarcomatous transformation is thought to occur in less than 1% of cases, but should be suspected in the presence of cortical destruction or a soft tissue mass.
- A common presentation is pain related to pathological fracture. It is important to carefully assess for its presence, especially in polyostotic disease.
- Polyostotic fibrous dysplasia may be unilateral or bilateral in distribution.

Differential Diagnosis

The following are potential differential diagnoses for multiple lytic bone lesions in a child or young adult:
- Langerhans' cell histiocytosis.
- Multiple enchondromas:
  - Calcified chondral matrix is dissimilar to the typical appearance of fibrous dysplasia.
  - Skeletal distribution may be similar.
- Neurofibromatosis:
  - Long bone involvement is rare but recognised.
  - Lesions are usually fibroxanthomas and therefore will be of low signal on all pulse sequences on MR imaging.
  - Clinical differentiation is often required.
- Multiple nonossifying fibromas (Jaffe–Campanacci syndrome):
  - May have café-au-lait spots
  - May be associated with neurofibromatosis.

- Hyperparathyroidism (brown tumours). The presence of the following favours hyperparathyroidism:
  - Subperiosteal bone resorption
  - Bone sclerosis
  - Soft tissue and vascular calcification.
- Malignancy:
  - Malignant disease is generally associated with "aggressive"-appearing bony lesions, that is, ill-defined with cortical destruction and irregular periosteal reaction.
  - For examination purposes at least, bony metastatic disease is unusual below the age of 40 years in the absence of a known primary lesion (e.g., neuroblastoma in a child).
  - Lymphoma and leukaemia can cause multiple lytic lesions in children and young adults, but again the lesions are generally aggressive-looking.
  - For these reasons, malignancy should not form a part of the differential diagnosis in this case.

Notes

- Polyostotic fibrous dysplasia may be associated with variable endocrine abnormalities and specifically the following syndromes:
  - McCune–Albright syndrome (predominantly in girls): polyostotic fibrous dysplasia (usually unilateral), café-au-lait spots, and endocrine dysfunction (especially precocious puberty)
  - Mazabraud's syndrome, a rare combination of fibrous dysplasia and soft tissue myxomas.
- The most common physical deformities are leg length discrepancy and "shepherd's crook deformity" of the proximal femur.

Bibliography

Fitzpatrick KA, Taljanovic MS, Speer DP, et al. Imaging findings of fibrous dysplasia with histopathologic and intraoperative correlation. AJR Am J Roentgenol 2004;182(6):1389–1398

Kransdorf MJ, Moser RP Jr, Gilkey FW. Fibrous dysplasia. Radiographics 1990;10(3):519–537

3.16 Lisfranc Injury

Clinical History

A 32-year-old woman presents with a painful foot following trauma (Fig. 3.16.1).

Ideal Summary

These are dorsopedal and oblique views of the foot. There is mild midfoot soft tissue swelling. There is malalignment of the second tarsometatarsal joint, with a small ossific avulsion fragment at the interval between the bases of the first and second metatarsals. On the oblique view, there is slight irregularity of the medial margin of the base of the third metatarsal. The remaining tarsometatarsal joints are normally aligned. No other fractures are seen. The cuboid bone appears normal. No vascular calcification is seen. The appearances are of a Lisfranc injury. CT of the foot is advised to assess tarsometatarsal alignment and exclude further fractures. Orthopaedic referral is advised.

These are the CT images you have asked for (Figs. 3.16.2 and 3.16.3).

These are axial and sagittally oriented reformats from a CT of the midfoot, demonstrating malalignment of the second tarsometatarsal joint with an intra-articular fracture at the base of the second metatarsal. This confirms the Lisfranc injury pattern.

Examination Tips

- On the dorsoplantar radiograph of the foot:
  - The lateral margin of the first metatarsal should align with the lateral margin of the medial cuneiform.

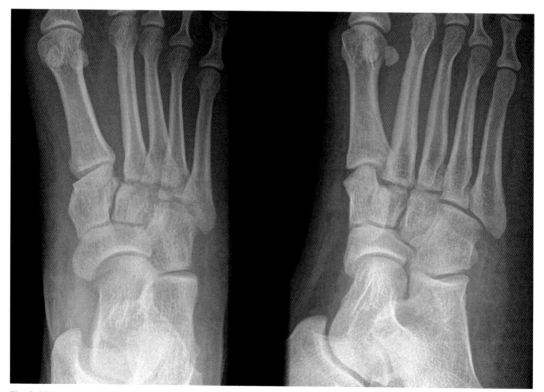

Fig. 3.16.1

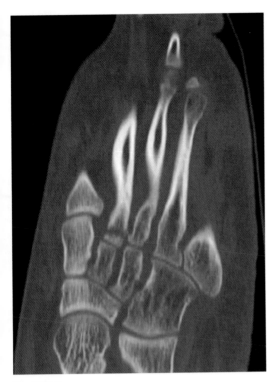

Fig. 3.16.2

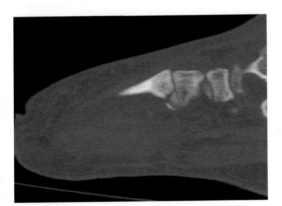

Fig. 3.16.3

- The medial margin of the second metatarsal should align with the medial margin of the intermediate cuneiform.
- On the oblique radiograph of the foot:
  - The lateral margin of the second metatarsal should align with the lateral margin of the intermediate cuneiform.
  - The medial margin of the third metatarsal should align with the medial margin of the lateral cuneiform.
- The most critical of these alignments is the medial margin of the second metatarsal and the intermediate cuneiform. Even a subtle step in this alignment is likely to be significant in a patient who has experienced midfoot trauma.

Differential Diagnosis

- The findings in this case are characteristic, and no differential diagnosis needs to be provided.
- In the absence of trauma, a similar pattern of injury can be seen in the presence of peripheral neuropathy, most commonly in diabetic patients (look out for vascular calcification). In the later stages, there are likely to be the classic features of a Charcot foot with sclerosis, bony fragmentation, collapse of the articular surface, and deformity, but in the early stages appearances may be quite similar to the case described here.

Notes

- The Lisfranc ligament originates at the lateral margin of the medial cuneiform and inserts on the medial margin of the second metatarsal base.
- Lisfranc injuries are characterised by malalignments and fractures at the tarsometatarsal joints that may be isolated to the second tarsometatarsal joint or extend across the whole midfoot.
- Lateral deviation of the metatarsals at the time of injury can result in a compression fracture of the cuboid between the metatatarsal bases and the calcaneum, known as a "nutcracker fracture."
- Lisfranc injuries commonly result in an unstable midfoot, even in radiographically subtle or occult cases.
- CT is important where midfoot injury is suspected as fractures and malalignments are usually underestimated radiographically, and surgical stabilisation is often required.

Bibliography

Hatem SF. Imaging of lisfranc injury and midfoot sprain. Radiol Clin North Am 2008;46(6):1045–1060

3.17 Sarcoidosis

Clinical History

*A 30-year-old woman presents with pain in the hands and feet (**Figs. 3.17.1** and **3.17.2**).*

Ideal Summary

The first set of images are dorsopalmer and oblique radiographs of the hand of an adult patient. There is soft tissue swelling of all the fingers predominantly centred at midphalangeal level. There is bony abnormality affecting virtually all of the phalanges. This is characterised by trabecular disruption, small cystic lucencies, and a "lace-like" reticular pattern. These changes are most severe in the middle phalanx of the middle finger, where there is also a well-defined lytic lesion identified on the ulnar margin with cortical disruption. Within this phalanx, there are small areas of periosteal new bone formation. The terminal tufts also show trabecular loss with early erosion consistent with some acro-osteolysis. The articular surfaces, metacarpals, and carpal bones are spared, with preservation of the joint spaces within the hand and wrist. With the exception of the middle phalanx of the middle finger, there is no periosteal reaction. There is no evidence of fracture, bony sequestrum, or soft tissue calcification.

The second set of images are dorsoplantar and oblique radiographs of the forefoot. Similar to the radiographs of the hand, there are lytic lucencies and early "lace-like" reticulation within the phalanges with soft tissue swelling. This is most notable within the distal phalanx of the first toe (here, with distal tuft erosion) and middle phalanx of the second toe. Again, the joint spaces are preserved and the periosteal reaction is absent.

Overall, the findings are in keeping with a diagnosis of sarcoidosis. A chest radiograph and referral to the respiratory physicians is recommended. I would also advise imaging of the other hand and foot.

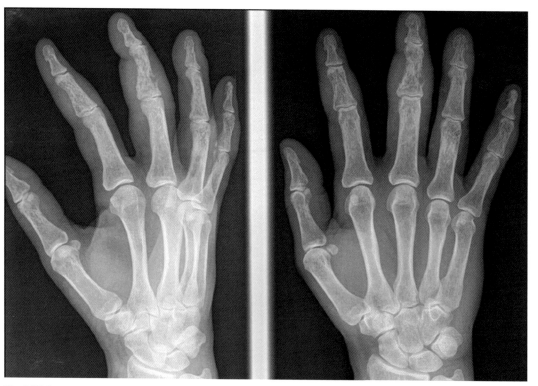

Fig. 3.17.1

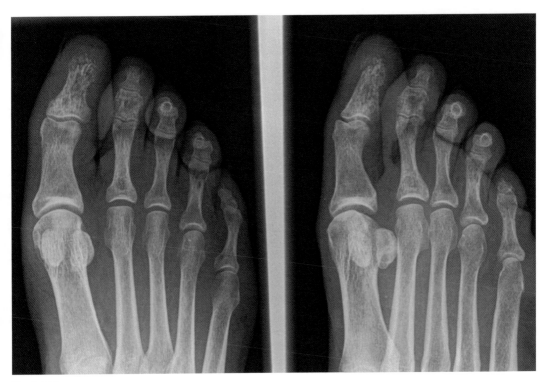

Fig. 3.17.2

*This is a gallium scintigraphy (gallium 67 citrate) study from the same patient (**Fig. 3.17.3**).*

Selected images confirm uptake in multiple areas of the distal aspects of both hands and feet. Uptake is also present within the mediastinum. These findings further support the diagnosis of sarcoidosis.

Examination Tips

- The abnormality in this case is within the bones, not the joints.
- The distribution of bony lesions in sarcoidosis is usually bilateral but asymmetrical. The hands are most commonly affected, especially the middle and distal phalanges, but any bone may be involved.
- Sarcoidosis of the extremities produces a typical "lace-like" trabecular pattern (see **Fig. 3.17.4**). Cystic lesions in the bones are also typical.
- Soft tissue swelling and soft tissue masses are common.
- Less commonly sarcoidosis can produce diffuse sclerosis or multiple focal sclerotic bony lesions.

- Soft tissue calcification and periosteal reactions are generally not present; if prominent, these signs should prompt consideration of alternative diagnoses.
- Joint involvement can also occur:
  - Acute polyarthritis produces nonspecific radiographic signs of periarticular soft tissue swelling and periarticular osteopaenia.
  - Chronic polyarthritis may be seen as soft tissue swelling, periarticular osteopaenia, joint space loss, and erosions.

Differential Diagnosis

The abnormal trabecular pattern with a "lace-like" reticular pattern involving multiple sites is characteristic of sarcoidosis. In this case, a differential diagnosis need not be given, but ambiguity may be encountered in the following:
- Scleroderma
  - If there is osseous destruction of the distal phalanges, appearances may be similar. The entities can be differentiated by the presence of soft tissue subcutaneous and periarticular

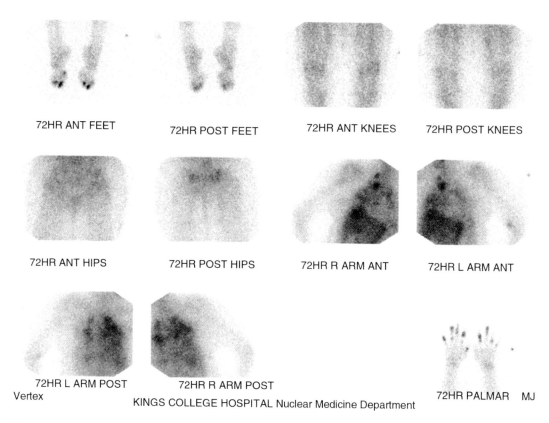

72HR ANT FEET   72HR POST FEET   72HR ANT KNEES   72HR POST KNEES

72HR ANT HIPS   72HR POST HIPS   72HR R ARM ANT   72HR L ARM ANT

72HR L ARM POST   72HR R ARM POST   72HR PALMAR   MJ

Vertex

KINGS COLLEGE HOSPITAL Nuclear Medicine Department

Fig. 3.17.3

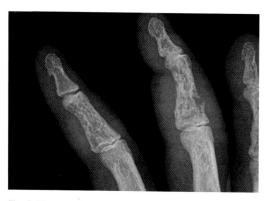

Fig. 3.17.4

calcifications; these are common in scleroderma but not evident in sarcoidosis.

- Gout
  - Occasionally, sarcoidosis may present with sharply marginated cyst-like areas with thin sclerotic margins, similar to gout. Extraosseous manifestations of sarcoidosis (pulmonary and skin) and gout (tophi), and biochemical testing (angiotensin-converting enzyme level for sarcoidosis, and uric acid level for gout), may help differentiate the entities.
- Hyperparathyroidism
  - In this entity, the typical site of involvement is the radial aspect of the middle phalanges with subperiosteal bone resorption. The presence of soft tissue calcification or brown tumours would also help differentiate this.
- Tuberculosis
  - This condition can manifest with soft tissue swelling, cortical thinning and a "lace-like" reticular pattern but, unlike sarcoidosis, this is usually confined to a single digit and is associated with a periosteal reaction.

Notes

- Osseous sarcoidosis is thought to be present in 5% of all patients with the disease.

- Osseous sarcoid is rare in the absence of clinical or radiological evidence of extraskeletal disease. Around 80 to 90% of patients with bony sarcoidosis have radiographic evidence of pulmonary disease, and almost all have skin disease (even if only subtle).
- The hands and feet are the usual sites of involvement, less common sites being the long bones, vertebrae (especially lower thoracic and upper lumbar), nasal bones, skull, and sternum.
- Bone pain can occur in up to 50% of patients. Symptomatic relief may be achieved by the use of corticosteroids, nonsteroidal anti-inflammatory agents or disease-modifying antirheumatic drugs; however, in the majority of cases, these will not normalise the bony abnormality.
- In rare cases of diagnostic uncertainty, it may be necessary to perform a biopsy to detect the presence of a noncaseating granuloma.

Bibliography

Hyzy MD, Kroon HM, Watt I, De Schepper AM. Chronic osseous sarcoidosis. JBR-BTR 2007;90(3):194–195

Yaghmai I. Radiographic, angiographic and radionuclide manifestations of osseous sarcoidosis. Radiographics 1983;3:375–396

3.18 Gout

Clinical History

*A 62-year-old man presents with recurrent pain in his forefeet (**Figs. 3.18.1** and **3.18.2**).*

Ideal Summary

This is a dorsoplantar radiograph of both feet. There are well-defined juxta-articular erosions with overhanging edges within the distal aspects of the left first and fifth metatarsals with overlying soft tissue swelling. Further juxta-articular erosion is seen at the right first

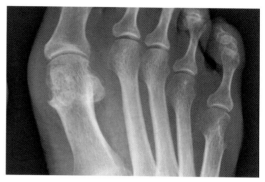

Fig. 3.18.2

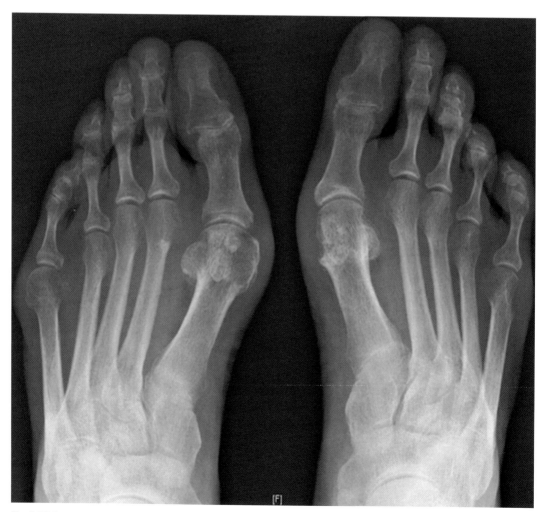

Fig. 3.18.1

proximal phalanx. There are subchondral lucencies in the right first and fifth metatarsal heads with overlying soft tissue swelling. The first metatarsophalangeal joints bilaterally show moderate joint space loss, and there is a bilateral hallux valgus. The remaining metatarsophalangeal joint spaces are preserved. The involved joints show some periarticular osteopaenia. There is no periosteal reaction or soft tissue calcification. In summary, the appearances are of a nonsymmetrical forefoot polyathropathy with juxta-articular erosions. These features would be typical for gout.

Examination Tips

- Early disease may show nonspecific radiographic features of periarticular soft tissue swelling and occasionally fine periosteal reaction. However, more specific radiographic signs may not be seen until as long as 10 years after the first attack.
- Characteristic features include tophi, soft tissue calcification, and erosions that are juxta-articular (rather than marginal or central). Erosions typically have new bone formation at their periphery, causing an "overhanging margin."
- Look for a tophus of chronic gout in the periarticular soft tissues, within the joints, or in the bone; these are calcified in 50%.
- Although the initial presentation of gout is usually monoarticular (involving the first metatarsophalangeal joint in 50%), as the disease progresses it typically becomes an asymmetrical polyarthropathy that can affect any joint, with a predilection for the peripheries and the lower extremities.
- The joint space is typically preserved until late on in the disease, and periarticular bone mineral density is typically preserved (although disuse osteopaenia may occur in late disease).

Differential Diagnosis

In this case, the features are characteristic. In a less characteristic case, the differential diagnosis of an asymmetrical erosive polyarthropathy would include:

- Psoriatic arthritis:
  - Much like gout, periosteal reactions, juxta-articular erosions, and soft tissue swelling are all recognised features. Disease distribution and skin changes should help differentiate the two entities.
- Erosive osteoarthritis:
  - Central intra-articular erosions
  - Rapid destruction and loss of joint space

- Hands being the most common site, especially the thumb carpometacarpal and trapezioscaphoid joint and the distal interphalangeal joints.
- Rheumatoid arthritis
  - Erosions that are typically marginal, ill-defined, and without marginal new bone formation
  - Joint space lost earlier in the disease process
  - Usually bilateral and symmetrical
  - Periarticular osteopaenia is typical.

Importantly, in a case of a monoarthropathy, septic arthritis may be the key differential diagnosis. Septic arthritis is usually associated with periarticular osteopaenia, early joint space loss, and ill-defined erosions without new bone formation. In such cases, joint aspiration for microbiology and crystal examination are mandatory.

Notes

- Gout is caused by the deposition of monosodium urate crystals. The condition can be primary, or secondary to conditions such as myeloproliferative diseases, renal failure, or hyperproliferative skin disorders.
- Analysis of synovial fluid aspirate is often undertaken: the presence of negatively birefringent crystals under polarised light microscopy confirms the diagnosis.
- Ultrasound examination can be used to guide direct needle aspiration for crystal analysis, detect erosions, or more clearly define tophi. A specific diagnostic feature on ultrasound is the "double-contour sign": this describes a hyperechoic, irregular band over the superficial margin of articular cartilage that is the result of crystal deposition.
- MRI is rarely required, but it may help differentiate gout from infection or neoplasm in cases with diagnostic uncertainty. Tophi are usually low-to-intermediate on T1-weighted imaging; signal can vary on T2-weighted imaging, with heterogeneous low-to-intermediate signal most commonly encountered.

Bibliography

Dhanda S, Jagmohan P, Quek ST. A re-look at an old disease: a multimodality review on gout. Clin Radiol 2011;66(10):984–992

Llauger J, Palmer J, Rosón N, Bagué S, Camins A, Cremades R. Nonseptic monarthritis: imaging features with clinical and histopathologic correlation. Radiographics 2000;20(Spec No:S263–S278)

3.19 Cervical Instability in Rheumatoid Arthritis

Clinical History

A 45-year-old woman presents with neck pain and paraesthesia (**Fig. 3.19.1**).

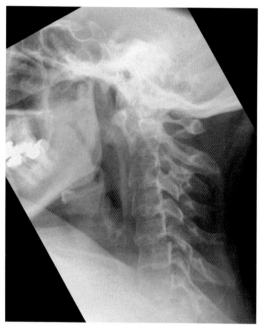

Fig. 3.19.1

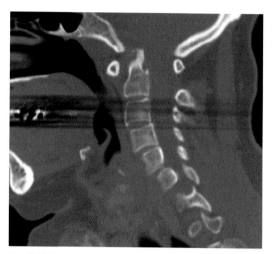

Fig. 3.19.2

Ideal Summary

This is a lateral radiograph of the cervical spine that demonstrates the skull base to C7 levels. There is marked widening of the anterior atlantodental interval consistent with atlantoaxial instability. Additionally, there is evidence of vertical atlantoaxial subluxation with superior displacement of C2 relative to the arch of C1. The odontoid peg is poorly visualised, and linear lucency at the base of the odontoid peg suggests a type 2 odontoid fracture. There is also evidence of minor subaxial subluxations with a "stepladder deformity" due to anterolistheses at all levels from C3 to C6. There is also erosion of one of the mandibular condyles. The appearances are of a rheumatoid cervical spine. There appears to be a fracture at the base of the odontoid peg. In addition, the atlantoaxial subluxation, particularly in the vertical

direction, indicates a high risk for cervical cord compression. I would immediately arrange for cervical immobilisation and neurosurgical review. I would arrange a cervical spine CT to assess for fractures, and MRI for further assessment of the cord.

This is a CT image of the same patient (**Fig. 3.19.2**).

This is a sagittal plane reformat from a cervical spine CT. This confirms erosion of the odontoid peg, and also the widened anterior atlantodental interval and vertical atlantoaxial subluxation, consistent with an unstable rheumatoid spine. There is, however, no fracture seen of the odontoid peg, although I would review the remaining CT images to confirm this.

The MRI showed no cord compression. The patient was then lost to follow-up and returned with increasing neurological signs 6 months later (**Fig. 3.19.3**).

This is a sagittal T2-weighted MR image of the cervical spine that demonstrates further basilar invagination, with the C1 arch now lying at the C2–C3 junction, and the C2 vertebral body completely invaginated into the foramen magnum. As a result, there is compression of the cervical cord. No cord signal change is seen on this single image. This unstable spine requires immediate cervical immobilisation and neurosurgical review.

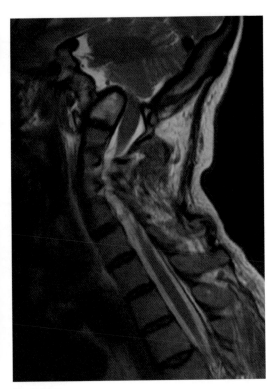

Fig. 3.19.3

Examination Tips

- The anterior atlantodental interval is measured on a lateral radiograph from the anterior border of the odontoid peg to the posterior border of the anterior arch of C1. In adults, this should measure 3 mm or less.
- The cervical canal should measure a minimum of 14 mm in anteroposterior depth throughout. A canal width of less than 14 mm is associated with risk for paralysis.
- Vertical atlantoaxial subluxation is measured by:
  - Protrusion of the tip of the odontoid peg more than 4.5 mm above McGregor's line (a line joining the hard palate to the inferior tip of the occiput). This may be difficult to assess if the odontoid peg is eroded.
  - Ranawat's method: the vertical distance between the centre of Harris ring (the sclerotic ring

at the body of C2) and a line joining the centres of the anterior and posterior arches of C1. The distance should be ≥ 13 mm in females and ≥ 15 mm in males.

Differential Diagnosis

No differential diagnosis needs to be given in this case as the appearances are characteristic. Other potential causes of atlantoaxial instability include:
- Trauma
- Seronegative arthritides
- Calcium pyrophosphate dihydrate deposition disease
- Gout
- Down's syndrome
- Marfan's syndrome

Notes

- Cervical subluxations are common in patients with rheumatoid arthritis.
- 50% of rheumatoid patients with cervical instability are asymptomatic.
- Cord compression is the cause of death in 10% of rheumatoid patients with cervical instability.
- Various types of cervical instability should be considered:
  - Atlantoaxial instability (50 to 70% of cervical subluxations in rheumatoid disease):
    - Horizontal plane instability between C1 and C2
    - Anterior atlantodental interval > 3 mm (adult)
    - Canal width < 14 mm
  - Subaxial subluxation (20 to 25%)
  - Vertical atlantoaxial subluxation (10 to 15%)
    - Also termed cranial settling or basilar invagination
    - The most severe form of cervical instability, with a high risk for cord and brainstem compression
  - Posterior, lateral, and rotatory instabilities are less common.

Bibliography

Roche CJ, Eyes BE, Whitehouse GH. The rheumatoid cervical spine: signs of instability on plain cervical radiographs. Clin Radiol 2002;57(4):241–249

3.20 Pigmented Villonodular Synovitis

Clinical History

A 30-year-old man presents with chronic right knee pain (**Figs. 3.20.1** and **3.20.2**).

Ideal Summary

These are anteroposterior radiographs of both knees and a lateral radiograph of the right knee. There is a large effusion in the right knee, seen on both the anteroposterior and lateral radiographs. On the anteroposterior radiograph, there are subtle lucencies in the distal femur around the intercondylar notch (**Fig. 3.20.1**, arrow). The notch is not widened, and the joint space is preserved. Periarticular bone mineral density is normal. The left knee demonstrates small sclerotic foci at the medial tibial and femoral condyles consistent with incidental bone islands. The left knee is otherwise normal. Assuming this is a monoarthropathy, septic arthritis may need to be excluded in the first instance by aspiration of the effusion. The differential diagnosis would include pigmented villonodular synovitis (PVNS) or gout. Further assessment with MRI may be helpful. The aspirate should routinely be sent for microbiological assessment and crystal examination.

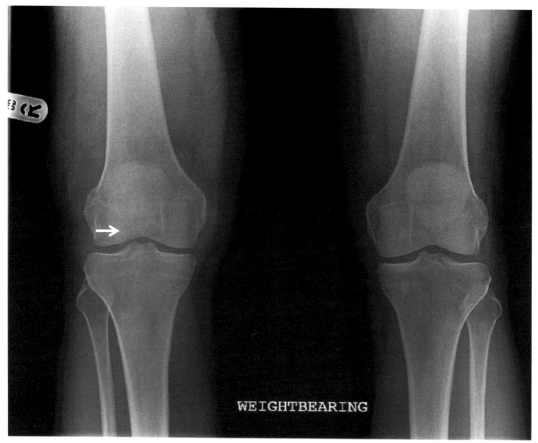

WEIGHTBEARING

Fig. 3.20.1

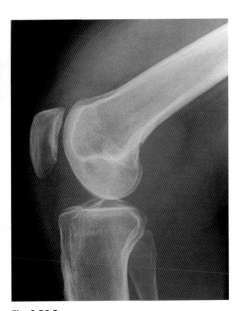

Fig. 3.20.2

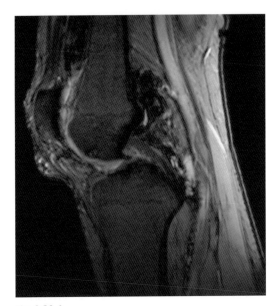

Fig. 3.20.4

These are the MR images from the same patient (**Figs. 3.20.3–3.20.5**).

These are sagittal fat-saturated proton density, sagittal gradient-echo, and coronal T1-weighted MR images of the right knee. There are multiple large intra-articular masses that are heterogeneous on proton density fat saturation, but contain areas of low signal on all sequences. On gradient-echo scanning, the low signal is more prominent and appears larger, consistent with "blooming" artefact, which is likely to be due to haemosiderin deposits. There is cartilage

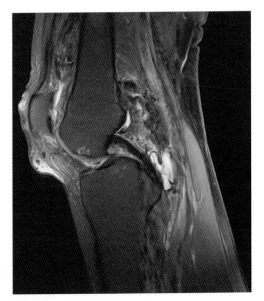

Fig. 3.20.3

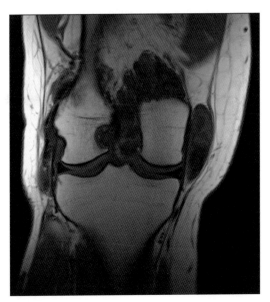

Fig. 3.20.5

loss from the retropatellar surface and a large, well-defined erosion laterally at the intercondylar notch of the femur. The features are typical of PVNS.

Examination Tips

- The radiographs show a joint-based pathology with features of an effusion and some subchondral lucencies. These findings are nonspecific and would produce a wide differential diagnosis. The key is to recognise that this is a *monoarthropathy* that has a short list of differential diagnoses, listed below.
- You cannot know for certain that this is a monoarthropathy as you have only been given two joints to review. Using the phrase "assuming this is a monoarthropathy" allows the examiner to redirect you if your assumption is wrong. It is a reasonable assumption, however, since:
  - You have been shown both knees and only one is abnormal.
  - In this case, it is the only finding that would enable you to reach a short differential list and examination cases tend to be chosen because, when correctly analysed, they lead to a relatively narrow differential list.
- The most important differential diagnosis for a monoarthropathy is septic arthritis, and you must show that you practise safely by saying that you would exclude this by joint aspiration.
- On MRI, haemosiderin deposits are typically identified in PVNS. Haemosiderin deposits are of low signal on all sequences and appear larger and blacker on gradient-echo sequences. This is known as the "blooming" artefact.
- Gradient-echo sequences may be recognised by the sharp edge appearance of cortical bone (as if the bones have been outlined with black pencil), or by the short repetition times (tens of milliseconds) if parameters are available.

Differential Diagnosis

The differential diagnosis of a monoarthropathy includes:
- Septic arthritis:
  - Very early on, there is periarticular osteopaenia and an effusion (which may result in a preserved or even widened joint space in some joints).
  - Subsequently, there is a rapidly progressive joint space loss with subchondral cysts and erosions.

- Synovial proliferative disorders including:
  - Pigmented villonodular synovitis
  - Synovial osteochondromatosis, which appears as multiple intra-articular bodies, are calcified in 70 to 75% of cases.
  - These conditions are typically associated with *preservation* of the joint space and periarticular bone density. There are often large subchondral cysts and erosions.
- Gout:
  - Soft tissue masses and calcification
  - Juxta-articular erosions with overhanging margins.
- Osteoarthritis:
  - This may affect a single joint, especially if there is an underlying traumatic cause.
  - Osteophyte formation, subchondral sclerosis, and early joint space loss should help distinguish this from other causes.
  - Any early inflammatory arthritis may affect a single joint initially.

Notes

- Pigmented villonodular synovitis is a benign disorder of unknown aetiology resulting in proliferation of the synovium.
- It may affect a joint, bursa, or tendon sheath (where it is known as a giant cell tumour of the tendon sheath).
- Within a joint, PVNS may affect the synovium diffusely or result in a single focal mass.
- The disease is usually seen in the second to fifth decades of life, with equal sex distribution.
- The disease is monoarticular, with the knee being the joint most commonly affected. It can also affect the hip and shoulder joint.
- Treatment of diffuse articular disease is usually by complete synovectomy, with recurrence associated with partial resection. If there is marked joint destruction, patients may also undergo arthrodesis or arthroplasty following synovectomy.

Bibliography

Murphey MD, Rhee JH, Lewis RB, Fanburg-Smith JC, Flemming DJ, Walker EA. Pigmented villonodular synovitis: radiologic-pathologic correlation. Radiographics 2008;28(5):1493–1518

Wong K, Sallomi D, Janzen DL, Munk PL, O'Connell JX, Lee MJ. Monoarticular synovial lesions: radiologic pictorial essay with pathologic illustration. Clin Radiol 1999;54(5):273–284

4.   Introduction to Neurological Imaging

Aarti Shah and Nagachandar Kandasamy

Anecdotal experience suggests that all candidates will be tested on neuroradiology as part of their viva, with MRI playing a larger role here than in other organ systems.

Basic approach to brain MRI:

1. Briefly look at all of the films to see what sequences were performed, in which plane, and whether there are any postcontrast images, as this may provide a clue to the pathology.
2. Remember that although the axial plane is the primary plane for neuroimaging, orientation may often be a clue to the underlying pathology; for example, coronal views are always performed when evaluating the sella as well as temporal lobe anatomy for refractory seizures. Sagittal views are useful for midline lesions (third ventricle, sella, pineal region, and corpus callosum) as well as the brainstem and cerebellar vermis.
3. On T1-weighted images, fat appears bright, and therefore the myelin sheaths of white matter appear brighter than grey matter. T1-weighted images are most useful for anatomical detail, and usually contrast-enhanced sequences tend to be T1-weighted. Do not assume that hyperintensity on a postcontrast sequence is enhancement; always check with the noncontrast images to confirm.
4. The signal intensity on T2-weighted imaging depends on water content and, as fat is darker than on T1-weighted imaging; white matter appears darker than grey matter on this sequence. T2-weighted images are most sensitive for detecting pathology, and therefore most basic protocols will include a T2-weighted and a fluid-attenuated inversion recovery (FLAIR) sequence. FLAIR images are T2-weighted with the cerebrospinal fluid (CSF) signal suppressed and are particularly helpful in the assessment of periventricular lesions.
5. Contrast does not enhance rapidly flowing blood, so different techniques such as gradient-echo and magnetic resonance angiography are used for the evaluation of vascular structures. Due to the magnetic susceptibility of blood, gradient-echo imaging has been shown to be a sensitive method of detection of chronic haemorrhage.
6. **Table 4.1** illustrates the signal characteristics of the evolution of haemorrhage with time.

In general, there are three types of cases that examiners tend to favour:

1. The "Aunt Minnie" cases (cases that are classic for a particular condition)
2. Cases where the abnormality is not immediately obvious and a systematic review is required
3. Cases where the abnormality is obvious and hence would merit a detailed discussion.

The "Aunt Minnies"

1. It is important to prepare for these cases as a candidate may potentially achieve a high score; this is especially true in cases with a classic constellation of findings. Neurocutaneous syndromes and congenital malformations are common examples.
2. If you are able to recognise the constellation of findings but unable to collate them into an unifying diagnosis, tell the examiner that you will arrive at a conclusion after seeking more information from the clinical details and referring to the appropriate literature.

Systematic Review (Computed Tomography)

1. Brain parenchyma:
   - Look for symmetry, normal grey–white matter differentiation, and any evidence of haemorrhage.
   - However, pathology can be symmetrical, for example, bilateral thalamic infarcts are often missed on CT.
2. Ventricles and subarachnoid spaces:
   - Look for symmetry and the presence of haemorrhage (commonly missed in the interpeduncular cistern, posterior Sylvian fissures, and dependent occipital horns).
   - Ensure the basal cisterns are not effaced.
3. Dura and subdural spaces:
   - The falx is normally denser than the brain parenchyma, but again asymmetry may give a clue to subdural haemorrhage adjacent to the falx (commonly missed in the parafalcine space, in the inferior frontal sulci, and along the convexities).

④ Bone and air spaces:
- Fluid, particularly an air–fluid level, within the paranasal sinuses, middle ear cavity, or mastoid air cells should raise the possibility of fractures within the adjacent bone.
- Sometimes looking at the scout view can demonstrate an obvious fracture.

⑤ Always mention that you would review on the appropriate window settings for each area; for example, a thin section bone algorithm to look for skull base fractures with the use of reformatted images where appropriate.

⑥ A candidate who demonstrates a systematic approach based on everyday experience will always reassure the examiner. When practising cases, try to review on "hard copy" format with multiple small images—up to 16 on each film—to get used to looking at smaller images without the luxury of "scrolling" up and down. However, the Royal College of Radiologists (RCR) has suggested that eventually the examination will be conducted with digital images and hard copy films will no longer be shown.

Approach to a Mass Lesion

① Age of the patient—as this alters the differential diagnosis
- Anatomical location—Where is the centre of the lesion? Is it intra- or extra-axial?

- Extent of disease—Is it solitary or multifocal?
- Distribution—Are they related to the grey–white matter junction? Do they follow a vascular territory? Does the lesion cross the midline?
- Signal characteristics.
- Assess mass effect—subtle effacement of the fourth ventricle and crowding at the foramen magnum may be due to low-lying tonsils or mass lesions that are often missed.

② Try to describe fully before launching into a list of differential diagnoses, and never exclude the possibility that the lesion could be simulating a tumour (e.g., abscess, aneurysm, white matter plaque, or vascular)

Table 4.1 Signal Characteristics of the Evolution of Haemorrhage

Stage of Haemorrhage	T1-Weighted	T2-Weighted
Hyperacute (h)	Isointense/Dark	Bright
Acute (1–2 days)	Isointense/Dark	Dark
Early subacute (2–7 days)	Bright	Dark
Late subacute (1–4 weeks)	Bright	Bright
Chronic	Dark	Dark rim

4.1 Sturge–Weber Syndrome

Clinical History

A 10-year-old boy presents with a history of seizures (**Figs. 4.1.1** and **4.1.2**).

Ideal Summary

These are axial CT images of the brain. There is extensive gyriform calcification within the right cerebral hemisphere, with atrophy of the affected parenchyma. The asymmetrical calcification is suggestive of a diagnosis of Sturge–Weber syndrome (SWS). I would like to take this case further by performing an MRI examination.

These are MR images from the same patient (**Figs. 4.1.3** and **4.1.4**).

These are coronal T2-weighted and fluid-attenuated inversion recovery MR images. They demonstrate volume loss in the right cerebral hemisphere with associated enlargement of the right lateral ventricle. There are multiple subcortical T2 hypointense lesions that appear to correspond to the calcification on the CT examination. I can also see numerous tiny flow voids within the extra-axial subarachnoid space on the right, in keeping with leptomeningeal collaterals. There are no features to suggest acute haemorrhage. Overall, the findings are pathognomonic for SWS. I would like to compare these scans with any previous images and ask whether there are any cutaneous manifestations.

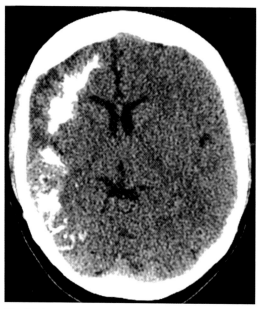

Fig. 4.1.1

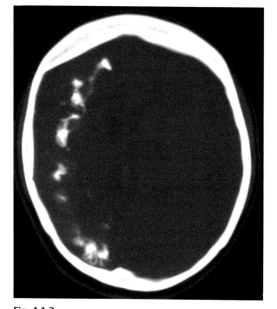

Fig. 4.1.2

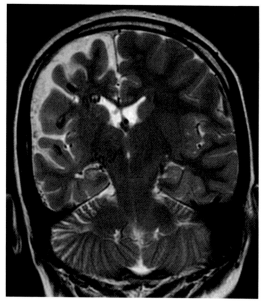

Fig. 4.1.3

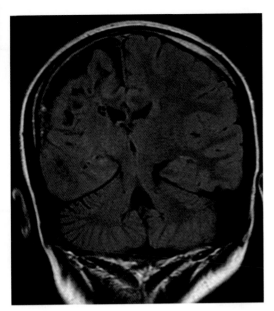

Fig. 4.1.4

Examination Tips

- The neurocutaneous syndromes have pathognomonic findings that should be described fluently when encountered in the examination.
- Findings on contrast-enhanced CT vary according to the chronicity of the disorder. Pial enhancement is typical among younger patients, but less evident in "burnt-out" disease, which is characterised by calcification and atrophy.
- Remember that enhancement can be difficult to appreciate in areas of heavy calcification on CT.
- In addition to the features listed above, look for enlargement of the ipsilateral choroid plexus.

- Thickening of the adjacent skull vault and orbit can also occur as a reaction to atrophy; this is termed the Dyke–Davidoff–Masson syndrome.

Differential Diagnosis

Gyriform calcification:
- Previous infarction
- Arteriovenous malformation
- Previous meningitis
- Leukaemia (following intrathecal chemotherapy or skull irradiation)

Notes

- Sturge–Weber syndrome is a rare, congenital, neurocutaneous disorder involving the vasculature of the face, the choroid of the eye, and the leptomeninges.
- It occurs with equal frequency among men and women and is usually sporadic.
- Contrast-enhanced MRI is the best modality for evaluation of the grey–white matter changes, vascular abnormalities, and parenchymal volume loss that may be present in SWS.
- All patients require ocular assessment as choroidal angiomas, which occur in around 40 to 50% of patients, increase the risk of glaucoma and retinal as well as choroidal detachment.

Bibliography

Herron J, Darrah R, Quaghebeur G. Intra-cranial manifestations of the neurocutaneous syndromes. Clin Radiol 2000;55(2):82–98

4.2 Multiple Sclerosis

Clinical History

A 32-year-old woman presents with tingling in her legs (**Figs. 4.2.1–4.2.3**).

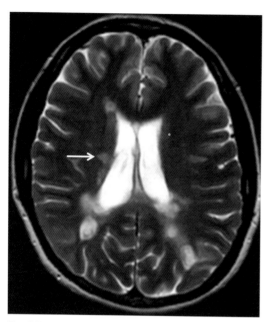

Fig. 4.2.1

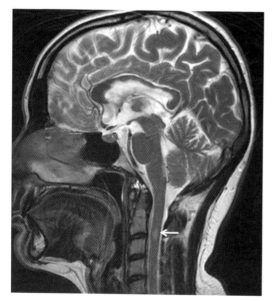

Fig. 4.2.2

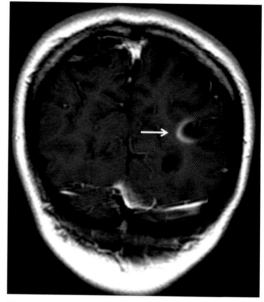

Fig. 4.2.3

Ideal Summary

These are axial and sagittal T2-weighted MRI and a coronal T1-weighted, contrast-enhanced image through the brain and upper cervical cord. There are multiple T2 hyperintense lesions in both cerebral hemispheres in a periventricular, deep white matter, and juxtacortical location. I can also see lesions within the corpus callosum in the callososeptal interface (**Fig. 4.2.1**, arrow) and there is a further lesion within the upper cervical spinal cord (**Fig. 4.2.2**, arrow). The postcontrast image shows an incomplete ring-enhancing lesion in the left parietal lobe (**Fig. 4.2.3**, arrow), which I would like to confirm by comparing to the noncontrast sequence. The morphology and distribution of these lesions is most in keeping with demyelination with multiple sclerosis (MS) as the likely diagnosis. I would like to ask if there is any previous imaging available for comparison, correlate with the results of cerebrospinal fluid (CSF) analysis for oligoclonal bands, and refer the patient to a neurologist. If there are symptoms attributable to lower spinal cord involvement, I would image the rest of the spine.

Examination Tips

- Think of the diagnosis in a young patient if there is a "relapsing–remitting" history involving different parts of the central nervous system.
- MRI is much more sensitive than CT, and lesions are characteristically hyperintense on T2-weighted images.
- The best sequences are T2-weighted and fluid-attenuated inversion recovery to demonstrate lesions as high-signal intensity foci in contrast to brain and CSF. The lesions are usually ovoid with their long axis oriented perpendicular to the ventricular margins, representing perivascular demyelination (Dawson's fingers).
- Typically, there is involvement of the periventricular white matter with a predilection for the temporal lobe, inferior aspect of the corpus callosum (callososeptal interface), and internal capsule.
- Always review the cervical cord for lesions on a sagittal image as spinal cord involvement is seen in up to 10% of cases.
- A contrast-enhanced sequence is useful to evaluate for "activity," with acute lesions demonstrating enhancement.

Differential Diagnosis

Causes of white matter lesions:
- Acute disseminated encephalomyelitis:
  - This usually affects a younger age group, has a viral prodrome, and is usually a monophasic illness.
  - There are usually fewer, larger lesions than in MS, with more frequent grey matter involvement.
  - Multifocal, sometimes confluent, T2 hyperintense lesions involve both cerebral hemispheres and are usually asymmetrical.
  - It does not usually involve the callososeptal interface, and may show punctuate or ring (either complete or incomplete) enhancement.
- Autoimmune-mediated vasculitis:
  - This can be seen in systemic lupus erythematosus, Behçet's syndrome, and polyarteritis nodosa.
  - Lesions are characterised by punctiform enhancement and usually spare the callososeptal interface (unlike in MS).
- Small vessel ischaemia:
  - This is seen in older patients.

- It is located in deep white matter and, in contrast to MS, which can be markedly asymmetrical, small vessel ischaemic changes are usually symmetrical with no predilection for the temporal lobes or corpus callosum.
- Lyme's disease:
  - This is usually associated with a rash and systemic symptoms (fever, myalgia, etc.).
  - Lesions can look very similar to those of MS.
  - Lyme's disease may also be associated with cranial nerve enhancement (most commonly of the VIIth).
- Susac's syndrome:
  - This is a self-limiting monophasic illness presenting with encephalopathy, retinal artery branch occlusion, and hearing loss (the classic triad).
  - There are multiple white matter lesions, almost always with callosal involvement (sparing the callososeptal interface, unlike MS).

Notes

- MS commonly occurs in the 20- to 40-year-old age range, with a peak onset at 30 years of age.
- CT is relatively nonspecific, demonstrating low-density white matter lesions, which may show nodular or irregular ring-like enhancement.
- According to the revised McDonald criteria for MS (2010), the diagnosis requires dissemination in time and space:
  - Dissemination in space can be demonstrated by the presence of more than one T2 lesion in two of the four following areas (excluding the symptomatic lesion in the event of a brainstem or spinal cord syndrome)
    - Periventricular
    - Juxtacortical
    - Infratentorial
    - Spinal cord
  - MRI is crucial to demonstrate multiplicity of lesions (dissemination in space), some of which can be clinically occult, and the contrast enhancement of some, but not all, lesions (dissemination in time).

Bibliography
Pretorius PM, Quaghebeur G. The role of MRI in the diagnosis of MS. Clin Radiol 2003;58(6):434–448

4.3 Tuberous Sclerosis

Clinical History

A 9-year-old girl presents with a history of seizures (**Figs. 4.3.1–4.3.3**).

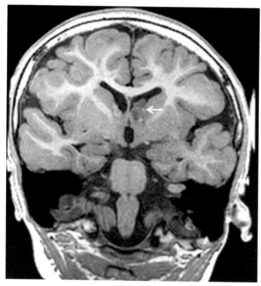

Fig. 4.3.1

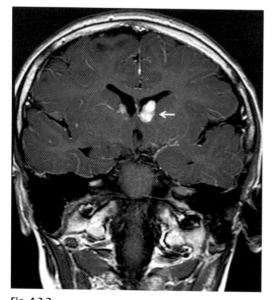

Fig. 4.3.2

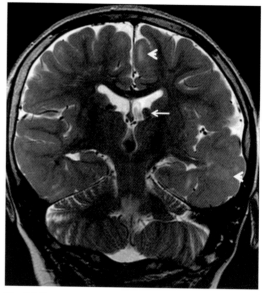

Fig. 4.3.3

Ideal Summary

These are T1 pre- and postcontrast and T2-weighted coronal images of the brain. The postcontrast images show two enhancing nodules within the lateral ventricle adjacent to the foramen of Monro (**Figs. 4.3.1** and **4.3.2**, arrow). The coronal T2 image shows further T2 hypointense, subependymal nodules along the walls of the lateral ventricles (**Fig. 4.3.3**, arrow). Furthermore, there are scattered areas of subcortical T2 hyperintense signal change expanding the left superior frontal gyrus (**Fig. 4.3.3**, arrowhead) and both temporal lobes (**Fig. 4.3.3**, arrowhead), more conspicuous on the left. There is no evidence of hydrocephalus. The hypointense subependymal nodules represent calcified subependymal hamartomas, and the cortical/subcortical white matter changes are tubers. The enhancing lesions in the region of the foramen of Monro are likely to represent subependymal giant cell astrocytomas; comparison with previous imaging is necessary to demonstrate growth. The features are consistent with tuberous sclerosis. I would compare these scans with previous imaging in the first instance to assess any interval increase in dimensions and suggest a neurosurgical opinion. In addition, tuberous sclerosis is a multisystem disorder and I would like to evaluate the kidneys, lung, and heart in a patient who is newly diagnosed.

Examination Tips

- The typical neuroimaging abnormalities of tuberous sclerosis are cortical tubers, subependymal nodules, subependymal giant cell astrocytomas (SGCAs), and white matter abnormalities.
- The appearance of the hamartomas varies depending on the degree of calcification. On CT, they are hypo- or isodense, with 50% eventually calcifying. When calcified, they are of low signal intensity on T1/T2-weighted imaging; if not, they are usually T2 hyperintense.
- The distinction between subependymal nodules and SGCAs relates to a progressive increase in size as they are indistinguishable histologically. Symptomatic SGCAs occur in approximately 10% of individuals with tuberous sclerosis; therefore, remember to look for hydrocephalus and an increase in size on serial imaging as these are indications for neurosurgical referral. Contrast enhancement alone is not a reliable predictor of malignancy as up to 80% of subependymal nodules may show enhancement.
- Regular screening with MRI is advised to monitor SGCAs.

Differential Diagnosis

The constellation of findings above is pathognomonical of tuberous sclerosis. However, the differential diagnoses for the following isolated abnormalities are:
- Periventricular calcification:
  - Cytomegalovirus. Periventricular and subependymal calcifications can mimic tuberous sclerosis.
  - Toxoplasmosis. Nodular calcifications are randomly seen in the periventricular, basal ganglia, and cerebral cortical areas.
- Mass within lateral ventricle:
  - Choroid plexus papilloma:
    - Typically arises from atrium of the lateral ventricle, not at the level of the foramen of Monro (as with subependymal giant cell astrocytomas) or in subependymal locations
    - Shows intense contrast enhancement.
  - Central neurocytoma:
    - Usually attached to the septum pellucidum, but can arise at the foramen of Monro
    - Necrosis and cyst formation are common.

- Germinoma:
  - Classically, has a central area of "engulfed" calcification
  - Can appear confusing as it arises in the midline near the third ventricle.
- Meningioma. Usually attached to choroid plexus.

Notes

- The classic clinical triad of facial angiofibromas, mental retardation, and seizures (Vogt's triad) is seen in less than a third of patients.
- The majority of patients do, however, have neurological abnormalities, including seizures, cognitive deficits, and learning disabilities.
- Tuberous sclerosis is characterised by the involvement of multiple organs:
  - Kidneys:
    - Angiomyolipomas. These can be multiple and bilateral. The risk of haemorrhage increases with size.
    - Cysts. Cysts are commonly single or multiple, but asymptomatic. Less commonly, tuberous sclerosis can coexist with polycystic kidney disease, and this has a poorer prognosis.
    - Renal cell carcinoma. This has a 1 to 2% risk in adults.
  - Lungs:
    - Lymphangioleiomyomatosis. Pulmonary manifestations of tuberous sclerosis can be indistinguishable from those of lymphangioleiomyomatosis, with uniform thin-walled cysts, chylous effusions, and pneumothorax.
  - Heart:
    - Rhabdomyoma. This is a benign tumour that is a characteristic cardiac manifestation of tuberous sclerosis.
  - Bones:
    - Cyst formation, periosteal reaction in the tubular bones with an "undulating appearance," and areas of sclerosis that can affect the entire skeleton.

Bibliography

Herron J, Darrah R, Quaghebeur G. Intra-cranial manifestations of the neurocutaneous syndromes. Clin Radiol 2000;55(2):82–98

4.4 Acute Cerebral Infarction

Clinical History

*A 54–year-old man presents with sudden-onset right-sided weakness (**Figs. 4.4.1–4.4.3**).*

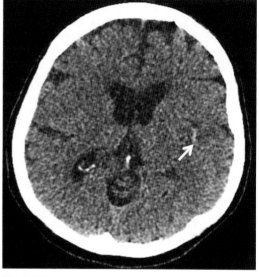

Fig. 4.4.3

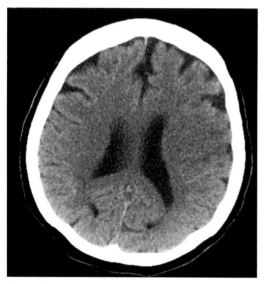

Fig. 4.4.1

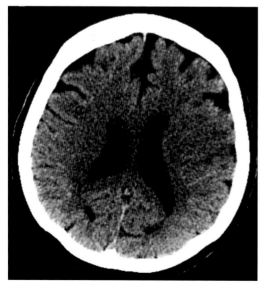

Fig. 4.4.2

Ideal Summary

These are selected axial images of a noncontrast CT. There is low cortical attenuation resulting in a loss of grey–white differentiation involving the left pre- and postcentral gyri. I note that **Fig. 4.4.2** has been "windowed," with a narrow window width. There is associated linear hyperdensity of the left middle cerebral artery (M2 segment) within the Sylvian fissure (**Fig. 4.4.3**, arrow), in keeping with acute thrombus. There is no acute intracranial haemorrhage on these images, but in my normal practice I would like to assess the remainder of the images for evidence of a contraindication to thrombolysis. These appearances are in keeping with an acute infarct. Depending upon the time of onset, the patient may be a candidate for intravenous thrombolysis.

*These are CT images of a different patient with right-sided weakness (**Figs. 4.4.4–4.4.8**).*

These are selected axial images of a noncontrast CT. (**Figs. 4.4.5 and 4.4.7** have a narrow window width.) There is low attenuation within the left caudate, lentiform nucleus, and insula, with presumptive involvement of the internal capsule making the Alberta

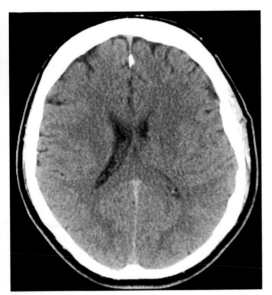

Fig. 4.4.4

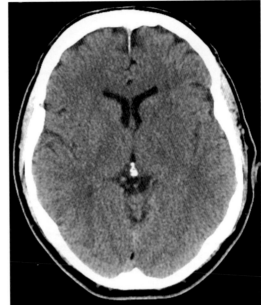

Fig. 4.4.6

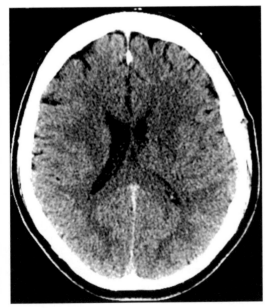

Fig. 4.4.5

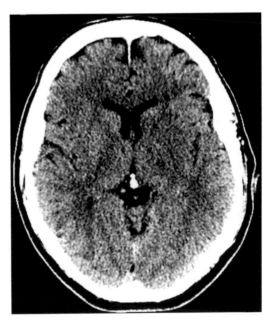

Fig. 4.4.7

Stroke Program Early CT Score (ASPECT) 6. Hyper-density representing thrombus is seen within the left M1 segment (**Fig. 4.4.8**, arrow). The appearances are in keeping with an acute infarct. An ASPECT score of 6 suggests the patient may not benefit from thrombolysis.

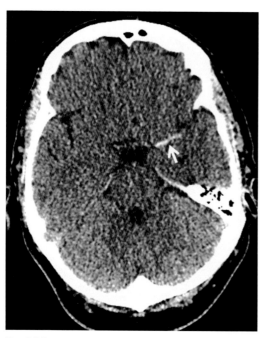

Fig. 4.4.8

Examination Tips

- Always review all the available images to ensure you are not missing another significant finding, such as haemorrhage.
- "Stroke" windows (W30 L30) were provided to improve detection of the loss of cortical high attenuation. Do not forget to say you would do this.
- Decide if contrast-enhanced imaging would be of value in the rare situation where the clinical history is not acute—it would be important to exclude a stroke mimic.
- Depending on the availability or otherwise of acute thrombolysis, each hospital will have a protocol outlining the indications for further imaging in acute stroke. Ensure you are familiar with your own. Additional imaging may be indicated when patients are above the 4.5-hour window following onset of symptoms or when the timing of onset is unknown.
- If there is a history of decreased consciousness, look for thrombus within the basilar artery.
- Comment on the presence of small vessel disease and previous infarction.

- Consider a venous infarct (usually secondary to venous sinus thrombosis) if the infarct does not conform to an arterial distribution.

Differential Diagnosis

No differential diagnosis should be offered for these examples.

Notes

The cortical branches of the middle cerebral artery (MCA) supply the lateral surface of the hemisphere, except for the medial frontal and parietal lobes (anterior cerebral artery), and the inferior temporal lobe (posterior cerebral artery). The deep penetrating branches of the MCA (lenticulostriate) supply the basal ganglia.

ASPECT Score
- This is a 10-point score that was devised by the Alberta Stroke Program to standardise the reporting of ischaemic low attenuation on CT.
- It is determined from evaluation of two standardised regions of the MCA territory: the basal ganglia level, where the thalamus, basal ganglia, and caudate are visible, and the supraganglionic level, which includes the corona radiata and centrum semiovale (see Pexman et al).
- A normal CT scan receives a score of 10, and a point is deducted for each area that appears ischaemic on the CT. Clinical trials show that patients with scores of 8 to 10 are more likely to benefit from intravenous thrombolysis, whereas those with scores 7 or lower may not.

The goal of early imaging in stroke is to exclude haemorrhage or stroke mimics, detect signs of early infarction, depict the extent of ischaemia, and guide treatment decisions.

CT and magnetic resonance (MR) perfusion studies are able to distinguish between brain tissue that is irreversibly infarcted and potentially salvageable tissue.

Diffusion-weighted MRI is more sensitive for acute ischaemia and, together with gradient–echo imaging to assess for haemorrhage, it is probably the study of choice in the acute setting. However, the availability of and patient intolerance to MRI in the acute setting means that CT with or without contrast remains the workhorse of acute imaging.

Bibliography

Merino JG, Warach S. Imaging of acute stroke. Nat Rev Neurol 2010;6(10):560–571

Pexman JH, Barber PA, Hill MD, et al. Use of the Alberta Stroke Program Early CT Score (ASPECTS) for assessing CT scans in patients with acute stroke. AJNR Am J Neuroradiol 2001;22(8):1534–1542

Srinivasan A, Goyal M, Al Azri F, Lum C. State-of-the-art imaging of acute stroke. Radiographics 2006;26(Suppl 1): S75–S95

4.5 Glioblastoma

Clinical History

*A 51-year-old man presents with a history of increasing confusion (**Fig. 4.5.1**).*

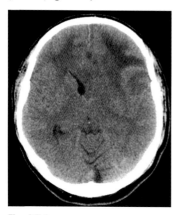

Fig. 4.5.1

Ideal Summary

This is a noncontrast axial CT of the brain. There is white matter hypodensity involving the anterior aspects of both frontal lobes, more prominent on the left. Irregular soft tissue low density is seen at the genu of the corpus callosum, with ill-defined borders. This is causing mass effect with effacement of the frontal horn of the left lateral ventricle and the sulci of the frontal lobes. I would be concerned about a high-grade glioma and would recommend further evaluation with MRI.

*These are MRI scans from the same patient (**Figs. 4.5.2–4.5.6**).*

The MRI examination comprises axial fluid-attenuated inversion recovery, coronal T2-weighted images, and axial T1-weighted images with and without contrast. These sequences show a heterogeneous T2 hyperintense lesion involving the anterior aspects of both frontal lobes, more extensive on the left, with callosal involvement. There is a cystic component in the superior left frontal white matter and an enhancing nodular component in the left paramedian aspect. There is an associated mass effect with gyral expansion and lateral ventricle effacement. No calcification or haemorrhage is shown on the available sequences. The findings are suggestive of a primary neoplasm, a "butterfly" glioma of a high grade, likely a glioblastoma multiforme.

Examination Tips

Questions to ask when assessing a "tumour":
- What is the patient's age? Glioblastoma multiforme (GBM) is mostly seen in older patients.
- Is the lesion intra- or extra-axial? What is the location of the "centre" of the mass?
- Is it a solitary lesion? If multiple, consider metastases and inherited disorders, such as the phakomatoses, before considering rarer possibilities.
- Are there specific CT or MRI findings: calcification, fat, cystic components, or signal characteristics? As most tumours are of low T1 and high T2 signal intensity, the converse may point to a specific diagnosis (melanoma, a haemorrhagic primary, or a metastasis).
- Is there evidence of contrast enhancement? Enhancement usually indicates a higher grade of

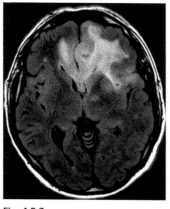

Fig. 4.5.2

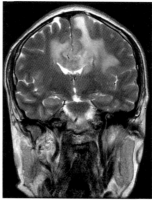

Fig. 4.5.3

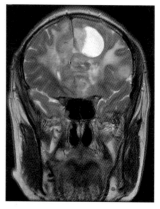

Fig. 4.5.4

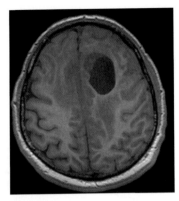

Fig. 4.5.5

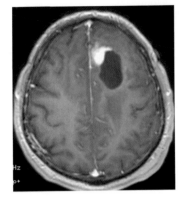

Fig. 4.5.6

malignancy, but with infiltrative tumours such as gliomas, it can underestimate the full extent of the tumour as enhancement only occurs in areas of breakdown of the blood–brain barrier.
- Be careful in describing the surrounding low density as vasogenic oedema—it is thought to represent tumour infiltration in glioblastoma.
- Comment on complications: haemorrhage and mass effect.
- Is this a tumour mimic?

Differential Diagnosis

- Abscess:
  - Ring enhancement is thinner than GBM, especially medially.
  - An abscess shows restricted diffusion restriction on diffusion-weighted imaging.
- Metastasis:
  - There are usually multiple lesions at the grey–white junction.
  - If single, it may be difficult to distinguish from glioblastoma.
- Tumefactive multiple sclerosis:
  - A solitary demyelinating lesion greater than 2 cm in size can mimic a tumour, but is usually in a characteristic (periventricular) location in a young patient.
  - There may be "horseshoe-shaped" enhancement that is open towards cortex, that is, incomplete ring enhancement.
- Lymphoma:
  - This is iso- or hypointense on T2 imaging due to a high nucleus-to-cytoplasm ratio, while GBM is heterogeneous and usually hyperintense on T2 weighting.
  - It usually has a periventricular location.

- Subacute ischaemia:
  - This is usually found in a vascular territory.
  - It may show mass effect and enhancement.

Notes

- Gliomas account for greater than 80% of primary central nervous system malignancies.
- "Glioma" is a generic term for tumours arising from glial cells (i.e., astrocytes, oligodendrocytes, and ependymal cells).
- A glioblastoma is a grade 4 astrocytoma, which demonstrates aggressive features, such as high mitotic rate and necrosis on histology. This is the most common primary intracranial neoplasm.
- Glioblastoma usually arises in the supratentorial white matter, with the occipital lobe being the least affected.
- For most patients presenting with a large mass or extensive neurological symptoms, histological diagnosis is obtained at the time of "debulking" surgery. However, for patients with a small tumour without a mass effect, with transient symptoms, or with a "tumour in eloquent cortex," watchful waiting with possible stereotactic biopsy may be an alternative to surgery with supportive chemotherapy and radiotherapy.
- The overall prognosis for glioblastoma is poor.
- GBM, anaplastic astrocytoma, meningioma, and lymphoma can disseminate along white matter, giving rise to a classic "butterfly" pattern of spread at the corpus callosum.

Bibliography

Rees JH, Smirniotopoulos JG, Jones RV, Wong K. Glioblastoma multiforme: radiologic-pathologic correlation. Radiographics 1996;16(6):1413–1438, quiz 1462–1463

4.6 Toxoplasmosis

Clinical History

A 33-year-old HIV-positive patient presents with a seizure (**Figs. 4.6.1–4.6.3**).

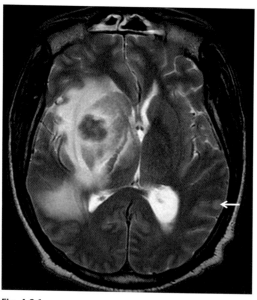

Fig. 4.6.1

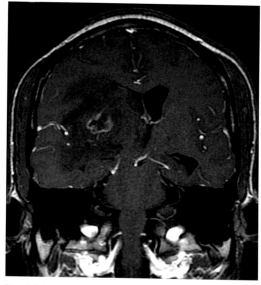

Fig. 4.6.3

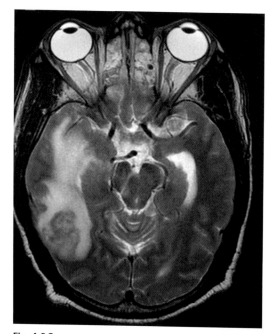

Fig. 4.6.2

Ideal Summary

These are axial T2-weighted images and a coronal T1 postcontrast image through the brain. The axial images show predominantly T2 hypointense lesions centred on the right basal ganglia and posterolateral right temporal lobe, with extensive surrounding white matter T2 hyperintensity. A further focus of T2 hyperintensity is also present in the left posterolateral temporal lobe (**Fig. 4.6.1**, arrow). There is associated mass effect with partial efface-ment of the right lateral ventricle and cerebral sulci and a shift of midline structures to the left. The postcontrast sequence shows irregular ring enhancement of the basal ganglia lesion. Given the clinical history of immune compromise, there are several differential diagnoses for these appearan-ces. The two most likely differentials include toxo-plasmosis and primary central nervous system (CNS) lymphoma. Other infective processes, such as tuberculosis or bacterial infection, are also in the differential. The signal characteristics and location in this case would favour toxoplasmosis. I would correlate with serology and advise interval imaging following initiation of treatment.

Examination Tips

Always ask for postcontrast images in the context of HIV/AIDS if these have not been provided. The most useful sign to look for in the context of a patient with immune compromise is the presence of mass effect:

- Lesions with mass effect:
  - Lesions usually demonstrate surrounding oedema and enhance with contrast administration.
  - Mass effect must be identified as lumbar puncture may be contraindicated.
  - The main differential diagnoses are infection and neoplastic lesions, commonly toxoplasmosis and primary CNS lymphoma (PCNSL). Tuberculosis and bacterial abscess should also be considered.
  - If the lesion is solitary and greater than 4 cm in size, think of PCNSL. If lesions are multiple and serology is positive for HIV, toxoplasmosis is most likely, although interval imaging will be prudent to assess change.
  - In practice, these features are not always reliable and biopsy often provides the definitive diagnosis.
- Lesions without mass effect:
  - These are usually nonenhancing.
  - The main differential diagnoses are progressive multifocal leucoencephalopathy, HIV encephalitis, and cytomegalovirus encephalitis.

The lesions in toxoplasmosis are located in the basal ganglia in 75%, followed by the thalamus and parietal/frontal lobes.

Differential Diagnosis

- PCNSL:
  - Solitary, large (> 4 cm) lesions are more suspicious for PCNSL, but solitary and multiple lesions occur with almost equal frequency.
  - Lesions that involve the corpus callosum or the periventricular areas are more likely to be due to PCNSL (in comparison, toxoplasmosis commonly involves the basal ganglia).
  - Calcification and haemorrhage are rare.
  - A thallium scan will be positive (whereas a thallium scan is negative in toxoplasmosis).
  - Differentiation between PCNSL and toxoplasmosis is difficult, and interval scanning is often used in the absence of single photon emission CT.
- Tuberculomas:
  - There are solitary or multiple ring or nodular enhancing lesions.
  - They are uncommon in the Western population, but consider them in the differential diagnosis if there is any history of travel to an endemic region.

Notes

On MRI, toxoplasmosis lesions are typically T1 low and T2 high signal, although the T2 signal can vary.

Bibliography

Offiah CE, Turnbull IW. The imaging appearances of intracranial CNS infections in adult HIV and AIDS patients. Clin Radiol 2006;61(5):393–401

4.7 Herpes Simplex Virus Encephalitis

Clinical History

A 13-year-old girl presents with sudden-onset fever, headache, and confusion (Figs. 4.7.1–4.7.4).

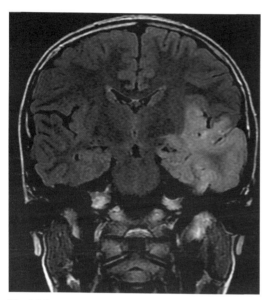

Fig. 4.7.1

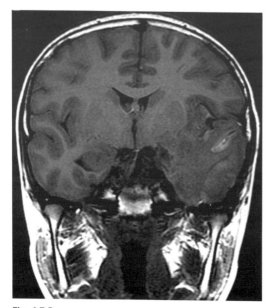

Fig. 4.7.2

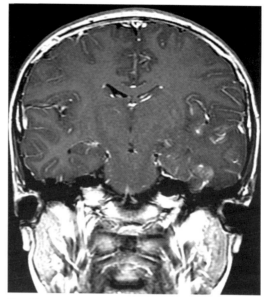

Fig. 4.7.3

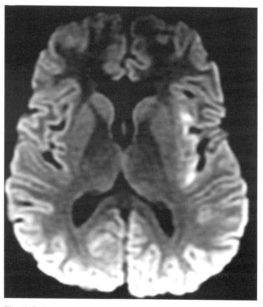

Fig. 4.7.4

Ideal Summary

These are coronal fluid-attenuated inversion recovery (FLAIR), pre- and postcontrast coronal T1-weighted, and axial diffusion-weighted images through the brain. The coronal FLAIR image (**Fig. 4.7.1**) shows confluent hyperintensity involving most of the left temporal lobe, extending to the hippocampus and insular cortex, with associated gyral swelling. The T1-weighted image (**Fig. 4.7.2**) shows diffuse hypo-intensity corresponding to the abnormality on the FLAIR sequence, with a loss of grey–white matter differentiation; there is also gyral T1 hyperintensity in keeping with haemorrhage. There is gyriform enhancement on the postcontrast T1 sequence (**Fig. 4.7.3**). The diffusion-weighted image (**Fig. 4.7.4**) shows patchy restricted diffusion involving the left insula. The cingulate gyrus and the right cerebral hemisphere appear normal. Given the clinical history, *Herpes simplex* virus (HSV) encephalitis is the most likely diagnosis. I would correlate with cerebrospinal fluid (CSF) findings, inform the clinicians so therapy can be initiated, and suggest interval imaging.

Examination Tips

- Always consider HSV encephalitis when there is involvement of the medial temporal and inferior frontal lobes, insula, and cingulate gyri (limbic system) with sparing of the basal ganglia.
- HSV encephalitis presents acutely and is typically bilateral and asymmetrical.
- Contrast enhancement (usually gyriform and occasionally meningeal) may occur.
- Early CT is often normal. MRI is the imaging test of choice, with the FLAIR sequence being most helpful to look for the hyperintense swollen cortex and subcortical white matter signal change.
- The pattern may be atypical in the paediatric age group, but abnormality of the limbic system should make the candidate think of HSV encephalitis.

Differential Diagnosis

- Cortical infarction:
  - Sudden onset
  - Confined to a vascular territory

- Transient postictal signal change:
  - Usually a clinical history of seizures
  - Can cause an abnormal T2/FLAIR cortical signal involving the temporal lobe in temporal lobe epilepsy with contrast enhancement, but no T1 signal change or haemorrhage
- Meningoencephalitis:
  - Other viral encephalitides, for example, from Epstein–Barr virus and *Varicella zoster* virus, can have a similar appearance but no predilection for the limbic system (as is the case with HSV encephalitis)
- Limbic encephalitis:
  - A rare paraneoplastic syndrome caused by a primary tumour (commonly of the lung)
  - Imaging features are similar to, and may be indistinguishable from, those of HSV encephalitis
  - Gradual onset of symptoms and absence of haemorrhage help differentiate it from HSV encephalitis
- Gliomatosis cerebri:
  - Diffusely infiltrating glial tumour that may involve more than one lobe
  - Clinical onset is usually indolent

Notes

- In adults, HSV type 1 causes greater than 90% of fatal cases of sporadic encephalitis. HSV type 2 accounts for the majority of cases in children and neonates.
- The gold standard for establishing the diagnosis is the detection of HSV DNA in the CSF by polymerase chain reaction, so a lumbar puncture should be performed.
- Empirical treatment is started before the diagnosis is confirmed.

Bibliography

Bulakbasi N, Kocaoglu M. Central nervous system infections of herpesvirus family. Neuroimaging Clin N Am 2008; 18(1):53–84, viii

4.8 Pituitary Fossa Mass

Clinical History

*A 50-year-old woman presents with headache and visual disturbances (**Figs. 4.8.1–4.8.3**).*

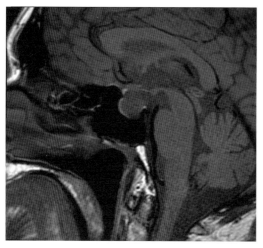

Fig. 4.8.1

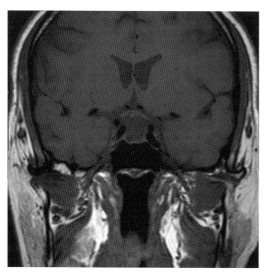

Fig. 4.8.2

Ideal Summary

This is a sagittal T1-weighted sequence and coronal pre- and postcontrast T1 sequences through the pituitary fossa. There is a T1 hypointense lesion

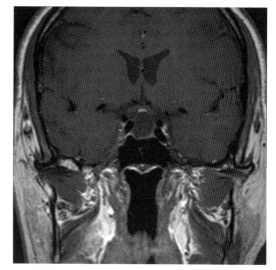

Fig. 4.8.3

within the sella, with minimal suprasellar extension and no parasellar extension. I cannot see any nodular component to the lesion. There is faint peripheral enhancement with no enhancing solid components, with both the pituitary infundibulum and optic chiasm displaced cranially. There is minimal expansion of the bony sella. I would like to review the rest of the available imaging, but the appearances are most in keeping with a cystic adenoma or a Rathke's cleft cyst. I would suggest correlation with pituitary function tests including prolactin, visual field testing, and referral to a multidisciplinary meeting. I would also compare with previous imaging if it is available.

*These are MRI scans from a different patient (**Figs. 4.8.4** and **4.8.5**).*

These are coronal pre- and postcontrast T1-weighted sequences. There is a large sellar mass that is homogeneous and of intermediate T1 signal intensity. The mass extends above the sella and encases just less than 50% of the circumference of the cavernous carotid arteries bilaterally. The mass enhances homogeneously on the postcontrast sequence. The optic chiasm is displaced superiorly. I would like to review the remainder of the images and any previous examinations. The imaging findings are in keeping with a pituitary macroadenoma.

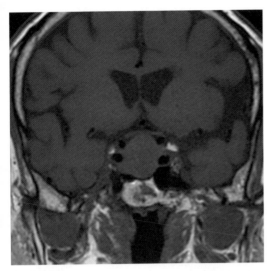

Fig. 4.8.4

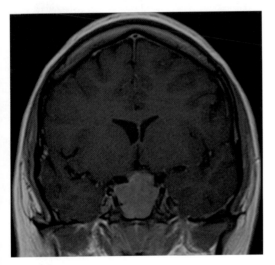

Fig. 4.8.5

Examination Tips

When dealing with a sellar mass, comment on the following:

- The epicentre of the lesion, that is, does it lie within, above, below, or lateral to the sella?
  - If the mass is intrasellar, is the sella enlarged?
- Can you identify the pituitary gland?
- Signal characteristics of the mass: is it calcified, cystic, or solid?
- Look for complications from mass effect, such as hydrocephalus and compression of the optic chiasm.
- Assess lateral extension into the cavernous sinus: look for encirclement of the internal carotid artery.

Always consider the possibility that a lesion in the region of the circle of Willis could represent a giant aneurysm. A flow void may provide a clue, and the pituitary gland should be visible separately from the eccentric mass.

Differential Diagnosis

- Intrasellar mass:
  - Pituitary hyperplasia
  - Pituitary microadenoma or macroadenoma
  - Rathke's cleft cyst
- Suprasellar mass—adult:
  - Pituitary macroadenoma
  - Meningioma
  - Aneurysm
  - Metastasis
- Suprasellar mass—child:
  - Craniopharyngioma
  - Hypothalamic hamartoma

Notes

- Meningioma:
  - Suprasellar epicentre and broad dural base
  - If intrasellar, the pituitary is visible separately
  - Can appear hyperdense, commonly calcifies, and may have associated hyperostosis
  - Uniform enhancement with contrast
- Pituitary macroadenoma:
  - Peak age 20 to 40 years; uncommon in children
  - More solid compared with craniopharyngiomas, with more intense, early enhancement
  - Calcification is rare
- Craniopharyngioma:
  - Although this arises from the suprasellar region, almost 50% have an intrasellar element
  - Cystic and solid enhancing components; calcification is more common
  - Comprises 50% of suprasellar tumours in children
- Rathke's cleft cyst:
  - Usually intrasellar and lies between the anterior and posterior pituitary. It can be indistinguishable from a microadenoma if it is small in size
  - Variable MRI signal depending on protein content; usually cystic with minimal peripheral or no enhancement.

Bibliography
Connor SEJ, Penney CC. MRI in the differential diagnosis of a sellar mass. Clin Radiol 2003;58(1):20–31

4.9 Cavernoma

Clinical History

*An 18-year-old woman presents with sudden-onset headache and a first seizure (**Fig. 4.9.1**).*

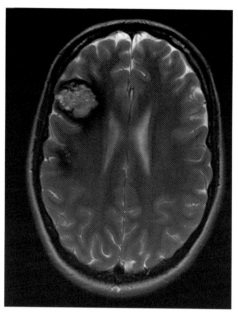

Fig. 4.9.2

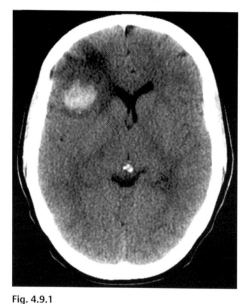

Fig. 4.9.1

Ideal Summary

This is a noncontrast axial CT image through the brain. There is a focus of high density seen within the right frontal lobe in keeping with acute haemorrhage. The surrounding white matter is of low attenuation with minimal associated mass effect. Given the age of the patient, haemorrhage secondary to an underlying neoplasm seems less likely. I would like to evaluate further with an MRI examination, ideally in 6 to 8 weeks depending on the clinical status, to exclude an underlying lesion. Vascular imaging (CT angiography or catheter angiography) can also be considered in the acute setting.

*These are MRI scans from the same patient at a later date (**Figs. 4.9.2–4.9.4**).*

These are axial T2-weighted and gradient-echo images, and sagittal T1-weighted sequences. There is a lobulated, heterogeneous, but predominantly T2 hyperintense lesion in the right middle frontal gyrus with a peripheral susceptibility artefact on the gradient-echo sequence. There are foci of T1 hyperintensity within the lesions in keeping with subacute

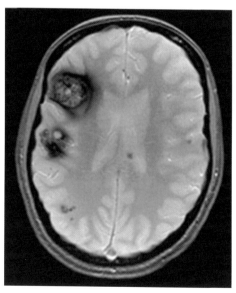

Fig. 4.9.3

haemorrhagic degradation products. The lesion can be described as "popcorn"-like. The gradient-echo sequence shows further lesions in the right frontal and parietal lobes and also within the left cerebral hemisphere. The appearances are in keeping with multiple cavernomas, and I would refer the patient to the neurosurgical team.

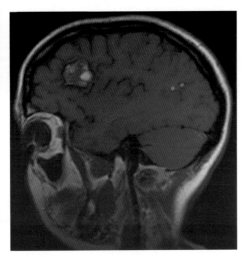

Fig. 4.9.4

Examination Tips

- If the typical "popcorn" appearance is present on MRI, this is considered diagnostic of a cavernoma. A cavernoma usually consists of a well-circumscribed, lobulated lesion with heterogeneous signal intensities on T1- and T2-weighted imaging due to the presence of evolving blood products.
- A surrounding ring of T2 low signal indicates haemosiderin deposition causing a susceptibility artefact on $T2^*$ gradient–echo images.
- Not all cavernomas demonstrate this typical appearance, the variations being due to differences in the evolution of blood products.
- There is minimal or negligible blood flow through the lesion, making contrast-enhanced sequences less useful. For the same reason, they are usually not visualised on angiography.
- There is a higher incidence of vascular malformations in patients with hereditary haemorrhagic telangiectasia or Osler–Weber–Rendu syndrome.

Differential Diagnosis

- Single "popcorn" lesion:
  - Capillary telangiectasia:
    - Moderately hypointense on gradient echo
    - Faint "brush-like" enhancement
    - Most commonly found in the pons, middle cerebellar peduncles, and dentate nuclei
    - Multiple lesions common
  - Arteriovenous malformation (AVM):
    - CT usually shows intraparenchymal haemorrhage, and the diagnosis can be difficult to make on CT in the setting of acute haemorrhage.
    - MRI is used to delineate the nidus of the AVM, often associated with a draining vein.
    - This is usually seen as dark flow voids on T1- and T2-weighted imaging.
    - Angiography is the gold standard for diagnosis.
- Multiple lesions with susceptibility artefact:
  - Amyloid angiopathy:
    - Elderly, normotensive patients
    - Usually subcortical, rarely involving the deep subcortical nuclei
  - Hypertensive microhaemorrhages
    - History of hypertension
    - Lesions in the deep white and grey matter

Notes

Types of congenital cerebral malformations
- Developmental venous anomalies:
  - These are the most common and may be encountered in up to 25% of patients with cavernomas.
  - They are composed of multiple radially arranged veins converging onto a dilated, central, venous trunk, which drains normal brain parenchyma.
  - This is represented as a "sunburst" pattern on T1-weighted contrast-enhanced MRIs.
  - They are usually incidental findings without clinical sequelae or any need for intervention.
- Cavernoma:
  - The term "cavernoma" is synonymous with cavernous malformation, cavernous angioma, or cavernous haemangioma.
  - Clinical presentation includes seizures or progressive neurological deficits.
  - If asymptomatic, it can be followed without intervention; otherwise may require surgery.
- Capillary telangiectasia:
  - It is usually an incidental finding without clinical consequence.
- AVM:
  - This most commonly present with haemorrhage, especially in children.
  - The choice of treatment depends upon multiple factors including the patient's age, size of lesion, location of lesion, and history of haemorrhage.

Bibliography

Hegde AN, Mohan S, Lim CCT. CNS cavernous haemangioma: "popcorn" in the brain and spinal cord. Clin Radiol 2012;67(4):380–388

4.10 Meningioma

Clinical History

*A 57-year-old patient presents with long-standing headache and a recent personality change (**Fig. 4.10.1**).*

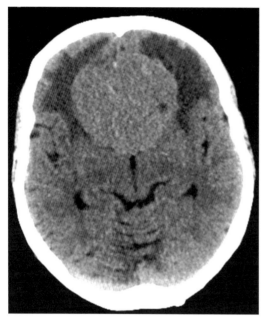

Fig. 4.10.1

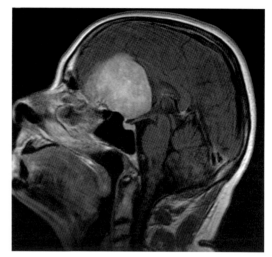

Fig. 4.10.2

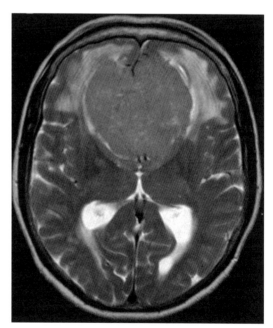

Fig. 4.10.3

Ideal Summary

This is an unenhanced axial CT image through the brain. There is a large space-occupying lesion centred on the inferior frontal region in the midline. I can see a few specks of calcification within the mass. Low density is seen around the lesion, which is predominantly of white matter distribution, and there is a mass effect with effacement of the sulci of the frontal lobes. I would like to review the remainder of the images and ask if a postcontrast CT was performed. The mass is most likely a primary malignancy, and I would take this forward by arranging an MRI examination.

*These are MRI scans from the same patient (**Figs. 4.10.2** and **4.10.3**).*

These are contrast-enhanced sagittal T1-weighted and axial T2-weighted images. The MRI shows a large, avidly enhancing extra-axial lesion centred on the midline adjacent to the floor of the anterior cranial fossa and extending to the tuberculum sellae. The lesion displaces the genu of the corpus callosum and the anterior cerebral arteries. There is bifrontal, perilesional white matter low attenuation. Given its location, size, and enhancement, the most likely diagnosis for an extra-axial mass is a meningioma. I would recommend comparison with old imaging if available and referral for a neurosurgical opinion.

Examination Tips

When evaluating a peripherally sited mass lesion, identifying the lesion to be extra or intra-axial is important. The following features help in the differentiation, remembering that evaluation of the lesion in all planes is important as some of the differentiating features may be seen in one plane only:

- Extra-axial masses by definition displace the underlying gyri, resulting in "white matter buckling" with maintenance of the grey–white interface, while an intra-axial mass expands the gyrus.
- Other signs that are helpful in the diagnosis of an extra-axial mass are paradoxical widening of the subarachnoid space (a cerebrospinal fluid cleft), displacement of the subarachnoid vessels, and bony reaction (hyperostosis).
- Thickened, enhancing tissue that surrounds the dural attachment of the tumour (dural tail) is present in approximately 65% of meningiomas, but although it is highly suggestive of meningioma, it is not specific. Remember that dural enhancement may also been seen in intra-axial lesions, although it is infrequent.

Differential Diagnosis

Convexity, parasagittal, and sphenoid wing meningioma:

- Metastases:
  - Breast, lung, prostate, and renal cell carcinomas are the most common primaries.
  - Features favouring metastases include multiplicity, heterogeneous enhancement, and bony invasion.
  - Hodgkin's lymphoma can spread haematogenously to the dura and meninges, and produces a well-circumscribed dural-based mass.
- Granuloma, for example, sarcoidosis:
  - Usually, sarcoidosis develops in the basal leptomeninges and can affect the hypothalamus, infundibulum, and cranial nerves.

- Lesions that can mimic a meningioma tend to occur in the cribriform plate, sphenoid wing, optic nerve, and cerebellopontine angle.
- Extramedullary haemopoiesis:
  - Rarely, this disorder can give multilobulated, extra-axial lesions.
  - Associated skull marrow changes and paranasal soft tissue masses may be a clue.

Notes

- Meningioma is the most frequent primary brain tumour.
- It can arise anywhere from the dura. Common sites include the parasagittal or lateral cerebral convexities, sphenoid ridge, olfactory grooves, and posterior cranial fossa.
- On CT, they are usually smooth, well-defined, and iso- or hyperdense to brain tissue. CT is particularly useful to demonstrate hyperostosis and calcification (15 to 20%).
- Typical MRI signal characteristics are that it is iso- or hypointense to grey matter on T1-weighted sequences, and iso- or hyperintense on T2-weighted with avid homogeneous contrast enhancement.
- Up to 15% can, however, show atypical features, such as heterogeneous enhancement or large cysts.
- MRI is particularly helpful for imaging the posterior fossa and juxtasellar region.
- Many are incidental findings in asymptomatic patients. If the patients remain asymptomatic and there is no evidence of tumour growth on surveillance, a conservative approach can be maintained.
- The indications for surgery include symptoms or, in the case of asymptomatic patients, growth, infiltration, or surrounding oedema. Therefore, reports of follow-up imaging should comment on these.

Bibliography

Buetow MP, Buetow PC, Smirniotopoulos JG. Typical, atypical, and misleading features in meningioma. Radiographics 1991;11(6):1087–1106

4.11 Chiari Malformation

Clinical History

*A 31-year-old woman presents with long-standing headache, new-onset nystagmus, and brisk knee reflexes on examination (**Figs. 4.11.1–4.11.5**).*

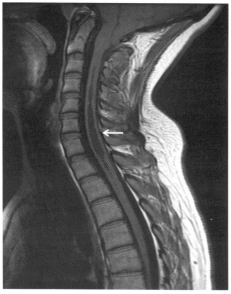

Fig. 4.11.1

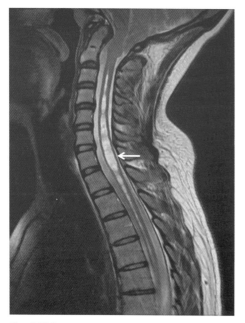

Fig. 4.11.2

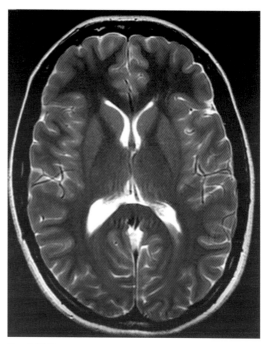

Fig. 4.11.3

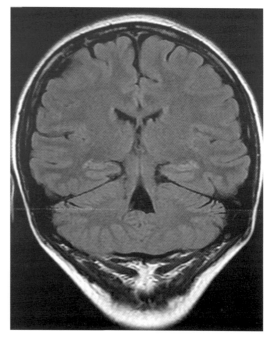

Fig. 4.11.4

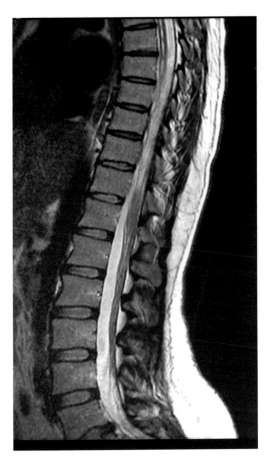

Fig. 4.11.5

Ideal Summary

These are sagittal T1-weighted and T2-weighted images of the cervical spine, a sagittal T2-weighted image of the lumbar spine, and axial T2-weighted and coronal fluid-attenuated inversion recovery (FLAIR) images of the brain. On the sagittal images, there is an extensive lobulated T1 hypointense/T2 hyperintense cavity extending from C3 to T5 with minor expansion of the spinal cord at C7/T1 (**Figs. 4.11.1** and **4.11.2**, arrow). There is ectopia of the cerebellar tonsils, with the inferior aspect appearing pointed. The axial image (**Fig. 4.11.3**) of the brain shows no hydrocephalus, and the locations of the remainder of the cerebellum, brainstem, and fourth ventricle are normal, as shown on the coronal FLAIR image (**Fig. 4.11.4**). No myelomeningocoele is seen on the sequence through the lumbar spine (**Fig. 4.11.5**). The appearances are in keeping with tonsillar ectopia and a diagnosis of Chiari type I

malformation with associated hydrosyringomyelia. I would suggest a neurosurgical referral.

Examination Tips

- The cerebellar tonsils may be found up to 5 mm below the level of the foramen magnum in adults.
- If the cerebellar tonsils are abnormally low-lying, narrow your differential diagnosis:
  - From above: intracranial space-occupying lesion.
  - At the level of the cerebellar tonsils: pointed tonsils (Chiari type I) and basilar invagination.
  - From below: following lumbar puncture, resulting in intracranial hypotension with a "sagging" brainstem.
  - If provided with spinal MRI scans only, always ask to review the brain to look for evidence of hydrocephalus or another cause for the raised intracranial pressure causing the tonsillar descent, such as a posterior fossa mass.
  - The size of the posterior fossa is important in distinguishing Chiari type I from Chiari type II malformations: a small posterior fossa is a hallmark of Chiari type II.
  - If the posterior fossa is enlarged, think of a Dandy–Walker malformation.

Differential Diagnosis

There are no differential diagnoses for the given imaging findings.

Notes

- Tonsillar ectopia refers to herniation of the cerebellar tonsils through the foramen magnum.
- To assess this, a measurement is made of the amount of displacement in millimetres below a line that is drawn from the basion (anterior) to the opsithion (posterior). A Chiari type I malformation is considered in an adult when this displacement is 5 mm or greater; in infants, however, up to 6 mm can still be normal.
- The presence of hydrosyringomyelia is usually an indication for surgery as this implies a change in cerebrospinal fluid flow dynamics. The aim of surgery is to prevent hydrocephalus and worsening symptoms.

Bibliography

el Gammal T, Mark EK, Brooks BS. MR imaging of Chiari II malformation. AJR Am J Roentgenol 1988;150(1):163–170

4.12 Subarachnoid Haemorrhage

Clinical History

*A 39-year-old patient presents with a sudden-onset severe headache (**Fig. 4.12.1**).*

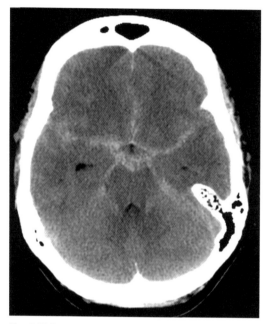

Fig. 4.12.1

Ideal Summary

This is a single axial image from a noncontrast CT. Diffuse high density is present within the basal cisterns, Sylvian fissures bilaterally, and anterior interhemispheric fissure, in keeping with extensive subarachnoid haemorrhage (SAH). Given the clinical history, I would perform an immediate CT angiogram to evaluate for the presence of an intracranial aneurysm.

*This is the investigation you asked for (**Fig. 4.12.2**).*

This is a selected CT angiographic maximum-intensity projection image. There is a saccular aneurysm arising from the right internal carotid artery at the origin of the right posterior communicating artery (**Fig. 4.12.2**, arrow). The neck appears narrow on this single view. The appearances are consistent with an aneurysmal SAH, secondary to right posterior communicating artery origin aneurysm rupture. I would recommend

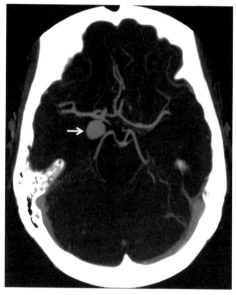

Fig. 4.12.2

referral to the vascular neurosurgeons and interventional neuroradiologists to facilitate further management, which should include consideration of coil embolisation of the aneurysm.

*These are further images from the same patient (**Figs. 4.12.3** and **4.12.4**).*

These are selected angiogram images showing the large saccular aneurysm and subsequent coil embolisation.

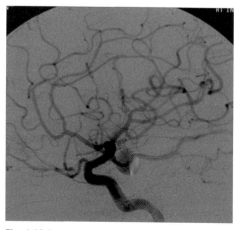

Fig. 4.12.3

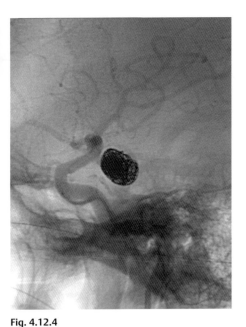

Fig. 4.12.4

Examination Tips

- In the presence of SAH on CT without a history of trauma, you should always ask for a CT angiogram.
- Always review the thin axial cuts, especially at the base of the skull, to improve the chances of detecting SAH.
- Carefully inspect the following sites for pooling of blood: interpeduncular fossa, posterior aspect of the Sylvian fissures, and occipital horns of the lateral ventricles.
- Comment on the distribution of subarachnoid blood, which may help locate the aneurysm:
  - Anterior communicating artery aneurysm: interhemispheric fissure and suprasellar cistern
  - Middle cerebral artery bifurcation aneurysm: ipsilateral Sylvian fissure
  - Posterior circulation aneurysm: interpeduncular cistern and peri-medullary cisterns.
- Remember that the sensitivity of CT for detection of subarachnoid blood decreases with time, falling to 50% at about 1 week, so a lumbar puncture (testing for xanthochromia) should be performed if SAH is suspected but CT is negative.
- Look for complications, such as intracerebral parenchymal haematoma, acute hydrocephalus, and global cerebral ischaemia.
- "Pseudo-subarachnoid haemorrhage" can occur in the context of severe cerebral oedema, in which normal vessels can appear spuriously hyperdense, mimicking SAH; the mechanism for this remains unclear.

Differential Diagnosis

Nontraumatic SAH:
- Arteriovenous malformations (AVMs):
  - Superficial AVMs can bleed into the cerebrospinal fluid space at the convexities, but it is unusual for SAH to be present without intracerebral haematoma.
  - In the spine, dural AVMs are the most common type of AVM, and those that cause SAH are usually within the cervical cord.
- Perimesencephalic haemorrhage:
  - This refers to blood confined to the cisterns around the midbrain with a normal angiogram.
  - It is thought to have a better prognosis than aneurysmal SAH.
- Intracranial arterial dissection:
  - This is more commonly seen with vertebrobasilar dissection.
- Septic aneurysms:
  - They are usually secondary to infective endocarditis.
  - They can occur in any location, not just those "typical" for saccular aneurysms.

Notes

- The most common cause of SAH is trauma.
- Intracranial aneurysms typically arise within or near the circle of Willis, with middle cerebral artery bifurcation and anterior communicating artery aneurysms accounting for nearly 60% of all sites.
- Other common sites include the posterior communicating and ophthalmic artery origins.
- Within the posterior circulation, the most common site is the basilar artery tip.
- MRI can detect SAH with a high sensitivity in patients that present subacutely, although there are a large number of causes of fluid-attenuated inversion recovery hyperintensity, such as meningitis, imaging under general anesthesia, and gadolinium administration.

Bibliography

Goddard AJ, Tan G, Becker J. Computed tomography angiography for the detection and characterization of intra-cranial aneurysms: current status. Clin Radiol 2005;60(12):1221–1236

4.13 Subdural Empyema

Clinical History

A 41-year-old presents with headache, fever, and vomiting (**Figs. 4.13.1–4.13.3**).

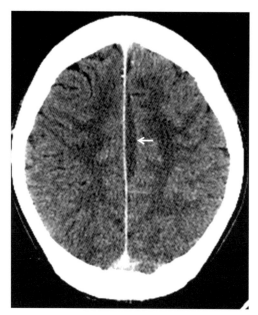

Fig. 4.13.1

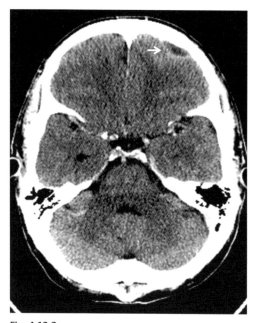

Fig. 4.13.2

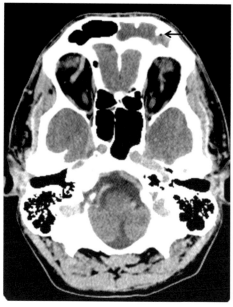

Fig. 4.13.3

Ideal Summary

These are axial postcontrast CT images through the brain. There are low-density extra-axial collections in the left parafalcine (**Fig. 4.13.1**, arrow) and anterior frontal (**Fig. 4.13.2**, arrow) regions. The left anterior frontal collection shows peripheral enhancement. In addition, there is opacification of the left frontal sinus (**Fig. 4.13.3**, arrow). The appearances are in keeping with subdural empyema secondary to frontal sinusitis. I would like to review the bone reconstructions to look for a bony defect or evidence of osteomyelitis. This is an emergency, and I would suggest referral to the neurosurgeon as a matter of urgency. An MRI examination should be performed to delineate the extent of involvement and to assess the underlying cerebral parenchyma.

These are MRI scans from a different patient with a similar history (**Figs. 4.13.4–4.13.6**).

These are T1 postcontrast and T2 axial images through the brain. There is a right-sided subdural collection, with a hyperenhancing rim upon administration of contrast (**Figs. 4.13.4** and **4.13.5**, arrow). There is opacification of the right ethmoid air cells (**Fig. 4.13.6**, arrow), likely representing the source of infection.

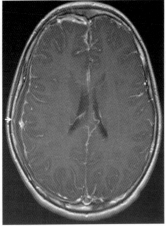

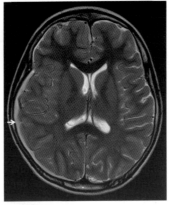

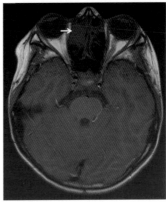

Fig. 4.13.4   Fig. 4.13.5   Fig. 4.13.6

Examination Tips

Always consider the possibility of intracranial complications in patients with sinus opacification and neurological symptoms. Look for the underlying aetiology and associated complications:

- Opacification of mastoid air cells (mastoiditis or otitis media) or sphenoid sinus (sinusitis).
- Erosion of mastoid bone or sphenoid or frontal sinus.
- Venous sinus thrombosis:
  - Unenhanced CT may demonstrate a hyperdense venous sinus ("cord sign") with the typical "empty delta" sign (filling defect within the lumen of the sagittal sinus with a thin, outlining rim of contrast) only seen in 20% of cases.
  - MRI shows loss of the normal flow void within the sinus.
  - CT venography demonstrating the thrombus as a filling defect is the best method for confirming the diagnosis.
  - Venous infarction: usually haemorrhagic, and the area of infarction does not conform to any arterial territory, distinguishing it from a stroke.
- Abscess formation: varies depending on the stage at the time of imaging. Later phases almost always show a rim-enhancing lesion. Diffusion-weighted imaging may show restricted diffusion (bright signal).

Differential Diagnosis

- Chronic subdural haematoma
  - Usually high signal intensity on T1-weighted imaging

- May show peripheral enhancement similar to an empyema
- Subdural hygroma:
  - Cerebrospinal fluid (CSF) density
  - Nonenhancing
- Metastases:
  - Typically breast or prostate
  - Diffuse nodular enhancement

Notes

- Extra-axial collections of pus can be subdural or extradural, with a predilection for the frontal convexities and parafalcine regions.
- A subdural empyema is typically crescentic and confined by the falx, whereas an extradural empyema is biconvex and often continuous along the midline.
- The majority of subdural empyemas are located intracranially, where they arise due to extension of infection from the paranasal sinuses or as a complication of meningitis.
- Most extradural empyemas are spinal, due to haematogenous spread or direct extension from adjacent vertebral osteomyelitis.
- Signs of empyema and its complications are often better appreciated on MRI than on CT.
- The T1-weighted MRI appearance is isointense relative to CSF and hyperintense on T2-weighted sequences, with evidence of restricted diffusion on diffusion-weighted imaging. These signal changes are typical of proteinaceous fluid.

Bibliography

Rich PM, Deasy NP, Jarosz JM. Intracranial dural empyema. Br J Radiol 2000;73(876):1329–1336

4.14 Medulloblastoma

Clinical History

*A 9-year-old boy presents with headache, vomiting, and visual deterioration (**Fig. 4.14.1**).*

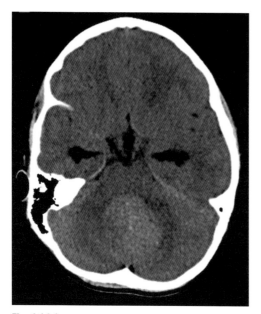

Fig. 4.14.1

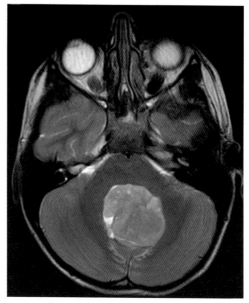

Fig. 4.14.2

Ideal Summary

This is an axial noncontrast CT image through the brain. There is a moderately hyperdense posterior fossa mass in the midline, with effacement of the fourth ventricle. No calcification of the lesion is present. The temporal horns are dilated, representing hydrocephalus. I would like to review postcontrast images if these are available to further characterise the mass and assess the degree of hydrocephalus. Given the age of the patient and the imaging findings, a medulloblastoma seems most likely. I would recommend MRI of the brain and spine to assess for "drop" metastases, and referral to the neurosurgical team for management of the hydrocephalus.

*These are MR images from the same patient (**Figs. 4.14.2–4.14.4**).*

These are axial T2-weighted, postcontrast T1-weighted, and apparent diffusion coefficient (ADC) map images through the posterior fossa. The lesion

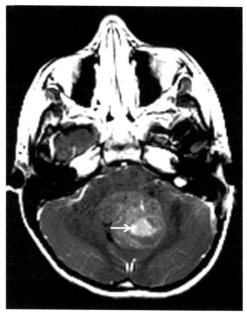

Fig. 4.14.3

is isointense to grey matter on the T2 sequence and shows heterogeneous enhancement. The avidly enhancing component demonstrates restricted diffusion on the ADC map (**Figs. 4.14.3** and **4.14.4**, arrow). The location and signal characteristics of this

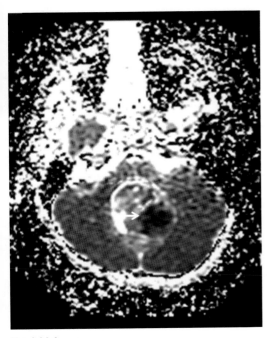

Fig. 4.14.4

lesion are typical for medulloblastoma. I would like to review the remainder of the neuraxis to check for "drop" metastases.

Examination Tips

Evaluation of posterior fossa mass lesions in children:
- The hyperdense appearance of medulloblastoma on CT, avid enhancement of the solid component, and restricted diffusion reflect densely packed cells.
- Comment on complications such as hydrocephalus, which will determine the emergent management. When the tumour arises from the roof of the fourth ventricle, it will usually displace this structure anteriorly. Look for the presence of a ventricular shunt.
- Sagittal images can be useful to see whether the tumour is arising from the roof (medulloblastoma) or floor (ependymoma) of the fourth ventricle. However, it may not be possible to see this if the lesion is large.
- The entire neuraxis must be imaged with contrast-enhanced studies to look for "drop" metastases as medulloblastoma is the most common cause of "drop" metastases and 10 to 30% of patients will have seeding along the cerebrospinal fluid pathways at the time of presentation.

- Remember that the differential diagnosis of a posterior fossa mass varies according to age of the patient.

Differential Diagnosis

Posterior fossa mass in a child:
- Ependymoma:
  - Usually arises from the floor of the fourth ventricle
  - "Squeezes" out of the foramen of Luschka and may extend around the anterior surface of the brainstem—so-called "plastic" ependymoma
  - Signal intensity on MRI is more heterogeneous than that with medulloblastoma due to haemorrhage and calcification (50%—higher than medulloblastoma)
- Pilocystic astrocytoma:
  - Typically a cyst with an enhancing nodule
  - Hypodense on CT (rather than hyperdense, as with medulloblastoma) due to the cystic component
  - Usually paracentral, that is, located in the cerebellar hemisphere
- Choroid plexus papilloma
- More common in the lateral ventricle, with a predilection for the trigone in children
- On CT, these are isodense to slightly hyperdense, well-defined, lobulated masses that can be described as "frond-like" or "cauliflower-like" and demonstrate homogenous enhancement
- May contain speckled calcification

Notes

- Medulloblastoma is the most common malignant paediatric tumour and occurs almost exclusively in the cerebellum.
- It is classified as a primitive neuroendocrine tumour.
- The typical clinical presentation reflects raised intracranial pressure.
- It can be associated with familial cancer syndromes such as basal nevus (Gorlin's) syndrome, Turcot's syndrome, and Gardner's syndrome.

Bibliography
Paldino MJ, Faerber EN, Poussaint TY. Imaging tumors of the pediatric central nervous system. Radiol Clin North Am 2011;49(4):589–616, v

4.15 Ruptured Dermoid

Clinical History

*A 55-year-old woman presents with severe headache and new-onset seizures (**Figs. 4.15.1–4.15.4**).*

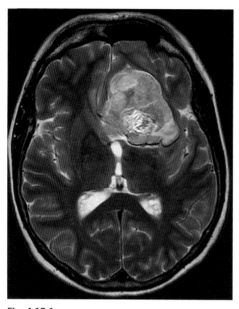

Fig. 4.15.1

Ideal Summary

These are axial T2-weighted and coronal T1-weighted precontrast and postcontrast sequences. A large intraparenchymal lesion is seen centred on the left inferior frontal region. The mass is heterogeneous and is high signal on both the T1- and T2-weighted sequences. There is some extension of the lesion across the midline with distortion of the third ventricle and displacement of the anterior cerebral arteries (A2 segments). On the coronal image, the lesion abuts the left optic hemichiasm. There are also multiple small foci of T1 hyperintensity within the sulcal spaces on the unenhanced T1 sequence (**Fig. 4.15.4**), more conspicuous on the left. There is no pathological contrast enhancement (**Fig. 4.15.3**). The signal characteristics are suggestive of a fat-containing lesion, and the T2 low signal margin along the posterior border of the mass appears to be secondary to chemical shift artefact. These features are typical of a dermoid, and the presence of T1 hyperintense foci within the sulcal spaces are in keeping with fat droplets secondary to rupture. I would recommend referral of the patient to the neurosurgical team for further management.

*These are CT images of the same patient (**Figs. 4.15.5** and **4.15.6**).*

These are selected unenhanced axial CT images. There is a large, low-density lesion centred on the left frontal lobe with peripheral calcification. The mass crosses the midline, but there is no surrounding oedema. There are multiple foci of low density seen within the sulcal spaces on the left. I would like to confirm if this is a fat density lesion by adjusting the window settings. If so, the findings are in keeping with a ruptured dermoid cyst, and I would recommend referral to the neurosurgical team.

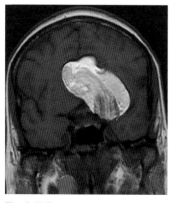

Fig. 4.15.2

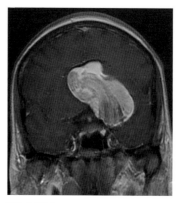

Fig. 4.15.3

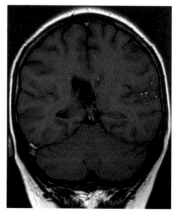

Fig. 4.15.4

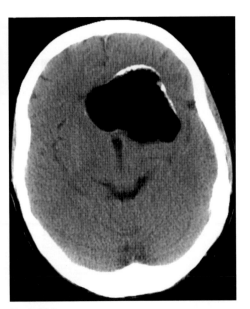

Fig. 4.15.5

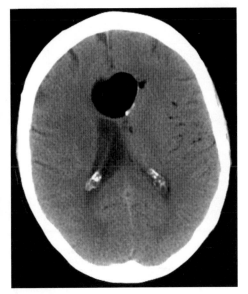

Fig. 4.15.6

Examination Tips

◉ Fat-suppressed MR sequences may be suggested to reach the diagnosis. This is especially useful as a dermoid cyst may appear hypo- or hyperintense on T2-weighted imaging.

◉ Fat droplets in the subarachnoid space or in the ventricles are virtually diagnostic of a ruptured dermoid cyst. A fat–fluid level within the cyst or the ventricles is commonly seen.

◉ Apart from minor peripheral enhancement, contrast enhancement is rare and should suggest an alternative diagnosis.

Differential Diagnosis

T1 hyperintense lesions:

◉ Lipoma:
   • These are more homogeneous than a dermoid.
   • They are less likely to exert a mass effect than a dermoid.
   • Lesions are more likely to have associated congenital abnormalities such as corpus callosum defects than dermoids.

◉ Acute or subacute haemorrhage or haemorrhagic tumour:
   • Lesions should be T2 hypointense (compare with a dermoid).
   • They will be associated with a mass effect and oedema.

◉ Teratoma:
   • In addition to fat, these contain calcium, soft tissue, and fluid components, and hence appear more heterogeneous.
   • Teratomas are often multicystic.
   • The soft tissue component will enhance with contrast.

◉ Epidermoid:
   • Epidermoids follow cerebrospinal fluid signal intensity on MRI. Rarely, high protein content can lead to a hyperintense appearance on T1-weighted imaging.
   • The use of a fat suppression technique or CT can help distinguish the two.

Notes

◉ Dermoids are not true tumours but epithelialised cysts containing ectodermal elements.

◉ The majority are benign, but they can rarely transform to squamous cell carcinoma.

◉ Larger lesions have a higher rate of rupture, which may lead to chemical meningitis resulting in vasospasm, infarction, and even death.

Bibliography

Osborn AG, Preece MT. Intracranial cysts: radiologic-pathologic correlation and imaging approach. Radiology 2006;239(3):650–664

4.16 Von Hippel–Lindau Syndrome

Clinical History

A   30-year-old   man   presents   with   ataxia
(**Figs. 4.16.1–4.16.4**).

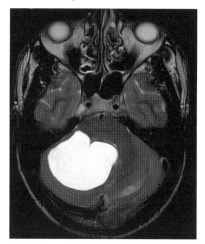

Fig. 4.16.1

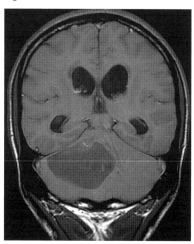

Fig. 4.16.2

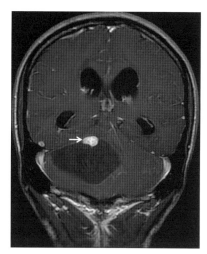

Fig. 4.16.3

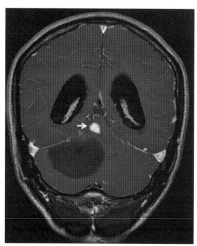

Fig. 4.16.4

Ideal Summary

These are axial T2-weighted and coronal T1-weighted
pre- and postcontrast MR images of the brain. There
is a large lesion centred on the right cerebellar hemisphere demonstrating fluid signal characteristics with
an avidly enhancing mural nodule in its superior
aspect (**Fig. 4.16.3**, arrow). Dilatation of the lateral
ventricles is present, in keeping with obstructive
hydrocephalus. A further enhancing nodule is seen

in the superior aspect of the vermis on the coronal
sequence (**Fig. 4.16.4**, arrow). The large cystic lesion
is typical of a haemangioblastoma. Given the age of
the patient and the multiplicity, this raises the possibility of von Hippel–Lindau (VHL) syndrome. Imaging
of the spine is suggested to exclude involvement. I
would suggest urgent neurosurgical referral in view
of the obstructive hydrocephalus.

This is the MRI of the cervicothoracic spine of the same
*patient (**Fig. 4.16.5**).*

This is a sagittal T1-weighted postcontrast image of
the upper spine. Multiple enhancing nodules are seen

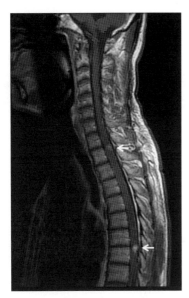

Fig. 4.16.5

along the spinal cord (**Fig. 4.16.5**, arrows). Overall, the features are consistent with VHL syndrome, with the cerebellar and spinal lesions likely representing haemangioblastomas. Further evaluation for other manifestations of VHL and genetic counseling in due course is also suggested.

Examination Tips

- The age of the patient is the most important clinical factor when faced with a cystic posterior fossa mass: pilocytic astrocytomas tend to occur in children and haemangioblastomas in adults, unless it is associated with VHL syndrome when they occur in younger adults.
- About two-thirds of haemangioblastomas have both cystic and solid components; the remainder can be entirely solid.
- If flow voids are seen on MR that are thought to represent feeding or draining vessels, this is highly suggestive of the diagnosis.
- While there may be enhancement of a thin uniform cyst wall, the presence of an irregularly thickened enhancing wall should raise the possibility of a more aggressive lesion, such as a metastasis or glioblastoma.
- Spinal haemangioblastomas are usually intramedullary and lie within the cervicothoracic spine. The imaging findings are those of cord expansion, an enhancing mass, and a dorsal draining vessel

that appear as flow voids. Commonly, there is an accompanying syrinx.

Differential Diagnosis

Cystic posterior fossa mass:
- Pilocytic astrocytoma:
  - The imaging appearance is similar, with a cystic mass and enhancing mural nodule, but unlike with haemangioblastomas, the nodule does not abut the pial surface, nor are there large vessels related to the enhancing nodule.
- Metastases:
  - These are the most common intra-axial posterior fossa mass in adults.
  - Usually solid rather than cystic and multiple.
- Arteriovenous malformation or cavernoma.
  - These can occasionally appear similar, but haemorrhage is rare in haemangioblastomas.
  - Multiple arteriovenous malformations can occur as part of a syndrome such as haemorrhagic hereditary telangiectasia.

Notes

VHL syndrome is an inherited, autosomal dominant syndrome that manifests clinically as benign and malignant tumours involving multiple organs. Although it is referred to as a neurocutaneous syndrome, there are no cutaneous manifestations:
- Central nervous system: haemangioblastomas of the brain and spine
- Retina: retinal angiomas
- Kidneys: clear cell renal carcinomas and renal cysts
- Adrenals: phaeochromocytomas (also extra-adrenal)
- Pancreas: serous cystadenomas, islet cell tumours, simple pancreatic cysts, rarely, adenocarcinomas

Around 25 to 40% of haemangioblastomas occur in association with VHL syndrome; the rest are solitary.

Patients with VHL syndrome require lifelong follow-up with screening, as those with one lesion are likely to develop others.

Surgical treatment is reserved for those lesions that are symptomatic or that show accelerated growth on follow-up, in an attempt to minimise intervention.

Bibliography

Leung RS, Biswas SV, Duncan M, Rankin S. Imaging features of von Hippel-Lindau disease. Radiographics 2008;28(1):65–79, quiz 323

4.17 Cerebellopontine Angle Mass

Clinical History

*A 38-year-old woman presents with progressive hearing loss and balance problems (**Figs. 4.17.1–4.17.4**).*

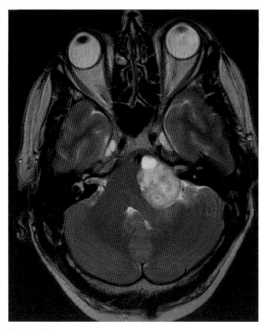

Fig. 4.17.1

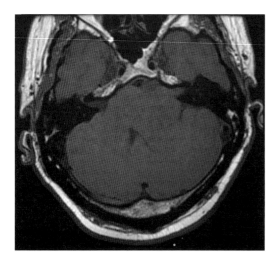

Fig. 4.17.2

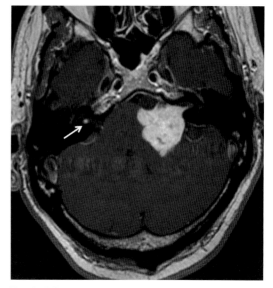

Fig. 4.17.3

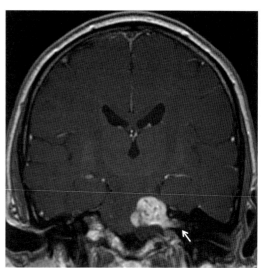

Fig. 4.17.4

Ideal Summary

These are axial T2-weighted, axial T1-weighted, and postcontrast axial and coronal T1-weighted images acquired at the level of the internal auditory meatus. There is a large heterogeneous mass centred on the left cerebellopontine angle. The mass is of T2 high and T1 intermediate signal, and it is avidly enhancing. A small fluid signal cyst is seen at the anterior aspect of the mass and does not enhance. On the coronal images, there is extension into the left intra-auditory meatus, which is expanded, with an "ice-cream cone" appearance (**Fig. 4.17.4**, arrow). There is a mass effect with distortion of the underlying middle cerebellar peduncle and partial effacement of the fourth ventricle. There is also a tiny enhancing nodule seen within the intra-auditory meatus on the right, which may represent an early similar lesion (**Fig. 4.17.3**, arrow). The imaging findings are in keeping with a vestibular schwannoma, and the presence of bilateral disease raises the possibility of neurofibromatosis type 2. I would compare with previous imaging to assess progression and recommend referral to a specialised neurosurgical unit (e.g., a neurofibromatosis clinic).

Examination Tips

- The finding of tumour extension into the intra-auditory meatus is highly suggestive of vestibular schwannoma as these represent over 90% of intracanalicular tumours, and intracanalicular meningiomas are very rare.
- Calcification is rare, but necrosis and cysts may be present in larger tumours.
- The appearance of these larger tumours is likened to an "ice-cream cone" with the intracanalicular part representing the cone, and the cerebellopontine angle component the ice-cream.
- Contrast enhancement is less helpful as both vestibular schwannoma and meningioma exhibit diffuse enhancement. Therefore, thin-section T2-weighted imaging will suffice for the detection of vestibular schwannoma, and contrast is not usually administered.

Differential Diagnosis

- Meningioma:
  - Calcification is present in 20 to 30%, resulting in low T2 signal intensity. Surrounding bone may show evidence of hyperostosis.

- It has a broad dural base making an obtuse angle with the petrous bone, and is usually eccentric to the internal acoustic meatus.
- Metastasis or lymphoma:
  - Lesions may also be bilateral, but they are more likely to feature leptomeningeal spread as opposed to a discrete mass.

Notes

- Vestibular schwannomas are also referred to as acoustic neuromas, acoustic schwannomas, or vestibular neurilemmomas.
- Bilateral vestibular schwannomas are one of the characteristic clinical features of neurofibromatosis type 2—an autosomal dominant disorder with lesions affecting the central nervous system, eyes (retinal hamartomas), and skin (schwannomas and plaques).
- The neurological manifestations can be summarised by the mnemonic MISME: multiple intracranial schwannomas, meningiomas, and ependymomas. Up to half of patients with neurofibromatosis type 2 have meningiomas, and although the incidence increases with age, neurofibromatosis type 2 should be considered when a meningioma is diagnosed in childhood.
- Of the spinal tumours, schwannomas with their characteristic "dumbbell" shape are the most common. Meningiomas tend to involve the extramedullary compartment while ependymomas are usually intramedullary.

Bibliography

Sriskandan N, Connor SE. The role of radiology in the diagnosis and management of vestibular schwannoma. Clin Radiol 2011;66(4):357–365

4.18 Neurocysticercosis

Clinical History

A 30-year-old patient was found fitting in bed (**Fig. 4.18.1**).

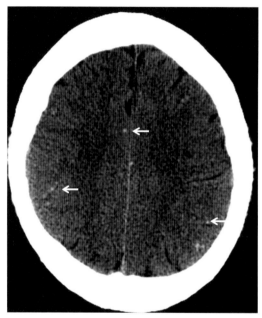

Fig. 4.18.1

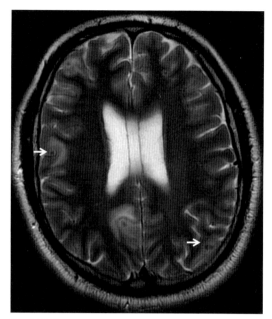

Fig. 4.18.2

Ideal Summary

This is a single noncontrast axial CT image through the brain. There are multiple tiny foci of calcification along the sulcal spaces over both cerebral convexities and parasagittal region (**Fig. 4.18.1**, arrows). I cannot see any signs of acute haemorrhage or a space-occupying lesion. The findings are nonspecific and may be related to previous infection or inflammation. I would like to review the remainder of the series and ask if any old images are available for comparison. I would take the case forward by arranging for an MRI.

These are MR images from the same patient (**Figs. 4.18.2** and **4.18.3**).

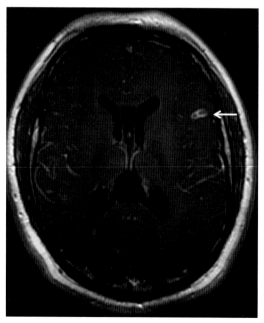

Fig. 4.18.3

These are axial T2-weighted and postcontrast T1-weighted MR sequences. On the T2-weighted image, there are multiple T2 hypointense lesions in a similar distribution to the CT (**Fig. 4.18.2**, arrows), with adjacent subcortical white matter T2 high signal change. The postcontrast image shows several possible enhancing lesions, one of which is ovoid in the left frontal lobe (**Fig. 4.18.3**, arrow). Low signal is seen within each of these lesions. I would like to compare this with the precontrast T1 sequence to confirm enhancement. The appearances are typical of neurocysticercosis, and the combination of the CT and MRI suggests these are lesions in different stages, both vesicular and calcified. I would suggest follow-up imaging following initiation of appropriate treatment to assess response.

Examination Tips

- Neurocysticercosis is most commonly found in the subarachnoid spaces of the convexities.
- T1-weighted and fluid-attenuated inversion recovery sequences may be helpful in the detection of intraventricular cysts.
- Gradient-echo sequences may be employed to identify a calcified scolex.
- Look for complications:
  - Hydrocephalus
  - Meningitis.

Differential Diagnosis

The appearances are typical of neurocysticercosis. The differential diagnosis would include fungal micro-abscess and tuberculosis.

Notes

- Neurocysticercosis is the most common parasitic infection of the CNS and is caused by the larval stage of the pork tapeworm *Taenia solium*. The most frequent clinical manifestations include seizures, focal neurological deficits, and headache.
- Imaging appearances vary according to the stage in the life cycle of the parasite. The live larvae appears as a hypodense cyst at the grey–white junction, with the scolex represented by an eccentric hyperdense nodule—"cyst with a dot." As the larvae die, there is formation of a granuloma, which causes breakdown of the blood–brain barrier, resulting in contrast enhancement and surrounding oedema. Finally, once the larvae are dead, the cysts and scolices appear as shrunken, densely calcified lesions.
- In 20 to 50% of patients, the lesion is solitary. When multiple, lesions are commonly seen at different stages in the same patient.
- MRI is more sensitive than CT, but CT is superior when demonstrating calcification. A reasonable approach is initially to investigate with a CT brain and serological tests. If the CT is inconclusive in the setting of high clinical suspicion, MRI may help identify small lesions and visualise the scolices. Identification of the scolex is the only pathognomonic radiological finding.
- There are characteristic plain radiographic findings of multiple, elongated, "cigar-shaped" calcifications in the skeletal muscles, and thus a radiograph of the soft tissues of the thigh can also confirm the diagnosis of intracranial neurocysticercosis.

Bibliography
Rahalkar MD, Shetty DD, Kelkar AB, Kelkar AA, Kinare AS, Ambardekar ST. The many faces of cysticercosis. Clin Radiol 2000;55(9):668–674

4.19 Spontaneous Intracranial Haemorrhage

Clinical History

A 55-year-old man was found unconscious (**Figs. 4.19.1** and **4.19.2**).

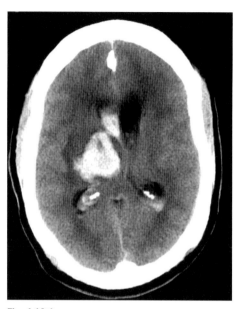

Fig. 4.19.1

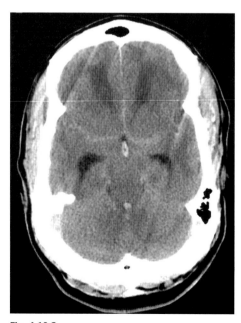

Fig. 4.19.2

Ideal Summary

These are axial unenhanced CT images through the brain. There is an area of high density centred on the right thalamus and lentiform nucleus, in keeping with acute haemorrhage. There is haemorrhagic extension into the lateral, third, and fourth ventricles and sub-arachnoid space, with associated hydrocephalus and some midline shift to the left. In addition, there is periventricular and deep white matter low attenuation most likely to represent transependymal inter-stitial oedema and almost complete effacement of the basal cisterns. The distribution of blood is typical of an acute hypertensive haemorrhage, and I would like to know if the patient is hypertensive. I would recommend an urgent neurosurgical referral in view of the intraventricular extension and hydrocephalus.

Examination Tips

- Hypertensive haemorrhage has a propensity for the areas of brain in close proximity to the higher vascular pressures of the circle of Willis, such as the basal ganglia, thalamus, pons, and cerebellum.
- Remember that patients under 45 years of age may harbour an underlying vascular lesion or venous thrombosis, and hypertension in a younger age group may be related to illicit drug use, for example of cocaine.
- Often the cause of a lobar haemorrhage is difficult to establish, and further imaging may be helpful if there is a clinical suspicion: MR for an underlying neoplasm or amyloid angiopathy; CT angiogram for the presence of an aneurysm.

Differential Diagnosis

- Amyloid angiopathy:
  - The patient is usually over the age of 65 years and normotensive
  - Predominantly lobar in distribution, parti-cularly in the parietal and occipital lobes and sparing the deep subcortical regions
  - Presence of T2 high signal in the white matter and microhaemorrhages on T2* gradient-echo imaging is suggestive of underlying amyloid angiopathy
  - Can coexist with hypertensive microangiopathy.

- Haemorrhagic transformation of an infarct:
  - Can be difficult to distinguish from primary intracerebral haemorrhage
  - An infarct is more likely if there is a wedge-shaped abnormality extending to the cortex or small area of hyperdensity within a larger low attenuation area.
- Arteriovenous malformation:
  - Multiple dilated veins and arteries separated by intervening brain tissue
  - MRI demonstrates multiple flow voids with serpentine contrast enhancement without significant brain parenchymal enhancement
  - Usually an incidental finding without preceding haemorrhage, but arteriovenous malformations do occur in the basal ganglia, and this can be difficult to distinguish.
- Venous infarction:
  - More commonly haemorrhagic than arterial infarction, and affects the white matter rather than the cortex
  - Sometimes, but not always, an adjacent thrombosed sinus can be seen.

- Haemorrhagic neoplasm:
  - Can be primary or secondary
  - Mixed signal intensities with enhancing components.

Notes

- Spontaneous intracranial haemorrhage is the second most common cause of stroke after ischaemic stroke and is usually hypertensive in aetiology in adults.
- On CT, hyperacute haematoma will appear of high density except in the context of severe anaemia.
- Over time, the density decreases, with the clot becoming isodense to brain over a period of weeks.

Bibliography

Dainer HM, Smirniotopoulos JG. Neuroimaging of hemorrhage and vascular malformations. Semin Neurol 2008; 28(4):533–547

4.20 Traumatic Brain Injury

Clinical History

A 20-year-old motorcyclist has been involved in a road traffic accident and has a Glasgow Coma Score of 3 (**Figs. 4.20.1–4.20.5**).

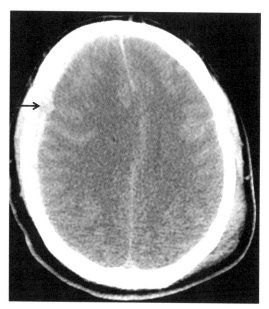

Fig. 4.20.1

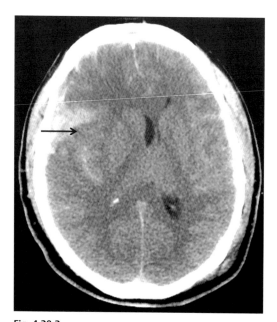

Fig. 4.20.2

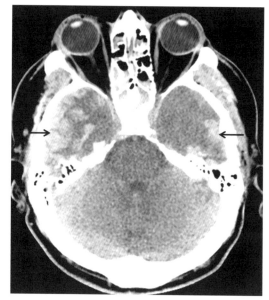

Fig. 4.20.3

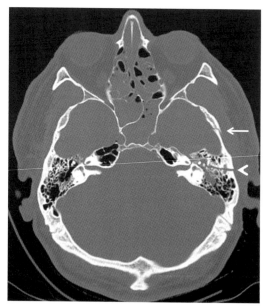

Fig. 4.20.4

Ideal Summary

These are unenhanced axial CT images on brain parenchymal and bony windows. There are extensive, bilateral, haemorrhagic contusions within the

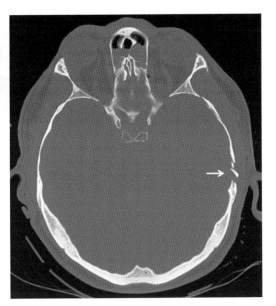

Fig. 4.20.5

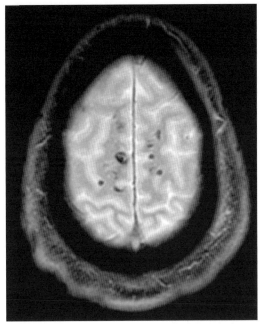

Fig. 4.20.6

temporal lobes (**Fig. 4.20.3**, arrows). In addition, there is a shallow acute subdural haematoma over-lying the right frontoparietal convexity (**Fig. 4.20.1**, arrow), with widespread subarachnoid blood. There is significant mass effect with midline shift to the left and effacement of the right lateral ventricle (**Fig. 4.20.2**, arrow). On review of the bony windows, there is a complex comminuted fracture through the left parietal bone that extends to involve the petrous temporal bone (**Figs. 4.20.4** and **4.20.5**, arrows). On closer inspection, there is apparent disruption of the left incudomalleal joint and haemotympanum (**Fig. 4.20.4**, arrowhead). There is high-density blood in the sinuses, and I would like to review the remaining images carefully for evidence of orbital fracture. The findings are in keeping with severe traumatic brain injury. In our institution, this pati-ent would be managed in a neurointensive unit with neurosurgical input.

These are MR images of a different patient who has been involved in a high-velocity road traffic accident (**Figs. 4.20.6** and **4.20.7**).

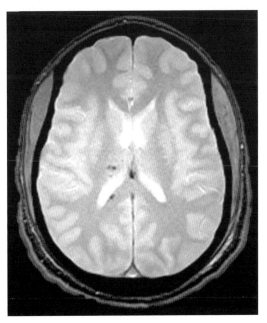

Fig. 4.20.7

These are selected gradient-echo sequences. The images show multiple foci of susceptibility involving the cortex, subcortical white matter, right thalamus, and splenium of the corpus callosum, in keeping with petechial haemorrhage. The distribution of haemorrhage is in keeping with shear or diffuse axo-nal injury.

Examination Tips

Traumatic brain injury may initially look daunting to a candidate who has little experience of this, but it can be easily broken down into a systematic description.

- Take your time and look at all of the available imaging. Do not be rushed into talking about the first thing that you notice and then altering your interpretation when something more important is evident.
- Describe each compartment of the head fully before moving onto the next section:
  - Brain parenchyma
  - Extra-axial compartment—subarachnoid and sub- and extradural layers
  - Bony skull
  - Soft tissue
    The order of the compartments is up to you; just make sure you are comfortable with each section before moving on.
- Comment on the primary abnormality and then the sequelae:
  - Intraparenchymal or extra-axial haemorrhage, which causes a mass effect (midline shift, and effacement of the ventricular system or basal cisterns)
  - Petrous temporal bone fractures, causing ossicular disruption.
- Remember the patterns of trauma:
  - Diffuse axonal injury = grey–white matter junction
  - Cerebral contusions = frontal and temporal lobes.
- Comment on complications:
  - Herniation—tonsillar, uncal, and subfalcine
  - Hydrocephalus
  - Possible ossicular disruption, cerebrospinal fluid (CSF) leak, and orbital entrapment.
- Always ask for imaging with bone windows if this has not already been provided; only comment on fractures when these images are available.
- Are there any abnormalities that require urgent intervention? If so, summarise and tell the examiner what you would recommend at your institution—usually neurosurgical referral.

Differential Diagnosis

There are no differentials for the above imaging findings in the context of trauma.

Notes

- CT is the mainstay of imaging in the assessment of head injury and is primarily used to identify patients who may require intervention, neurosurgical or otherwise.
- MRI may subsequently be employed to identify further lesions where the clinical–radiological image does not match, or to characterise unexplained abnormalities initially found on CT.
- Subarachnoid haemorrhage:
  - This is seen on CT as high density in the subarachnoid spaces.
  - On MRI, blood may be isointense with brain parenchyma, producing a "dirty" CSF picture.
  - Fluid-attenuated inversion recovery sequences are more sensitive than CT in the detection of small-volume subarachnoid blood.
- Cerebral contusions:
  - These occur in typical locations where the brain parenchyma lies adjacent to a "rough" bony surface or a dural fold.
  - Classic locations are the temporal lobes (temporal pole, inferior surface), frontal lobes (frontal pole, inferior surface), and parasagittal parenchyma.
  - Look for contusions underlying a skull fracture.
- Diffuse axonal injury:
  - The initial CT is normal in 50 to 80%.
  - Typical locations at the grey–white matter junction of the frontotemporal lobes, corpus callosum, and upper brainstem.
  - MRI is more sensitive than CT for the detection of lesions—gradient-echo imaging is the sequence of choice in many institutions.

Bibliography

Provenzale JM. Imaging of traumatic brain injury: a review of the recent medical literature. AJR Am J Roentgenol 2010;194(1):16–19

5 Introduction to Urogynaecological Imaging

Diana Bosanac and Dean Huang

The Specialty Training Curriculum for Clinical Imaging, published by the Royal College of Radiologists of the United Kingdom, sets out the skills required to undertake the practice of clinical imaging.[1] The syllabus provides an insight into the levels of expertise generally expected for success in any postgraduate imaging examination. Clinical conditions (and the imaging thereof) featured in the syllabus that are essential to any examination candidate's knowledge include haematuria, renal failure (acute or chronic), renovascular hypertension, lower urinary tract symptoms, a renal, pelvic, and scrotal mass or pain, dysmenorrhoea, infertility (male and female), and trauma to the kidneys and adrenal glands. Key skills expected include providing expert advice on appropriate imaging and interpretation of imaging findings.

To achieve these goals, a clear understanding of the specific imaging protocols used in urogynaecological imaging is essential. Over the past decade, important advances have been made in the imaging of urogynaecological conditions, with which the examination candidate should be acquainted. The examiner is very likely to show newer imaging techniques, as these are often of interest (mainly to the examiner!), but the classical imaging and established techniques should also be familiar to the candidate.

Some basic imaging principles in urogynaecological imaging are discussed below.

Renal Tract Imaging

CT is the key imaging modality used to evaluate the urinary tract, the "triple"-phase scan now being commonplace. A complete CT urogram can provide comprehensive evaluation of the urinary system for detecting renal calculi, renal masses, and urothelial abnormalities. Typically, the various phases of acquisition are defined as the nonenhanced, nephrographic, and urographic (or excretory) phases:

- Nonenhanced CT images play a role beyond defining the presence of renal calculi. In cases of high-attenuation renal cysts, it is often the nonenhanced study that aids recognition of these lesions. The nonenhanced study also provides

the baseline attenuation; a cyst does not enhance, and the attenuation should not increase by more than 10 to 20 HU.
- Nephrographic-phase imaging is often the "best" phase for characterising lesions (true cyst versus tumour) and detecting the smaller lesions. This is also the phase used for evaluating the renal vein and inferior vena cava.
- Urographic phase is "the" imaging sequence for diagnosing urothelial malignancies, congenital anomalies, calculi, and abnormalities of the collecting systems. Static assessment for any obstructive uropathy can also be made (a MAG3 renogram would be the modality of choice for functional assessment of obstructive uropathy).

When interpreting renal tract images, it is important to appreciate the strengths and limitations of the various phases of image acquisition. Examination candidates would be expected to understand the current applications of CT in the evaluation of renal abnormalities, including understanding the current role of imaging in the diagnosis and management of renal cell carcinoma and other solid renal lesions. In addition, candidates should be able to describe the various appearances of benign urinary tract abnormalities and transitional cell carcinoma of the upper and lower urinary tracts.

Adrenal Masses

Candidates should be able to describe the principles and adrenal applications of chemical shift MRI and optimised CT imaging protocols (for enhanced and washout ratio) used to differentiate between benign adrenal adenoma and other adnexal abnormalities.

The Retroperitoneum

Candidates should be confident in describing the anatomical boundaries of the retroperitoneum and pelvic extraperitoneal spaces. It is important to demonstrate ability in identifying the typical features of retroperitoneal fibrosis, and apply them to aid differentiation from malignancy.

Adnexal Abnormalities

The imaging evaluation of adnexal masses can pose a diagnostic challenge. Transvaginal ultrasonography (TVUS) remains the procedure of choice for the initial evaluation of adnexal masses. When findings on ultrasonography are indeterminate, further evaluation is performed with MRI, with excellent soft tissue differentiation and a high level of accuracy in the diagnosis of malignancy, especially when gadolinium-enhanced techniques are used. CT, with poor tissue discrimination, is of limited use in the interrogation of adnexal masses, except for lesions that contain fat and calcium. However, CT can be used to assess the extent of disease before and after treatment for ovarian malignancy.

Trauma

Candidates should be familiar with the elements of the trauma scale for grading renal parenchymal injuries. It is important to be able to distinguish the various types of bladder rupture, and recognise the implications and management of active haemorrhage from renal parenchymal injury.

Finally, there are many "classic signs" (or "Aunt Minnies") associated with a variety of pathological conditions in urogynaecological imaging.[2] When these "classic signs" are invoked, they may have specific diagnostic and pathological implications. Examination candidates should be familiar with these signs; they should also be confident in describing the pathophysiological characteristics associated with the radiological findings and, if appropriate, applying these classic signs across imaging modalities. These are the cases that need to be described in a faultless manner.

References

1. Royal College of Radiologists. Specialty Training Curriculum for Clinical Radiology. Update. 2012. http://www.rcr.ac.uk/content.aspx?PageID=1805 (accessed August 2012)
2. Dyer RB, Chen MY, Zagoria RJ. Classic signs in uroradiology. Radiographics 2004; 24(Suppl 1):S247–S280

5.1 Testicular Epidermoid Cyst

Clinical History

*An 18-year-old man presents with a painless lump in his left testis (**Figs. 5.1.1** and **5.1.2**).*

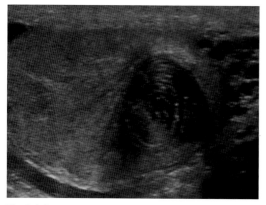

Fig. 5.1.1

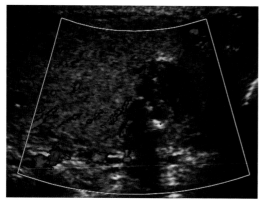

Fig. 5.1.2

Ideal Summary

These are B-mode and colour Doppler ultrasound images of a testis. There is a round, well-circumscribed focal intratesticular lesion with prominent alternating hypoechoic and hyperechoic rings, giving the lesion an "onion-skin" or "target" appearance. This lesion is completely confined within the testis and does not breech the tunica albuginea. No further focal intra- or extratesticular lesions are shown on the single image, and no features suggestive of testicular atrophy or microlithiasis are visible. A small left-sided varicocoele is present. The colour Doppler image study demonstrates no internal vascularity in the lesion. With no vascularity demonstrated within the lesion, the ultrasound appearances of this lesion would be most in keeping with an epidermoid cyst. I would complete the examination by scanning the contralateral testis. I would also recommend tumour marker screening and ultrasound follow-up.

Examination Tips

Remember that, in an adult patient, a focal intratesticular lesion on ultrasound should be managed as a malignant lesion until proven otherwise. A cautious approach is warranted. Look for and comment on:

- Vascularity of the lesion. The presence of vascularity usually indicates malignancy. Lack of vascularity is suggestive of benign disease (epidermoid cyst, haematoma, focal infarction, or abscess) if supported by the sonographic features and a relevant clinical history.
- Any background testicular abnormality. Specifically, look for testicular atrophy (increased risk of primary testicular malignancy) or the presence of microlithiasis (associated with an increased prevalence of testicular tumour).
- Focal testicular lesions with concentric "onion skin/target" appearances are characteristic of epidermoid cysts. However, these appearances are not pathognomonic, and comment should be made on the need for negative tumour markers to increase diagnostic confidence, and a follow-up ultrasound to demonstrate a lack of progression in the appearance.

Differential Diagnosis

- Testicular germ cell tumours. A teratoma may have internal echoes and poor vascularisation, and may mimic an epidermoid cyst.
- Testicular abscess. Look for features of epididymo-orchitis—enlargement of the testis with a vividly increased colour Doppler signal reflecting hypervascularity.

- Segmental testicular infarction. This may be wedge-shaped or round and demonstrate a lack of vascularity.
- Intratesticular haematoma. Look for a history of trauma. There will be a reduction in size on serial ultrasound examinations as the haematoma retracts.
- Rete testis. This may resemble a hyperechoic mass in a cross-sectional view, so scan in all planes.

Notes

- Histologically, epidermoid cysts are true cysts, filled with a cheesy, laminated material.
- In addition to the classic "onion skin" appearances, other appearances of epidermoid cysts have been described, including a densely calcified mass with an echogenic rim, or a cyst with a rim and either peripheral or central calcification.
- MRI: epidermoid cysts may appear as target lesions with a high T1 and T2 signal (cystic content), with low T1 and T2 signal fibrous capsules, and may contain low T1 and T2 signal calcified centres.
- Epidermoid cysts have no malignant potential, and treatment is usually with enucleation.
- Unnecessary orchiectomy could be avoided with accurate ultrasound evaluation in the absence of raised tumour markers.

Bibliography

Atchley JTM, Dewbury KC. Ultrasound appearances of testicular epidermoid cysts. Clin Radiol 2000;55(7): 493–502

5.2 Retroperitoneal Fibrosis

Clinical History

A 55-year-old woman presents with long-standing left-sided back and flank pain (**Figs. 5.2.1–5.2.3**).

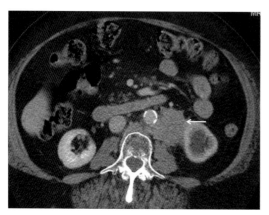

Fig. 5.2.1

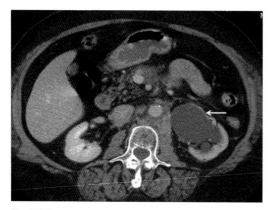

Fig. 5.2.2

Ideal Summary

These are selected venous- and urographic-phase CT images of the abdomen and pelvis in the axial and coronal planes. There is a left-sided, well-demarcated, but irregular para-aortic mass, which is isodense with surrounding muscle (**Fig. 5.2.1**, arrow). This is associated with left-sided pelvicalyceal dilatation without dilatation of the upper left ureter (**Fig. 5.2.2**, arrow). There is no contrast opacification of the left

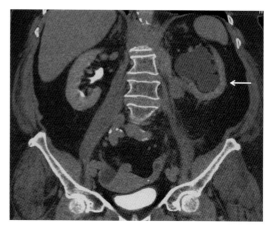

Fig. 5.2.3

renal collecting system on the urographic phase. In addition, there is global thinning of the left renal cortex, suggesting a chronic obstructive uropathy (**Fig. 5.2.3**, arrow). The aorta is encased by soft tissue, but is of normal calibre. There is no evidence of bone destruction. Mild mesenteric fat stranding and small-volume mesenteric lymph nodes are present, but no significant nodal enlargement is demonstrated elsewhere.

The differential diagnosis for this solid retroperitoneal mass includes retroperitoneal fibrosis, retroperitoneal nodal enlargement, and retroperitoneal haematoma. There are no convincing "aggressive" features to suggest malignancy. Given the likely long-standing nature of the left-sided renal obstruction, retroperitoneal fibrosis would be the most likely diagnosis. I would refer the patient to the urology team and recommend biochemical screening for acute renal deterioration and evidence of renal infection. This would determine the need for an urgent left-sided nephrostomy. I would also like to review any previous images that are available for comparison.

Examination Tips

- If shown a retroperitoneal mass, look for and comment on the location and morphology of the mass, and its effect on adjacent organs and bony and vascular structures.

Some features, although not entirely specific, have been described that may indicate underlying malignancy:

- A malignant retroperitoneal mass has a tendency to be bulkier, displaying a mass effect and displacing the aorta and inferior vena cava anteriorly from the spine and the ureters laterally. In contrast, the purely fibrotic process involved in retroperitoneal fibrosis results in "tethering" of these structures to the underlying vertebrae, with the classic "maiden waist deformity," with medial deviation of the middle third of the ureters.
- The presence of malignancy may result in a mass with peripheral nodularity and lobulation, whereas benign retroperitoneal fibrosis has a tendency to manifest as a plaque-like mass without peripheral changes.
- Osseous involvement may occur secondary to underlying malignancy. Benign retroperitoneal fibrosis is not known to produce local bone destruction.
- Enhancement (pre- and postcontrast images are required): both a malignant mass and retroperitoneal fibrosis can demonstrate enhancement. Retroperitoneal fibrosis is known to enhance to varying amounts depending on the degree of inflammation. If no enhancement is demonstrated, the possibility of a retroperitoneal haematoma or fluid collection should be raised.

Comment on any ancillary features that may allude to the underlying causes of retroperitoneal fibrosis or to the differential diagnosis for the appearances, such as abdominal aortic aneurysm with periaortic haematoma inflammation relating to pancreatitis or mesenteric lymphadenopathy, bowel strictures or wall thickening relating to Crohn's disease, and features of pulmonary tuberculosis.

Differential Diagnosis

Although the diagnosis of retroperitoneal fibrosis may be established on the basis of the clinical history and radiological observations, in some cases the diagnosis may only be established on histology. Other conditions to be considered include:

- Tumours: lymphoma, sarcomas, pancreatic malignancies, and metastatic disease
- Other causes of ureteric obstruction, for example, pelvic surgery and radiation therapy
- Retroperitoneal abscess
- Aortic aneurysm or periaortic haematoma

Notes

Causes of retroperitoneal fibrosis include:

- Idiopathic
- Secondary:
  - Desmoplastic reaction to malignancy
  - Drugs
  - Haemorrhage (post-trauma, abdominal aortic aneurysm)
  - Inflammatory conditions (Crohn's disease, diverticulitis, pancreatitis)
  - Infection (tuberculosis, histoplasmosis, actinomycosis, urinary tract infections)
  - Postradiotherapy
  - Amyloid

Bibliography

Cronin CG, Lohan DG, Blake MA, Roche C, McCarthy P, Murphy JM. Retroperitoneal fibrosis: a review of clinical features and imaging findings. AJR Am J Roentgenol 2008;191(2):423–431

5.3 Renal Papillary Necrosis

Clinical History

*A 28-year-old woman presents with abdominal pain and haematuria (**Fig. 5.3.1**).*

Ideal Summary

This is a post-micturition radiograph from an intravenous urogram series. There are poorly defined calyces adjacent to multiple contrast-filled papillary cavities bilaterally. In addition, there is evidence of calyceal widening, most marked in the right upper polar region, giving an "egg-in-cup" appearance. The ureters are of normal calibre. On review of the bones, there are no features to suggest sickle cell disease, or any evidence of underlying arthropathy. I would like to complete my evaluation by reviewing the control radiograph of this intravenous urogram series to look for renal calcification. The urographic appearances

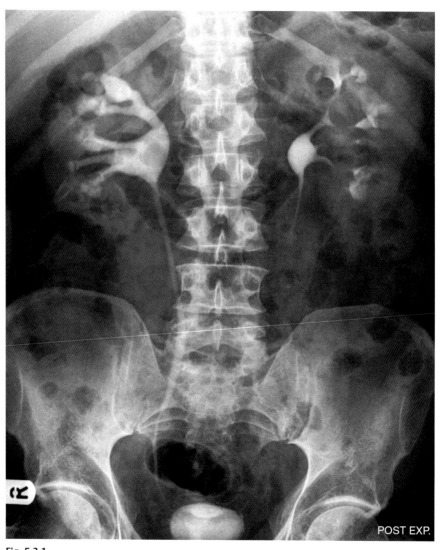

Fig. 5.3.1

are in keeping with renal papillary necrosis. No ancillary signs are present to indicate the underlying cause for these appearances.

Examination Tips

The following descriptive terms are often used referring to the radiographic patterns of papillary excavation seen with papillary necrosis:

- "Lobster claw." This calyceal deformity is produced when contrast fills the papillary excavation, resulting from necrosis, extending from the calyceal fornices.
- "Egg-in-cup." This term describes the appearance where contrast material fills central excavations in the papillae, reflecting shrinkage and sloughing of the papillae with forniceal widening and calyceal clubbing.
- "Signet ring." The necrotic papillary tip may remain within the excavated calyx. On the intravenous urogram, there is contrast filling of the papillary excavation and calyx surrounding a central filling defect caused by a necrotic papilla.

Differential Diagnosis

- Pelvocalyceal diverticula. Similar to the cavities in papillary necrosis, pelvocalyceal diverticula may manifest as contrast material-filled fluid collections adjacent to the calyces. However, these two entities can be distinguished on the basis of location: pelvocalyceal diverticula are not found in papillae, but adjacent to the calyceal fornices, infundibulum, or renal pelvis.

- Pyelotubular backflow. Retrograde flow of contrast out of the collecting system into the papillary ducts. This may appear as a striated area or blush extending from a calyx. The sharp calyceal margin is preserved, and this is usually considered a normal phenomenon.

Notes

- In renal papillary necrosis, there is ischaemic necrosis of the medulla secondary to either interstitial nephritis or vascular obstruction.
- Papillary necrosis is often associated with factors described by the mnemonic NSAIDs: nonsteroidal anti-inflammatory drugs, sickle cell anaemia, analgesic nephropathy, infection (especially tuberculosis), and diabetes mellitus. Look for and comment on features that may allude to these underlying causes:
  - Sickle cell disease: gallstones or cholecystectomy clips, skeletal manifestations, or lack of a splenic silhouette
  - Features suggestive of long-term analgesia use, such as severe arthropathy in the hip joints
  - Renal calcification: calcification of necrotic papillae being more common in patients with analgesic nephropathy than in those with other causes.

Bibliography

Jung DC, Kim SH, Jung SI, Hwang SI, Kim SH. Renal papillary necrosis: review and comparison of findings at multidetector row CT and intravenous urography. Radiographics 2006;26(6):1827–1836

5.4 Ureterocoele

Clinical History

A 44-year-old patient presents with right-sided flank pain (**Fig. 5.4.1**).

Ideal Summary

This is a post-micturition image from an intravenous urogram series. There is dilatation of the right pelvicalyceal system, with marked bulbous dilatation of the distal right ureter with a surrounding radiolucent halo, seen within the contrast-filled bladder. No filling defects are seen within the distal right ureter, and the surrounding lucent halo is well defined. There is delayed contrast clearance from the right renal collecting system relative to the left. The left renal collecting system decompresses normally, but the distal left ureter appears prominent. There is no evidence of a duplex collecting system on the right or on the left. The "cobra head" appearance of the right distal ureter is consistent with the diagnosis of a large, right-sided ureterocoele. This is complicated by a right-sided obstructive uropathy and a possible further small, uncomplicated ureterocoele on the left. In my routine practice, I would like to

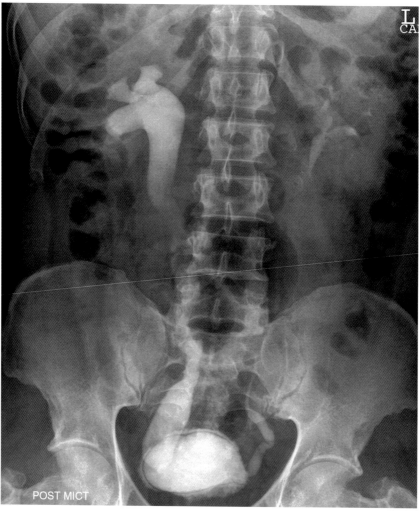

Fig. 5.4.1

review the control film and the remainder of the series.

Examination Tips

- The "cobra head" sign, when present, allows the diagnosis of an ureterocoele. This sign refers to dilatation of the distal ureter surrounded by a thin lucent line. The lucent hood represents the combined thickness of the ureteral wall and prolapsed bladder mucosa, outlined by contrast material within the bladder lumen.
- When large, ureterocoeles can cause obstruction of the bladder neck, along with obstruction of either the ipsilateral or contralateral ureter.
- Ectopic ureterocoeles are found in association with duplex ureters, and almost always arise from the upper pole ureter.
- The control radiograph and rest of the series should be assessed before completing the evaluation of any intravenous urogram series as ureterocoeles can be complicated by stone formation within the dilated distal ureters.

Differential Diagnosis

"Pseudo-ureterocoele" should be considered with any thickening, irregularity, loss of definition of the lucent line surrounding the dilated distal ureter, or filling defects within the ureterocoele. A pseudo-ureterocoele can result from oedema related to stone impaction, recent stone passage, or, more importantly, urothelial tumour. If the appearance is not convincing for an ureterocoele, cystoscopic evaluation should be performed.

Notes

- Ureterocoeles are classified as either intravesical or ectopic:
  - An intravesical, also termed orthotopic, ureterocoele arises from a ureter with a normal insertion into the trigone.
  - An ectopic ureterocoele lies in the submucosa of the bladder, and some part of it may extend into the bladder neck or urethra.
- Ectopic ureterocoeles are almost always seen in association with duplex ureters and arise from the upper pole ureter.
- Ultrasound may demonstrate the wall of the ureterocoele projecting into the lumen of the bladder.

Bibliography

Chavhan GB. The cobra head sign. Radiology 2002;225(3): 781–782

5.5 Ureteric Calculus

Clinical History

*A 54-year-old man presents with acute-onset right loin-to-groin pain and haematuria (**Figs. 5.5.1** and **5.5.2**).*

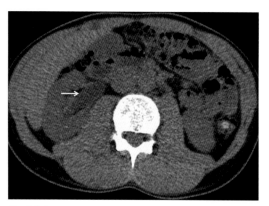

Fig. 5.5.1

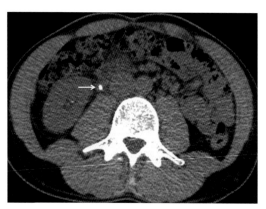

Fig. 5.5.2

Ideal Summary

These are selected axial images from an unenhanced CT of the abdomen. There is right-sided hydronephrosis (**Fig. 5.5.1**, arrow). I can see a small calculus within the right proximal ureter with ureteric wall thickening and periureteric stranding (**Fig. 5.5.2**, arrow). The appearances are in keeping with an obstructive uropathy secondary to a small right proximal

ureteric stone. In my routine practice, I would complete my assessment by reviewing the entire CT study in soft tissue, bony, and lung parenchymal window settings, and to exclude any further abnormality that may account for the patient's clinical symptoms. I would also like to ask if there are any markers of infection, which may necessitate decompressing the dilated right-sided collecting system with a nephrostomy.

Examination Tips

There are several well-recognised CT signs of urolithiasis. In addition to the detection of a high-attenuation calculus, look for:

- The "soft tissue rim sign." This is caused by oedema of the ureteral wall surrounding a calculus at its site of impaction. This may help distinguish a calculus in the ureter from a phlebolith in an adjacent vein.
  - It should be noted, however, that the soft tissue rim sign may be absent with large calculi or when a calculus is impacted at the vesicoureteric junction.
- The presence of hydronephrosis or hydroureter
- Asymmetric perinephric stranding
- Renal enlargement
- Reduced renal contrast enhancement as a consequence of delayed arrival of contrast
- The "comet sign." This may aid in the differentiation of a phlebolith from a calculus in the ureter. The phlebolith represents the "comet" nucleus and the adjacent tapering; the noncalcified portion of the vein is the comet tail.

Differential Diagnosis

No differential diagnoses should be offered for the above imaging appearances.

Notes

- Renal calculi are common. If a person experiences acute flank pain, they have a 67 to 95% chance of having a renal stone.
- If a calculus is less than 4 mm, there is an 80% chance that it will pass spontaneously.

- Nephrostomy or urological intervention is indicated if obstruction is present in a solitary or infected pelvicalyceal system, or a calculus is too large to pass or is not passing despite conservative management.
- Complications of urinary tract calculus disease include:
  - Abscess formation or urosepsis
  - Diminished renal function secondary to infection or long-standing obstruction

- Urinary fistula formation
- Ureteral scarring, stenosis, or perforation.

Bibliography

Heidenreich A, Desgrandschamps F, Terrier F. Modern approach of diagnosis and management of acute flank pain: review of all imaging modalities. Eur Urol 2002; 41(4):351–362

5.6 Xanthogranulomatous Pyelonephritis

Clinical History

*A 45-year-old woman presents with a 2-month history of progressive flank pain (**Fig. 5.6.1**).*

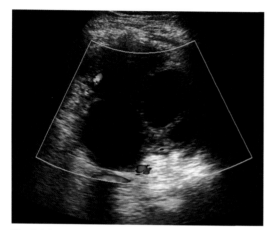

Fig. 5.6.1

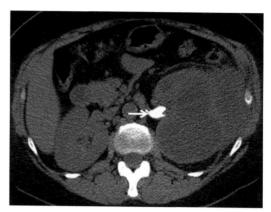

Fig. 5.6.2

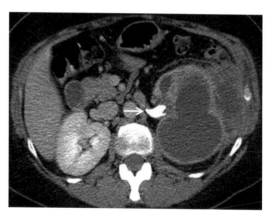

Fig. 5.6.3

Ideal Summary

This is a single ultrasound image of the left kidney with a colour Doppler overlay. There are multiple hypoechoic masses seen within the left kidney, with only residual normal renal parenchyma or cortex. The appearances are those of a multicystic abnormality, indistinguishable from long-standing renal obstruction. The common causes of this appearance beside long-standing renal obstruction include a multicystic renal neoplasm and xanthogranulomatous pyelonephritis. In view of the extent of this abnormality on the ultrasound examination, and to ascertain involvement of the surrounding structures, I would take this further by recommending a pre- and postcontrast enhanced CT examination of the abdomen.

*These are CT images from the same patient (**Figs. 5.6.2** and **5.6.3**).*

These are pre- and postcontrast axial CT images through the kidneys. These images demonstrate evidence of replacement of the renal parenchyma by low-attenuation fluid collections, which exhibit marginal enhancement. A central area of calcification,

likely a "stag-horn" renal calculus (**Figs. 5.6.2** and **5.6.3**, arrows), is seen within a contracted renal pelvis. Gerota's fascia on the left is thickened. An irregular perirenal fluid collection is well demonstrated lateral to the kidney, representing extrarenal spread of the process. The most likely diagnosis is xanthogranulomatous pyelonephritis, and I would like to review a delayed-phase CT and/or a nuclear medicine study to evaluate the function of the left kidney.

*These are nuclear medicine study images from the same patient (**Fig. 5.6.4**).*

This is a MAG3 renogram demonstrating good tracer uptake by the right kidney, which handles the tracer normally and contributes 98% to the divided function. There is virtually no uptake on the left.

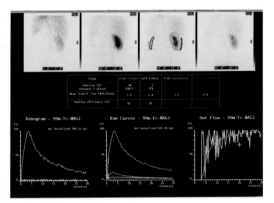

Fig. 5.6.4

This confirms a nonfunctioning left kidney as a consequence of the underlying xanthogranulomatous pyelonephritis. I would recommend urology referral.

Examination Tips

It may be difficult to determine the origin of a large mass in a renal or suprarenal location, particularly on ultrasound. If imaging features are not typical for a renal-based abnormality, consider an adrenal or retroperitoneal origin.

- The classic triad of CT features of xanthogranulomatous pyelonephritis are:
  - An enlarged, nonfunctioning kidney
  - Replacement of the renal parenchyma by hypoattenuating fluid collections arranged in a "bear's paw" pattern, which replaces the normal renal parenchyma
  - A centrally placed calculus. This is present in most, but not all, cases.
- Complex renal masses should be evaluated with at least a dual-phase (pre- and postcontrast) CT:
  - Precontrast scans will demonstrate calculi and provide a baseline for determining enhancement.
  - Postcontrast (nephrographic-phase) images allow evaluation of the degree of enhancement

of renal abnormalities. This also allows for evaluation of the remaining abdomen for the extent of local invasion by the lesion, and any distant lesions if malignancy is present.
- In some cases, additional delayed (urographic) phase images are useful to assess the renal pelvicalyceal systems for function and obstruction and to distinguish paracalyceal cysts from hydronephrosis.

Differential Diagnosis

- Multicystic renal cell carcinoma (lymph nodes, vascular invasion, and distant metastatic deposits)
- Renal tuberculosis (may be suggested by lung upper lobe fibrosis and calcified nodules)
- Renal abscess

Notes

- Xanthogranulomatous pyelonephritis is a chronic destructive granulomatous process that is a consequence of an incomplete immune response to subacute bacterial infection.
- Patients have no specific risk factors, although diabetes mellitus is present in 10%.
- The most common causal organisms are *Proteus mirabilis* and *Escherichia coli.*
- The renal parenchyma is normally diffusely involved, but focal extension into the perirenal fat is commonly seen.
- Although the focal form may be indistinguishable from a renal cell carcinoma, the more commonly seen diffuse process has characteristic imaging features detailed above.
- The presence of gas is rare.

Bibliography

Craig WD, Wagner BJ, Travis MD. Pyelonephritis: radiologic-pathologic review. Radiographics 2008;28(1):255–277, quiz 327–328

5.7 Emphysematous Pyelonephritis

Clinical History

A 58-year-old woman presents with left flank pain and fever (**Figs. 5.7.1** and **5.7.2**).

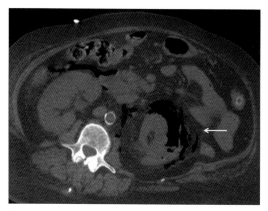

Fig. 5.7.1

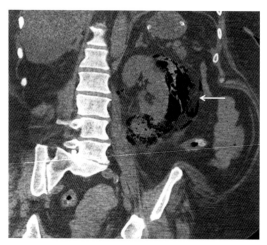

Fig. 5.7.2

Ideal Summary

These are selected unenhanced axial and coronal CT images. There is extensive free gas in the left retroperitoneal region, predominantly anterolateral to the left kidney (**Figs. 5.7.1** and **5.7.2**, arrows). The contour of the left kidney is distorted. There is an associated fluid collection along the posterior border of the left kidney, with associated minor perinephric stranding, mainly along the medial border of the left kidney. I can see further free gas in the left para-aortic region and also anterior to the right kidney. The appearances would be compatible with a diagnosis of left-sided emphysematous pyelonephritis. I would like to review the remainder of the series. If this is not available, I would perform enhanced CT imaging to demonstrate any asymmetrical renal enhancement, which may represent areas of necrosis or abscess formation. This is a surgical emergency, and urology referral is indicated.

Examination Tips

- CT is the investigation of choice for the evaluation of emphysematous pyelonephritis.
- CT findings include:
  - Enlargement and destruction of the renal parenchyma
  - Streaky or mottled gas collections, or bubbly/loculated gas within the parenchyma or collecting system
  - Fluid collections often surrounding the kidney
  - Gas–fluid levels when infection is extensive
  - Focal tissue necrosis with or without abscess formation.
- When presented with a case, look for and comment on potential risk factors for pyelonephritis including:
  - Renal calculi
  - A thick-walled bladder suggestive of outflow obstruction
  - Prostatic hypertrophy.
- Always ask if the patient has diabetes mellitus.

Differential Diagnosis

- Retroperitoneal gas:
  - Duodenal perforation: look for duodenal wall thickening and a possible defect adjacent to the pocket of free gas. The free gas may become distant from the perforation with time
  - Emphysematous pancreatitis
  - Retroperitoneal abscess with gas-forming organisms (e.g., psoas abscesses)

- Colonic or cutaneous fistula into a retroperitoneal collection
- Recent history of penetrating trauma or retroperitoneal surgery

Notes

- Emphysematous pyelonephritis is a life-threatening necrotising infection of the kidneys characterised by gas formation within or surrounding the kidneys.
- The majority of patients have poorly controlled diabetes mellitus. Other predisposing factors are an immunocompromised state and underlying malignancy.
- Conventional radiography may demonstrate gas bubbles overlying the renal fossa, or a diffusely mottled kidney with radially oriented gas corresponding to the renal pyramids. In addition, renal calculi may be identified with an abdominal radiograph.
- Intravenous urography may demonstrate a persistent, striated nephrogram on the affected side secondary to delayed excretion of contrast. The ipsilateral psoas shadow may be obscured. There may be evidence of an obstructive uropathy, with a dilated pelvicalyceal system.

- Ultrasound may demonstrate an enlarged kidney with nondependent hyperechoic shadowing, often with low-level posterior "dirty" acoustic shadowing, within the renal parenchyma or collecting system. Areas of hypoperfusion may be identified on colour Doppler ultrasound.
- *Escherichia coli* is the causative bacterial source in approximately 70% of cases, with *Klebsiella*, *Candida*, and *Pseudomonas* species isolated less frequently.
- Possible nonsurgical management options for emphysematous pyelonephritis include:
  - Aggressive intravenous antimicrobial therapy
  - Treatment of any renal tract obstruction
  - Surgical or CT-guided percutaneous drainage.
- Patients with a fulminant clinical course, unsuccessful drainage, and failed conservative therapy often require nephrectomy.

Bibliography

Craig WD, Wagner BJ, Travis MD. Pyelonephritis: radiologic-pathologic review. Radiographics 2008; 28(1):255–277, quiz 327–328

Grayson DE, Abbott RM, Levy AD, Sherman PM. Emphysematous infections of the abdomen and pelvis: a pictorial review. Radiographics 2002; 22(3):543–561

5.8   Testicular Microlithiasis

Clinical History

A 26-year-old man presents with dull scrotal pain (**Fig. 5.8.1**).

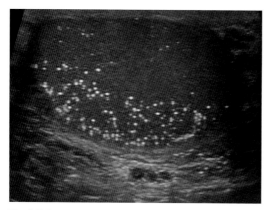

Fig. 5.8.1

Ideal Summary

This is a single ultrasound image of a testis. There are numerous small hyperechoic foci throughout the testis without evidence of posterior acoustic shadowing. These hyperechoic foci do not cause distortion of the testicular parenchyma, there is no testicular atrophy, and there are no focal hypoechoic intratesticular lesions. The appearances are in keeping with testicular microlithiasis (TM). No testicular tumour is demonstrated on this single view. In my normal practice, I would complete the ultrasound investigation by examining the contralateral testis to document any other abnormalities. There is an increased prevalence of primary testicular tumours with TM, and I would recommend urology review and follow-up.

Examination Tips

- ⊙ Testicular microlithiasis has characteristic ultrasound findings of:
  - Multiple high reflectivity foci with no acoustic shadowing
  - Foci measuring 1 to 3 mm
  - Random scattering throughout the testicular parenchyma

- "Classical" TM is described as more than five microliths per ultrasound field, and "limited" TM as less than five microliths per ultrasound field.
- ⊙ When evaluating testicular calcification, look for and comment on:
  - The morphology of the calcifications: micro- or macrocalcification, diffuse or clustered
  - Additional abnormalities: focal hypoechoic lesions or testicular atrophy
  - Whether it is unilateral or bilateral: assess the contralateral testis.

Differential Diagnosis

No differential diagnosis should be put forward for the above case, which is a classic example of TM. However, the finding of focal testicular calcification should alert you to the following as possible causes:
- ⊙ Testicular tumour:
  - The calcification associated with a germ cell tumour is more focal and irregular, and is seen in association with a hypo- or hyperechoic mass.
  - Embryonal and mixed germ cell tumours and teratomas are more likely to calcify.
  - Some benign tumours, such as epidermoid cysts, may also contain central or rim calcifications.
- ⊙ Macrocalcification:
  - If a large calcified focus with posterior acoustic shadowing is present, consider a "burnt-out" testicular tumour. Cases of testicular retroperitoneal metastatic disease with testicular macrocalcification and absence of a testicular tumour have been reported.
- ⊙ Testicular infarction:
  - The area of infarction is avascular and more commonly peripheral or wedge-shaped, and the calcification is often linear.
- ⊙ Granulomatous diseases:
  - May demonstrate multiple hypoechoic lesions with or without coarse macrocalcification. Evidence of granulomatous disease in other organs would confirm the diagnosis.

Notes

- ⊙ Testicular microlithiasis is usually discovered incidentally on ultrasound.

- There are several reported associations with TM, including cryptorchidism, infertility, testicular torsion, Klinefelter's syndrome, pulmonary alveolar microlithiasis, neurofibromatosis, AIDS, and primary testicular tumours.
- The association between TM and testicular tumour has been proposed based on several studies showing that the *prevalence* of testicular tumour is higher in patients with TM. However, many of these patients had other risk factors for tumour development, and several long-term follow-up studies since have not shown a definite causative association. As a result, it is unclear whether TM predisposes to the later development of testicular tumours. Currently, many institutions advise follow-up, especially in those with other risk factors.

Bibliography

Miller FN, Sidhu PS. Testicular microlithiasis: does it really matter? Clin Radiol 2002;57:883–890

Miller FN, Rosairo S, Clarke JL, Sriprasad S, Muir GH, Sidhu PS. Testicular calcification and microlithiasis: association with primary intra-testicular malignancy in 3,477 patients. Eur Radiol 2007;17(2):363–369

5.9 Testicular Tumour

Clinical History

*A 31-year-old man presents with a painless lump in his testis (**Figs. 5.9.1** and **5.9.2**).*

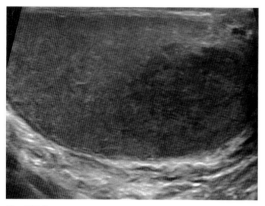

Fig. 5.9.1

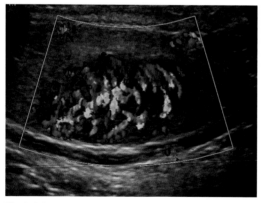

Fig. 5.9.2

Ideal Summary

These are B-mode and colour Doppler ultrasound images of a testis. There is a heterogeneous, but predominantly hypoechoic, intratesticular mass. This abuts, but does not appear to breach, the tunica albuginea. No calcification is seen within the lesion. There are no other masses on the given view. The colour Doppler ultrasound image demonstrates an increase in colour Doppler signal in comparison to the background testis, indicating that this is a vascular abnormality. The presence of internal vascularity within the lesion combined with the B-mode appearances would indicate a testicular malignancy. I would complete the examination by scanning the contralateral testis. I would recommend urgent referral to the urology multidisciplinary cancer meeting. Further imaging with a staging CT should be performed for treatment planning.

Examination Tips

Whenever an intratesticular mass is encountered, a primary testicular tumour must be considered malignant until proven otherwise. Look for and comment on:

- The presence of vascularity within the lesion. Lack of vascularity within the lesion suggests a benign cause, such as a segmental infarction, haematoma, abscess, or an epidermoid cyst.
- Although the ultrasound appearances of testicular tumours are variable, certain features may predict tumour type:
  - Seminomatous lesions are more commonly seen as a solid uniform mass of low reflectivity, with no foci of calcification.
  - Mixed germ cell tumours (nonseminomatous) are often seen as complex cystic masses with heterogeneous echogenicity and calcification.
- Any background testicular abnormality, such as testicular atrophy or the presence of microlithiasis, should be commented on, as these are risk factors for tumour development.

Differential Diagnosis

The following entities may present as focal testicular lesions. However, no vascularity should be demonstrated within the lesion:

- Testicular abscess (look for features of epididymo-orchitis)
- Segmental testicular infarction (may be wedge-shaped or round)
- Intratesticular haematoma (history of trauma, with a reduction in size as the haematoma retracts over time)

Notes

There are a variety of testicular tumours:

- Germ cell primary tumours
  - These account for the majority of testicular neoplasms. They are almost uniformly malignant.
  - Seminoma is the most common pure germ cell tumour and occurs in an older population.
  - Of the nonseminomatous germ cell tumours, mixed germ cell tumours are much more common than any of the pure histological forms.
- Non-germ cell primary tumours of the testis derive from the sex cords (Sertoli cells) and stroma (Leydig cells). These tumours are interstitial cell tumours, and 90% of non-germ cell tumours are benign.
- Non-primary tumours
  - Lymphoma, leukaemia, and metastasis can all manifest in the form of a testicular mass.

- Testicular lymphoma is the most common testicular neoplasm in men aged over 60 years.
- Metastases to the testes, which are rarely the presenting complaint, are most commonly seen in widespread prostate and lung malignancy.

Primary testicular tumours spread to para-aortic and left pararenal regions, liver, and lungs via lymphatic and haematogenous routes. A full staging CT is required for treatment planning. Serum tumour markers must always be obtained before treatment, so that if any are elevated this may be used as an indirect marker of tumour response to treatment.

Bibliography
Woodward PJ, Sohaey R, O'Donoghue MJ, Green DE. From the archives of the AFIP: tumors and tumorlike lesions of the testis: radiologic-pathologic correlation. Radiographics 2002;22(1):189–216

5.10 Horseshoe Kidney

Clinical History

A 40-year-old woman presents with increasing central and lower abdominal pain (**Figs. 5.10.1– 5.10.3**).

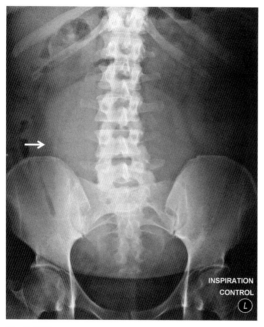

Fig. 5.10.1

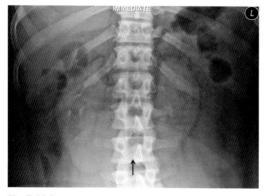

Fig. 5.10.2

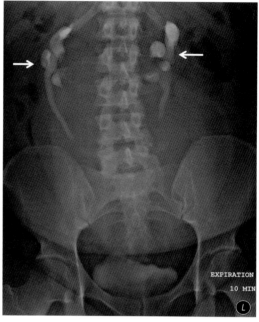

Fig. 5.10.3

Ideal Summary

These are selected images from an intravenous urogram series. On the control radiograph, there is a large, homogeneous, round, soft tissue opacity that appears to arise from the pelvis (**Fig. 5.10.1**, arrow). On the nephrogram phase of the urogram, the lower poles of the kidneys are fused across the midline (**Fig. 5.10.2**, arrow). This is suggestive of a horseshoe kidney. The 10-minute, full-length radiograph demonstrates malrotated collecting systems on both sides (**Fig. 5.10.3**, arrows). There appears to be calyceal clubbing, and the upper ureters are prominent. The bowel loops are displaced from the centre of the abdomen, but no dilated bowel loops are seen. There are no bony abnormalities. Overall, the appearances are in keeping with a renal fusion anomaly, likely a horseshoe kidney. The most likely differential for the abdominal mass is a fibroid uterus, although malignancy should be considered. This is causing some partial obstruction to the renal collecting system. I would like to check the patient's renal function and recommend cross-sectional imaging with CT or MRI to further characterise both the kidneys and abdominal mass.

Examination Tips

For the purpose of diagnosis of renal fusion anomalies, an intravenous urogram is usually the first-line investigation. Look for and comment on:

- Types of renal fusion anomaly:
  - "Horseshoe": fusion of the lower renal poles, which produces an isthmus (fused portion) of tissue crossing the midline. The axis of the kidneys is tilted such that the upper poles are lateral relative to the lower poles, and the lower pole calyces lie medial to the ureters.
  - "Crossed-fused ectopia" kidneys: one of the kidneys is abnormally sited to the contralateral side and is fused to the opposing kidney. The ureter of the ectopic kidney crosses the midline to enter the bladder in its normal position.
  - The "disc (pancake)" or "doughnut" kidney: fusion of both the upper and the lower poles.
- Complications relating to renal fusion anomalies include:
  - Varying degrees of obstruction of the renal moieties
  - An increased prevalence of stone formation
  - Infection.
- Features suggestive of associated congenital anomalies, for example, abnormal vertebral bodies
- As with all evaluations of intravenous urograms, do not forget to comment on any additional abnormalities observed outside the urinary track (in this case, a large pelvic mass).

Differential Diagnoses

- Purely from the nomenclature point of view: crossed-fused ectopia and other types of fusion anomalies; that is, not all fusion anomalies are "horseshoe" kidneys.
- On ultrasound, care must be taken to not mistake a horseshoe kidney for a midline retroperitoneal mass.

Notes

- "Horseshoe" describes the shape of the most common congenital renal fusion anomaly.
- Unless aware of the typical appearances of a horseshoe kidney, the abnormally rotated and inferiorly located kidney results in poor visualisation of the inferior pole and underestimation of the length of the kidney.
- Both CT and MRI demonstrate renal tissue of normal appearance but with an abnormal configuration.
- CT angiography imaging with three-dimensional reconstruction may demonstrate the vascular and collecting system anatomy for presurgical planning.
- Nuclear medicine imaging may demonstrate whether the isthmus contains functioning tissue.

Bibliography

Dyer RB, Chen MY, Zagoria RJ. Classic signs in uroradiology. Radiographics 2004;24(Suppl 1):S247–S280

5.11 Prostatic Tuberculosis

Clinical History

A 68-year-old man presents with low-grade fever, pelvic pain, and severe dysuria (Fig. 5.11.1).

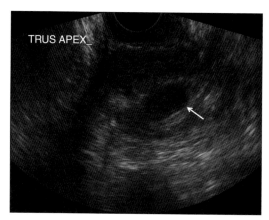

Fig. 5.11.1

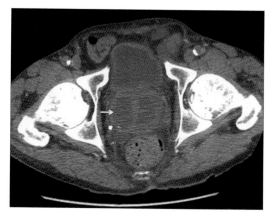

Fig. 5.11.2

Ideal Summary

This is a single B-mode transrectal ultrasound image of the prostate. There is a well-defined hypo-echoic area with some ill-defined internal echoes within the prostate gland close to the prostatic apex (**Fig. 5.11.1**, arrow). There is no posterior acoustic enhancement, making a cystic lesion unlikely. There is a well-defined hyperechoic rim surrounding this abnormality. The ultrasound appearances of the focal abnormality are nonspecific, and a colour Doppler ultrasound study may help differentiate between a prostatic abscess and a focal malignancy. Given the history of global pelvic pain, CT imaging would be more useful.

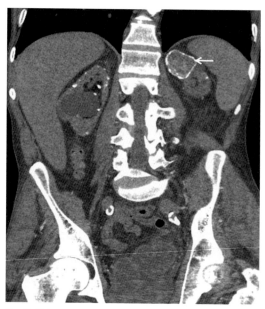

Fig. 5.11.3

*These are CT images from the same patient (**Figs. 5.11.2** and **5.11.3**).*

These are enhanced axial and coronal CT images through the abdomen and pelvis. The prostate is markedly enlarged and contains a multiloculated lesion with thick septations, extending superiorly (**Fig. 5.11.2**, arrow). No intraprostatic calcifications are seen. There is minor fat stranding surrounding the prostate. The bladder is thick-walled but is incompletely distended. There are multiple areas of calcification present in both kidneys, and a calcified rim in the upper pole of an atrophic left kidney (**Fig. 5.11.3**, arrow). Low-density cysts are also present in both kidneys.

There are no free pelvic fluid or enlarged lymph nodes on the given images. Given the clinical presentation, the appearances of a chronic prostatic abscess and renal calcification, the possibility or tuberculous infection is raised. I would like to assess the lungs for evidence of pulmonary tuberculosis.

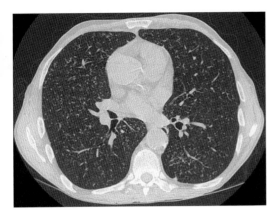

Fig. 5.11.4

*This is an image from the CT of the chest of the same patient (**Fig. 5.11.4**).*

This is an axial CT image through the chest of the same patient. There are multiple small, centrilobular nodules connected to linear branching opacities throughout both lungs. There are no cavitating lesions or evidence of enlarged lymph nodes. The combined imaging features of the kidneys and chest are suggestive of tuberculosis infection, and the abnormality within the prostate most likely represents a tuberculosis abscess.

Examination Tips

For features of genitourinary tuberculosis, look for and comment on the following:
- Kidneys:
  - Around 75% of renal tuberculous involvement is unilateral.
  - The earliest abnormality is a "moth-eaten" calyx on an intravenous urogram due to infective erosions, which progresses to papillary necrosis.
  - Dilated calyces (hydrocalycosis) related to infundibular strictures may be present at one or more sites within the collecting system.
  - Hydronephrosis may develop and tends to have irregular margins and filling defects owing to caseous debris.
  - Renal parenchymal cavitation may be detected as irregular pools of contrast material.
  - The involved kidney often becomes shrunken or scarred over time.
  - Calcification is common in the late stages and varies from punctate foci to dense calcification of the entire kidney.

- Characteristic calcifications in a lobar distribution are often seen in end-stage tuberculosis (tuberculous autonephrectomy).
- Prostate:
  - Contrast-enhanced CT imaging demonstrates hypoattenuating prostatic lesions, which represent foci of caseous necrosis and inflammation.
  - Sloughing and irregular cavitation of the prostate may eventually result in a smooth-walled cavity that replaces the prostate.
  - Tuberculous prostatic cavities or abscesses may discharge into the surrounding tissues, forming sinuses or fistulas to the perineum or rectum. These changes are best demonstrated on MRI.
  - Plain radiographs or CT imaging may show dense calcification within the prostatic bed.
  - An aspiration or biopsy is often required for accurate diagnosis; however, this may potentially risk fistula formation. Ancillary imaging signs pointing towards tuberculous infection should guide management.

Differential Diagnosis

- Nontuberculous pyogenic prostatic abscesses. These have a similar CT imaging appearance. In many cases, biopsy or culture specimens are needed to yield the definitive diagnosis, in the absence of other ancillary signs of tuberculosis.
- Prostatic malignancy. A search should be made for evidence of metastases elsewhere, particularly for pelvic nodal enlargement and sclerotic bone lesions.

Notes

- The genitourinary tract is the most common extrapulmonary site for tuberculous infection.
- Prostate tuberculous infection usually results from haematogenous spread.
- Approximately 85% of patients with prostate involvement also have renal tuberculous infection.
- MRI is the gold standard modality for the evaluation of intraprostatic abnormalities. However, a history of global pelvic pain should prompt a recommendation for CT assessment.

Bibliography

Jung YY, Kim JK, Cho KS. Genitourinary tuberculosis: comprehensive cross-sectional imaging. AJR Am J Roentgenol 2005;184(1):143–150

5.12 Urethral Injury

Clinical History

*A 24-year-old man presents with road traffic accident injuries (**Figs. 5.12.1** and **5.12.2**).*

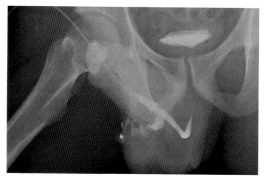

Fig. 5.12.1

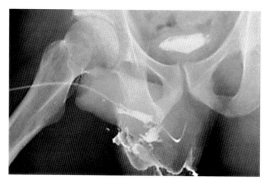

Fig. 5.12.2

Ideal Summary

These are selected oblique images of a retrograde urethrogram. There is contrast extravasation at the level of the distal bulbous urethra. Contrast is seen in the urethra proximal to this point and within the bladder, indicating that there is not a complete urethral transection. No obvious pelvic fractures are seen on the given views. The appearances would be in keeping with an anterior urethral injury without complete transection of the urethra. This may be related to a straddle or compression injury. I would discuss these findings with the urology team.

Examination Tips

If shown a urethral injury, look for and comment on:
- The anatomical location of the injury, and its implications:
  - Bladder neck. There is a risk of incontinence, as this is the site of the internal sphincter, which is the primary continence sphincter.
  - Intact, but "stretched" posterior urethra. There is rupture of the puboprostatic ligaments, but the continuity of the urethra is maintained.
  - Rupture of the membranous urethra *with contrast extravasation only into the pelvis and not into the perineum.* The membranous urethral is torn above an intact urogenital diaphragm.
  - Rupture of the membranous urethra *with contrast extravasation not only into the pelvic extraperitoneal space, but also into the perineum.* There is laceration of the urogenital diaphragm. This may be associated with incontinence related to traumatic damage to the external sphincter.
  - Injury at the bulbous portion of the anterior urethra. This is usually caused by straddle injuries where the bulbous urethra is compressed between a hard object or surface and the inferior aspect of the pubic bones. In general, this is not associated with pelvic bone injuries.
- The appearances of the bladder:
  - "Pear-shaped." This is indicative of perivesical haematoma.
  - "Pie in the sky." Complete disruption of the urethra may result in dislocation of the bladder out of the pelvis, which appears as a "pie in the sky" on urography performed through a suprapubic catheter.
  - Scrutinise for pelvic bone injuries. Posterior urethral injury is associated with crushing pelvic trauma and, in particular, pelvic fractures and bladder injuries.

Differential Diagnosis

Beware not to misinterpret normal structures as injury or extravasation:
- The verumontanum is seen as an ovoid filling defect in the posterior part of the prostatic urethra.
- Cowper's glands are two pea-sized glands that lie within the urogenital diaphragm on each side of the membranous urethra. The ducts of the

Cowper's glands are 2 cm long and empty into the bulbous urethra on either side of midline.

- Periurethral Littre's glands lie at the dorsal aspect of the penile urethra and in the bulbous urethra.
- Vascular opacification: increased pressure during contrast injection may result in opacification of the corpora and draining veins.

Notes

The male urethra is divided into anterior and posterior portions, each of which is subdivided into two parts:

- The anterior urethra is divided into the penile and bulbous parts at the penoscrotal junction. The penile portion terminates in the glans penis to form the fossa navicularis.
- The posterior urethra is divided into the prostatic and membranous urethra. The distal end of the verumontanum marks the proximal boundary of the membranous urethra, which is approximately 1 cm long and is the portion of the urethra that passes through the urogenital diaphragm.

Bibliography

Kawashima A, Sandler CM, Wasserman NF, LeRoy AJ, King BF Jr, Goldman SM. Imaging of urethral disease: a pictorial review. Radiographics 2004;24(Suppl 1):S195–S216

5.13 Angiomyolipoma

Clinical History

A 37-year-old woman presents with right upper quadrant pain (Figs. 5.13.1 and 5.13.2).

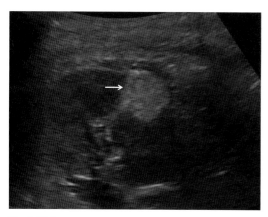

Fig. 5.13.1

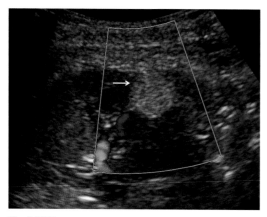

Fig. 5.13.2

Ideal Summary

These are a B-mode ultrasound image and a colour Doppler ultrasound image. There is a uniformly hyperechoic lesion in the mid-aspect of the kidney that demonstrates no increase in colour Doppler signal, suggesting a poorly vascularised abnormality (**Figs. 5.13.1** and **5.13.2**, arrows). The remainder of the kidney has a normal appearance on this single view. No free fluid surrounds the kidney, and there is no evidence of pelvicalyceal dilatation. The sonographic

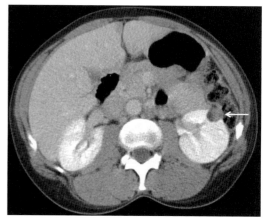

Fig. 5.13.3

appearances of this lesion would suggest an angiomyolipoma (AML). Other possible causes for this appearance to be considered include a renal cell carcinoma. In my routine practice, I would make references to any previous cross-sectional imaging of the kidney. If this lesion has not been previously characterised, I would recommend a CT to further evaluate this lesion.

*This is a single CT image of the same patient (**Fig. 5.13.3**).*

On this single venous-phase CT image, there is a low attenuation abnormality over the anterior aspect of the left kidney, which enhances less than the surrounding renal parenchyma (**Fig. 5.13.3**, arrow). Ideally, I would also review any arterial phase imaging and place a cursor over the lesion to ascertain the fat content on an unenhanced CT image. However, with the ultrasound image demonstrating a hyperechoic lesion, this is likely an AML. I would recommend a urology review and ultrasound follow-up.

Examination Tips

When shown a hyperechoic lesion on ultrasound in the kidney, particularly in the upper aspect of the kidney, consider and comment on the following:
- First, consider all possible anatomical origins of the lesion: renal, adrenal, hepatic/splenic, or retroperitoneal.
- Ultrasound characteristics of the lesion. An AML is classically described as the most hyperreflective

renal lesion with acoustic shadowing, a result of the multiple tissue interfaces between the fatty and non-fatty components of the mass.

- Colour Doppler assessment of an AML will rarely demonstrate colour signal, whereas often a malignant lesion will demonstrate some colour Doppler flow.
- However, up to 12% of renal cell carcinomas have been found to mimic AMLs sonographically. Conversely, there is a subset (5%) of AMLs with minimal fat components that appear isoechoic with renal parenchyma due to the lack of fat–muscle interfaces that produce the classical features. The assessment should be continued with a CT or an MRI.
- The diagnosis of an AML can be made if an unenhanced CT demonstrates a renal lesion with internal fat attenuation (between –10 and –30 HU) with interspersing soft tissue density.
- Multiple AMLs raise the possibility of underlying tuberous sclerosis (Bourneville's disease); AMLs also occur in 15% of patients with lymphangioleiomyomatosis, so check the lungs for a reticular pattern on the chest radiograph, or well-defined lung cysts on CT.

Differential Diagnosis

- Extrarenal: adrenal myelolipoma, or retroperitoneal lipoma or liposarcoma.
- Renal: the most important differential diagnosis of a fat-containing tumour in the kidney includes AML, renal cell carcinoma, and oncocytoma.

Notes

- Angiomyolipomas are benign renal tumours, isolated and sporadic in 80% of cases and most common in middle-aged women.
- Angiomyolipomas can be associated with tuberous sclerosis, in which case they are likely to be larger, bilateral, and prone to faster growth, with a need for earlier surgical treatment.
- Angiomyolipomas account for approximately 25% of spontaneous perirenal haematomas. The propensity for haemorrhage in AMLs is multifactorial, and the defects in the elastic tissues can lead to the development of aneurysms. The diagnosis should be suspected on ultrasound in the correct clinical setting, when a hyporeflective or perinephric collection is seen adjacent to a hyperreflective heterogeneous renal mass. The assessment should be continued with a CT examination in the acute setting.
- Classically, 4 cm is suggested as the limit above which elective treatment of an AML should be considered. In addition, the size of associated intralesional aneurysms may also be significant, with an aneurysm size of 5 mm predictive of rupture.

Bibliography

Halpenny D, Snow A, McNeill G, Torreggiani WC. The radiological diagnosis and treatment of renal angiomyolipoma – current status. Clin Radiol 2010;65(2):99–108

Logue LG, Acker RE, Sienko AE. Best cases from the AFIP: angiomyolipomas in tuberous sclerosis. Radiographics 2003;23(1):241–246

5.14 Renal Cell Carcinoma

Clinical History

A 65-year-old man presents with painless haematuria (**Figs. 5.14.1** and **5.14.2**).

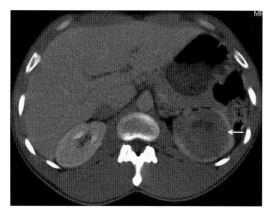

Fig. 5.14.1

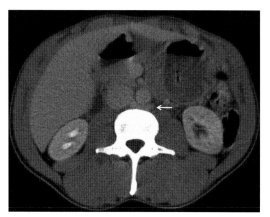

Fig. 5.14.2

Ideal Summary

These are selected axial nephrographic phase CT images through the upper abdomen. There is a well-circumscribed, hypoenhancing, central left renal mass (**Fig. 5.14.1**, arrow). It contains an area of low attenuation and distorts the calyceal system, but there is no evidence of pelvicalyceal obstruction. The mass appears to be confined to the left kidney. Incidental note is made of circumaortic left renal veins (**Fig. 5.14.2**, arrow), but there is no renal vein invasion. There are no enlarged lymph nodes. Allowing for the late venous phase of the scan, the remainder

of the study is unremarkable. The main differential diagnosis for the left renal mass is a renal cell carcinoma (RCC). Given the central low density within the mass, an oncocytoma is also a possibility, but this cannot be differentiated from an RCC on imaging. I would like to review the remainder of the study and recommend a CT chest to complete the staging.

These are further CT images from the same patient (**Figs. 5.14.3** and **5.14.4**).

These are two images from an arterial-phase CT scan of the chest and corticomedullary-phase images of the upper abdomen. I can see a large destructive soft tissue mass centred on the left scapula (**Fig. 5.14.3**, arrow). Within the upper abdomen, there is an enhancing retrocaval mass that demonstrates peripheral enhancement with central low attenuation (**Fig. 5.14.4**, arrow). Overall, the findings are most in keeping with left RCC metastasising to the left scapula and right

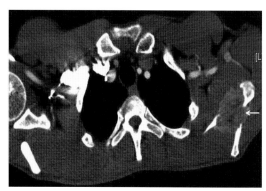

Fig. 5.14.3

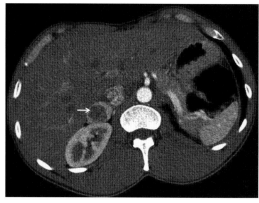

Fig. 5.14.4

adrenal gland. I would advise an urgent review at the urology multidisciplinary meeting.

Examination Tips

When presented with a focal renal mass, different enhancement phases should be carefully interpreted and commented on:
- An unenhanced scan. This is important for distinguishing hyperdense cysts from solid tumours. Fat density (between −10 and −30 HU) within a focal lesion suggests an angiomyolipoma.
- Corticomedullary phase (25 to 70 s following contrast injection):
  - Maximal opacification of the renal arteries and veins occurs. Allows diagnosis of venous extension of tumour (filling defect within the vein, abrupt change in the calibre of the renal vein, clots in collateral veins, heterogeneous enhancement of thrombus, and direct continuity of the thrombus with the primary tumour).
  - Hypervascular metastases to the liver, spleen, and pancreas are most conspicuous on the corticomedullary-phase scans.
- Nephrographic phase (80 to 180 s following contrast injection):
  - Most sensitive for tumour detection.
- Excretory phase (begins around 180 seconds after injection of contrast):
  - Evaluation of urothelial abnormalities (filling defects within the opacified collecting system).
  - Washout of contrast from a lesion could allow differentiation between renal neoplasms and hyperdense cysts.

The following staging features should be looked for and commented on:
- Perinephric tumour spread (T3a). Presence of enhancing nodules or stranding in the perinephric space.
- Adrenal glands. Visualisation of a normal adrenal gland on CT is associated with a high negative predictive value for tumoural spread. By contrast, if adrenal enlargement, displacement, or non-visualisation is demonstrated, adrenalectomy should be performed.
- Venous spread of tumours. Extension of RCC into the renal vein alone or including the infradiaphragmatic inferior vena cava (T3b) or supradiaphragmatic inferior vena cava (T3c).
- Regional lymph node metastases are reported on nodal enlargement of greater than 1 cm in short-axis diameter. However, nodal enlargement is caused by benign inflammatory changes in over 50%.
- Local extension and distant metastases:
  - Direct extension of RCC outside Gerota's fascia into the neighboring organs (stage T4a) is suggested when there is loss of tissue planes and irregular margins between the tumour and the surrounding structures.
  - RCC metastasises most frequently to the lungs and mediastinum, bones, and liver.

Differential Diagnoses

- Renal oncocytoma
  - Usually only differentiated from an RCC histologically
  - Can contain a central hypodense scar (30%)
  - No evidence of metastatic disease
- Renal lymphoma
  - Consider if lesions are bilateral
  - Lesions often are infiltrative and usually "encase," rather than replace, the renal parenchyma
  - Look for additional evidence of splenomegaly and nodal enlargement
- Central transitional cell carcinoma
  - Often the two can only be differentiated histologically
  - Significant ureteric involvement is more suggestive of a transitional cell carcinoma

Notes

- Usually affects men aged 50 to 70 years.
- Around 25 to 40% of RCCs are found incidentally on abdominal imaging.
- Calcification may be seen in 10% of cases of RCC.

Bibliography

Prasad SR, Humphrey PA, Catena JR, et al. Common and uncommon histologic subtypes of renal cell carcinoma: imaging spectrum with pathologic correlation. Radiographics 2006;26(6):1795–1806, discussion 1806–1810

Sheth S, Scatarige JC, Horton KM, Corl FM, Fishman EK. Current concepts in the diagnosis and management of renal cell carcinoma: role of multidetector CT and three-dimensional CT. Radiographics 2001;21 (Spec No):S237–S254

Zhang J, Lefkowitz RA, Bach A. Imaging of kidney cancer. Radiol Clin North Am 2007;45(1):119–147

5.15 Ovarian Dermoid

Clinical History

*A 66-year-old woman presents with left flank and left iliac fossa pain (**Fig. 5.15.1**).*

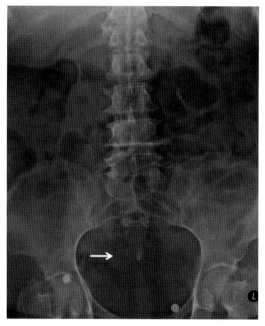

Fig. 5.15.1

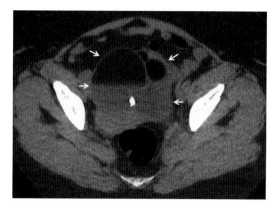

Fig. 5.15.2

*This is a selected CT image from the same patient (**Fig. 5.15.2**).*

This is an axial unenhanced CT image of the same patient. There is a well-defined, multilobulated central pelvic mass anterior to the uterus (**Fig. 5.15.2**, arrows). I can see a fat–fluid level within the main body of the lesion. There is a focus of internal calcification corresponding to the plain film appearances. The mass does not appear to invade adjacent structures, and there is no surrounding fat stranding or free fluid. The CT appearances confirm the plain film findings and are typical for an ovarian dermoid cyst. Given the size of the lesion and the associated risk of torsion, I would recommend gynaecology referral.

Ideal Summary

This is a plain abdominal radiograph of an adult patient. I can see no calcification in the line of the renal tracts. However, there is a coarse focus of calcification projected over the coccyx in the midline surrounded by a large area of well-defined low density (**Fig. 5.15.1**, arrow). The focal calcification itself appears "tooth-like." The bowel gas pattern is within normal limits, and there is no evidence of perforation or obstruction. Minor degenerative changes are noted in the lumbar spine, with disc space narrowing, end-plate sclerosis, and lateral osteophytes. The plain radiographic appearances are most in keeping with an ovarian dermoid, as evidenced by a "tooth-like" calcific density, possibly surrounded by fat. I would investigate this further by recommending a CT for characterisation.

Examination Tips

On any imaging modality, dermoid cysts (or mature teratomas) demonstrate a broad range of findings because they are composed of mature tissue from all three germ cell layers—ectoderm (skin and brain), mesoderm (muscle and fat), and endoderm (mucinous or ciliated epithelium). Imaging findings that suggest a dermoid cyst include:

- On conventional radiographs, a large mass with "tooth-like" calcifications and fat density
- On CT, fat attenuation within a cyst, with or without calcification in the wall, which is diagnostic for an ovarian dermoid cyst
- Ultrasound appearances that are nonspecific because dermoid cysts are derived from the three germ cell layers, so images can be cystic, solid, or complex

- On MRI, high signal fat or sebum on the T1-weighted sequence, with suppression on the fat saturated sequences

Look for complications of dermoid cysts:
- The following features are suggestive of torsion:
  - Deviation of the uterus to the twisted side
  - Engorged blood vessels on the twisted side
  - Mature cystic teratomas affected by torsion are larger than average (mean diameter 11 cm versus 6 cm)
- Malignant degeneration (1 to 3%)
- Rupture (rare, but causes granulomatous peritonitis)
- Hydronephrosis (extrinsic distal ureteric obstruction)

Differential Diagnosis

No differential diagnosis should be offered for the above imaging findings. However, while the CT appearances of a mature cystic teratoma are diagnostic, if a lesion is fat-poor consider:
- Immature cystic teratoma. This is usually larger, with more prominent solid components, is ill-defined, and has a perforated capsule.

- Ovarian tumour. Look for evidence of local invasion, peritoneal deposits, and distant (liver, lung, or bone) spread to indicate the malignant nature of the lesion.
- Tubo-ovarian abscess. A complex cystic or solid mass with enhancing thick walls and a possible thick-walled tubular structure (hydro- or pyosalpinx) is seen.

Notes

- Ovarian dermoid is usually asymptomatic and incidental.
- It is the most common ovarian tumour.
- Dermoids may be bilateral in 20%.

Bibliography

Outwater EK, Siegelman ES, Hunt JL. Ovarian teratomas: tumor types and imaging characteristics. Radiographics 2001;21(2):475–490

Jung SE, Lee JM, Rha SE, Byun JY, Jung JI, Hahn ST. CT and MR imaging of ovarian tumors with emphasis on differential diagnosis. Radiographics 2002;22(6):1305–1325

5.16 Renal Trauma

Clinical History

*A 48-year-old man was involved in a high-speed road traffic accident (**Figs. 5.16.1–5.16.3**).*

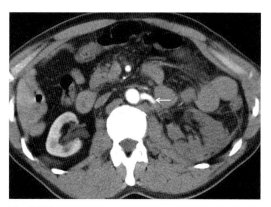

Fig. 5.16.1

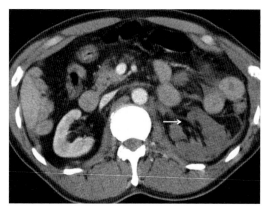

Fig. 5.16.2

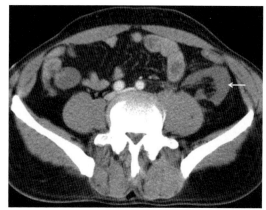

Fig. 5.16.3

image, I can still see part of the left kidney at the level of the pelvis (**Fig. 5.16.3**, arrow), and I would like to check if this is continuous with the upper pole. There are multiple thickened loops of small bowel in the left flank, anterior to the left kidney, with stranding of the adjacent small bowel mesentery. There is a small amount of associated free fluid, but no free air. I can also see fat stranding around the head of the pancreas and a small amount of free fluid around the liver. These findings are in keeping with significant intra-abdominal trauma with a devascularised left kidney and likely small bowel injury. I would expect more intra-abdominal blood from this injury, so I suspect that there is spasm of the left renal artery. I would like to review the remainder of the images on soft tissue and bone windows to fully assess the left kidney, as well as look for pancreatic injury and evidence of bony trauma. I would recommend an urgent surgical opinion if this has not already been done.

*This is a further CT image from the same patient (**Fig. 5.16.4**).*

This is a sagittal oblique reformat CT image. This demonstrates a devascularised and transected left kidney with the lower pole having "fallen" into the pelvis (**Fig. 5.16.4**, arrow). There is also a significant volume of perisplenic fluid. The appearances are most in keeping with a left renal transection and pedicle avulsion with the left lower renal pole lying in the pelvis. There is no active bleeding, presumably due to the spasm of the left renal artery. The perisplenic fluid may be related to a splenic injury.

Ideal Summary

These are selected axial arterial- and venous-phase CT images. The left kidney is nonenhancing compared with the normal right kidney, and there is surrounding perinephric fat stranding. The left renal artery is truncated in its proximal third, and there are no enhancing vessels in the region of the left renal hilum (**Figs. 5.16.1** and **5.16.2**, arrows). There is no ongoing contrast extravasation. On the caudal

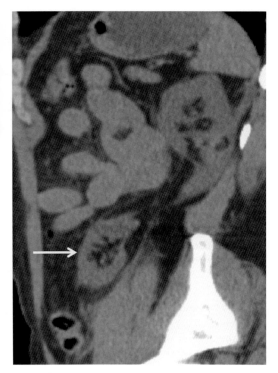

Fig. 5.16.4

In my routine practice, I would carefully examine the whole biphasic CT (including a single-phase CT) of the chest and head and neck (likely to be indicated given the mechanism of injury). In particular, I would look for any solid organ and bony injuries. I would alert the interventional radiologist and the urologist to plan the patient's further management.

Examination Tips

In practice, complex trauma imaging can involve thousands of images and require prolonged careful inspection to identify every single abnormality. As such, it would be unrealistic to expect a candidate to perform such a laborious task. However, it is reasonable to expect a worthy candidate to assess for significant injuries rapidly, prioritise, and decide on an appropriate management plan. To this end, the following points should be borne in mind when dealing with major trauma imaging:

- Listen to the history! The injuries you expect from a stabbing are different from those from a road traffic accident. Absorb every bit of help from the examiners you can.
- If there is a striking abnormality, describe the pattern and extent of the injury.
- Think about the mechanism of injury and anatomy. If there is a liver laceration, every adjacent structure is also at risk. Remember that the bowel and kidneys may move, and these injuries may appear distant from the primary abnormality.
- Look for significant injuries that require immediate intervention, such as ongoing haemorrhage, tension pneumothorax, unstable spinal fractures, and perforated bowel.
- Never forget about the pancreas and the bowel, as these structures are associated with morbidity.
- If there is an unusual finding, do not ignore it. The explanation will either be on the current film or on the subsequent film the examiner is holding.
- Always ask to review all of the images at the end, ask for reformats and bone windows.
- Although haematuria is present in over 95% of cases, its absence does not exclude significant renal injury as, for example, in cases of ureteropelvic junction injury or renal artery thrombosis.

Differential Diagnosis

No differential diagnosis should be offered.

Notes

Categories of traumatic renal injuries:
- Category I—minor injury:
  - Renal contusion, intrarenal and subcapsular haematoma; minor laceration with limited perinephric haematoma without extension to the collecting system or medulla; small subsegmental cortical infarct.
- Category II—major injury:
  - Major renal laceration through the cortex extending to the medulla or collecting system with or without urine extravasation; segmental renal infarct.
- Category III—catastrophic injury:
  - Multiple renal lacerations; vascular injury involving the renal pedicle.
- Category IV—ureteropelvic junction injury:
  - Avulsion or laceration (incomplete tear).

Bibliography

Kawashima A, Sandler CM, Corl FM, et al. Imaging of renal trauma: a comprehensive review. Radiographics 2001; 21(3):557–574

5.17 Bladder Rupture

Clinical History

A 17-year-old adolescent boy fell from a height (**Figs. 5.17.1–5.17.3**).

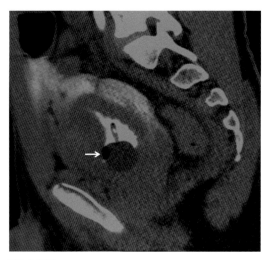

Fig. 5.17.1

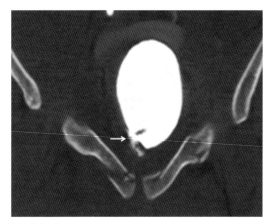

Fig. 5.17.2

Ideal Summary

These are selected coronal, sagittal, and axial images of the pelvis. The urinary catheter is in a satisfactory position (**Fig. 5.17.1**, arrow). On the coronal

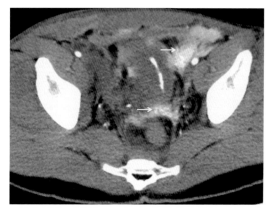

Fig. 5.17.3

view, the bladder is fully distended with contrast, and there is a defect in the inferior bladder wall on the right with contrast extravasation (**Fig. 5.17.2**, arrow). There are also multiple pubic rami fractures evident on the coronal image. There is extraperitoneal contrast on the axial (**Fig. 5.17.3**, arrows) and sagittal images, and there is no definite intraperitoneal component or evidence of significant vascular injury, although I would like to review all of the images to confirm this. The images are in keeping with extraperitoneal bladder rupture secondary to pelvic floor fractures. I would like to review the remainder of the images and recommend urgent urological review.

Examination Tips

- Accurate classification of bladder injury is critical for proper treatment:
  - Intraperitoneal bladder rupture requires laparotomy with surgical repair of the bladder defect and diverting vesicostomy.
  - Contusions and interstitial injuries are managed conservatively with bladder catheterisation.
  - Most extraperitoneal bladder ruptures may be treated with catheter drainage if the bladder neck is not injured; otherwise, formal surgical repair is necessary.

- Filling the bladder with a minimum of 250 to 300 mL of contrast material is necessary to safely rule out a bladder wall tear.
- Urographic (delayed) phase CT improves sensitivity in detecting bladder injury by enabling further bladder distension when compared with venous-phase images alone. Even allowing for the delay, antegrade bladder filling may be inadequate due to poor renal excretion.
  - A CT cystogram is an alternative that allows retrograde filling of the bladder with a sufficient volume of contrast; however, bladder catheterisation should only be performed after urethral continuity has been determined. If in doubt, catheterisation should be performed by a urologist under direct visualisation.
- In intraperitoneal bladder rupture, CT cystography demonstrates intraperitoneal contrast material around bowel loops, between mesenteric folds, and in the paracolic gutters.
- As in all CT examinations for a multitrauma patient, it is essential to look for and comment on any additional injuries—in this case, multiple pelvic fractures.

Differential Diagnosis

There is no differential diagnosis for these appearances. It is essential to detail all of the visible injuries and inform the examiner that you would always review all of the available images.

Notes

Classification system for bladder injury based on findings from CT cystography:
- Type 1—bladder contusion. Bladder contusion is defined as an incomplete or partial tear of the bladder mucosa with normal cystogram findings.
- Type 2—intraperitoneal rupture. This occurs in 10 to 20% of major bladder injuries, usually at the weakest portion, the bladder dome. It is typically associated with blunt injuries, and there is increasing bladder injury with increasing bladder distension.
- Type 3—interstitial bladder injury. Manifestations of interstitial injury include intramural haemorrhage and submucosal extravasation of contrast material without transmural extension.
- Type 4—extraperitoneal rupture. Simple rupture with contrast confined to the perivesical space versus complex extraperitoneal ruptures with contrast beyond the perivesical space dissecting into various fascial planes and spaces.
- Type 5—combined bladder injury. Combined intra- and extraperitoneal rupture usually demonstrates extravasation patterns that are typical for both types of injury.

Bibliography

Vaccaro JP, Brody JM. CT cystography in the evaluation of major bladder trauma. Radiographics 2000;20(5): 1373–1381

5.18 Phaeochromocytoma

Clinical History

A 57-year-old man presents with high blood pressure (**Figs. 5.18.1** and **5.18.2**).

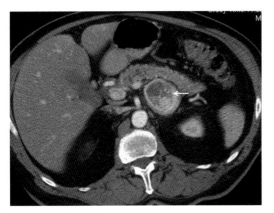

Fig. 5.18.1

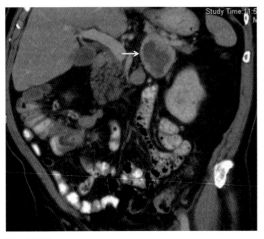

Fig. 5.18.2

Ideal Summary

These are selected venous-phase axial and coronal images of the abdomen. There is a well-circumscribed heterogeneously enhancing left upper retroperitoneal mass with minimal surrounding fat stranding and central low density. It arises from the medial limb of the left adrenal gland (**Figs. 5.18.1** and **5.18.2**, arrows). There is no intralesional calcification. I can see no evidence of local invasion. The spleen and the upper pole of left kidney are separate from the mass. Small-volume para-aortic and coeliac lymph nodes are present. On these images, no focal liver or bone lesions are demonstrated, although I would like to evaluate the whole scan, including the chest and the right adrenal gland, to look for a primary and to exclude distant lesions. Given the history of hypertension and nonadenomatous morphology of the lesion, the most likely differential diagnosis is phaeochromocytoma. I would like to confirm this with urinary catecholamine levels, and the patient may require an MIBG study.

Examination Tips

When dealing with an adrenal mass, consider the following:
- Establish that the mass is actually of adrenal origin:
  - Can you see one of the limbs of the involved adrenal gland?
  - Think about the anatomy: the mass may originate from the kidney (renal cell carcinoma), liver, or lymph node or may be a peritoneal deposit.
- Are you dealing with a single nodule, nodularity, or bilateral disease?
- What is the density of the lesion?
  - The most common adrenal lesion is a benign adenoma. Of these, 70% are lipid-rich and are of low density (< 10 HU) on unenhanced CT.
  - The lipid-poor adenomas demonstrate rapid contrast washout:
    - Absolute washout of over 60% = adenoma
    - Absolute washout (%) is calculated by (Enhanced – Delayed) / (Enhanced – Unenhanced) × 100.
  - Comment on ancillary features such as areas of haemorrhage, necrosis, and calcification.
- Phaeochromocytoma demonstrates homogeneous enhancement if it is solid, but heterogeneous enhancement in the presence of necrosis and haemorrhage.
- A phaeochromocytoma is typically greater than 3 cm in size.

- Always look for the presence of a primary as adrenal metastases may demonstrate a similar appearance.

Differential Diagnosis

The differential diagnosis for nonadenomatous adrenal lesions includes:

- Metastasis:
  - Often in the presence of a known malignancy
  - Lung and breast carcinoma and melanoma are the most common primary tumours
  - Usually well-defined, small, and with variable enhancement
- Adrenocortical carcinoma:
  - Rare, so place it lower on the differential diagnosis list
  - 90% unilateral
- Adrenal haemorrhage:
  - Usually bilateral
  - Nonenhancing; therefore, a precontrast scan is useful to differentiate it

Notes

- Phaeochromocytomas are paragangliomas arising from the adrenal medulla.
- Phaeochromocytomas are sometimes called the "10% tumour" because:
  - There is a 10% risk of malignancy.
  - 10% show bilateral disease.
  - 10% are hormonally inactive.
  - 10% are extra-adrenal.
- If an adrenal lesion is indeterminate and increases in size over 6 months, it is suspicious for malignancy. However, adrenal haemorrhage, myolipomas, and adenomas can sometimes enlarge.
- Adrenal multinodularity with preservation of outline indicates benign disease.

Bibliography

Johnson PT, Horton KM, Fishman EK. Adrenal mass imaging with multidetector CT: pathologic conditions, pearls, and pitfalls. Radiographics 2009;29(5):1333–1351

5.19 Pelvic Inflammatory Disease

Clinical History

A 23-year-old woman presents with a history of pelvic pain and fever (Figs. 5.19.1–5.19.4).

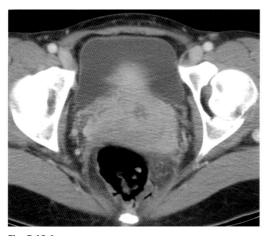

Fig. 5.19.1

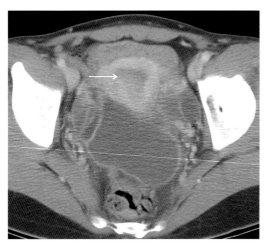

Fig. 5.19.2

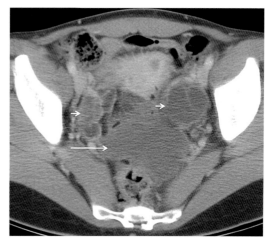

Fig. 5.19.3

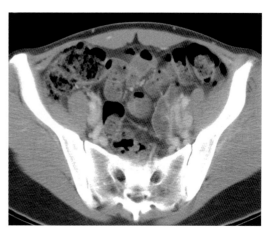

Fig. 5.19.4

Ideal Summary

These are axial CT images through the pelvis. The uterine cavity is fluid-filled (**Fig. 5.19.2**, arrow) with no contraceptive device, but the uterus otherwise appears unremarkable. The unprepared bowel is normal. There are tubular fluid density collections in both adnexae (**Fig. 5.19.3**, short arrows), with a large collection in the pouch of Douglas (**Fig. 5.19.3**, long arrow). The collections are homogeneous with enhancing walls and surrounding fat stranding. There is no gas within the collections. I cannot see the ovaries separately on these images. The most likely diagnosis is pelvic inflammatory disease (PID) complicated by bilateral pyosalpinx (**Fig. 5.19.3**, short arrows) and an abscess in the pouch of Douglas (**Fig. 5.19.3**, long arrow). I would like to review the rest of the images for potential complications such as hydronephrosis. I would recommend gynaecology referral and correlation with inflammatory markers.

Examination Tips

It is often difficult to evaluate the pelvis on CT against a background of inflammation, but try to establish the anatomical origin of the pelvic mass:
- Ovarian: will often cause the anterior displacement of the broad ligament
- Colon: look for evidence of diverticulosis or bowel obstruction
- Appendix: the tip may lie within the pelvis, and the diagnosis will be missed if this is not considered
- Renal tract: look for associated hydronephrosis and bladder wall thickening.

Look for and comment on:
- Pelvic free fluid and its density: high-density or layered free fluid may indicate a haemoperitoneum; the differential diagnosis will include:
  - Ectopic pregnancy (a gynaecological emergency)
  - Rupture of a haemorrhagic adnexal cyst
  - Endometrioma.
- The presence of tubular fluid-filled structures in the adnexae is highly suggestive of hydrosalpinx.
- Any intrauterine contraceptive device needs to be removed if there is evidence of PID.
- Consider ovarian torsion in any ovarian cyst or mass over 5 cm in size.
- Complications relating to pelvic abscess are:
  - Bowel obstruction
  - Hydronephrosis
  - Fistulous tracts with the bladder or bowel—look for intraluminal gas.
- Any peritoneal nodularity or abnormal enhancement may indicate disseminated infection or malignancy.

Differential Diagnosis

The differential diagnosis for ovarian masses includes:
- Haemorrhagic corpus luteum cyst. These have thicker walls that may be irregular and usually demonstrate internal echoes on ultrasound due to haemorrhage. On CT, these appear as a unilocular complex mass.
- Endometrioma. Around 80% occur in the ovaries and may appear as complex solid or cystic masses on CT and ultrasonography. They demonstrate minimal internal vascularity.
- Cystadenoma. This is a benign tumour that is predisposed to torsion.

Notes

- Pelvic inflammatory disease can appear subtle in the early stages, with mild stranding of the pelvic fat and increased enhancement of the fallopian tubes or ovaries.
- More advanced PID may present as pyosalpinx and/or tubo-ovarian abscesses.
- Consider a tubo-ovarian abscess in any pelvic collection where the cause is not apparent.
- Initial imaging and follow-up should involve transvaginal ultrasound, with CT imaging for complicated cases.
- Treatment involves antibiotics with or without image- or surgically guided drainage of any collections.

Bibliography

Kim SH, Kim SH, Yang DM, Kim KA. Unusual causes of tubo-ovarian abscess: CT and MR imaging findings. Radiographics 2004;24(6):1575–1589

Potter AW, Chandrasekhar CAUS. US and CT evaluation of acute pelvic pain of gynecologic origin in nonpregnant premenopausal patients. Radiographics 2008;28(6): 1645–1659

Sam JW, Jacobs JE, Birnbaum BA. Spectrum of CT findings in acute pyogenic pelvic inflammatory disease. Radiographics 2002;22(6):1327–1334

5.20 Renal Infarction

Clinical History

*A 57-year-old man presents with an acute onset of left upper quadrant and left flank pain (**Fig. 5.20.1**).*

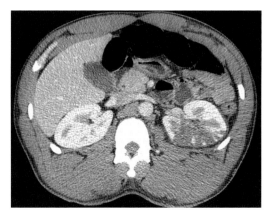

Fig. 5.20.1

Ideal Summary

This is an axial venous-phase CT image through the upper abdomen. There is a well-defined hypodense stellate area within the posterior left renal interpolar region. No hydronephrosis is present. There is no significant perinephric stranding. The visualised left renal vein and artery are patent. The visualised right kidney, liver, pancreas, and unprepared bowel appear unremarkable. No enlarged para-aortic lymph nodes are demonstrated. The appearances are in keeping with a segmental left renal infarct. However, focal pyelonephritis or an infiltrative neoplasm, such as a lymphoma, also needs to be considered. I would like to review the remainder of the images for other areas of infarction and ask if there is an arterial-phase scan available to assess the vessels. If the lesion is isolated, I would recommend referral to the renal team.

Examination Tips

◉ In renal infarcts, the low-density areas are usually well defined with a sharp transition

between abnormally and normally enhancing renal parenchyma.
◉ If subacute, the "cortical rim sign" may be present. This signifies the preserved subcapsular perfusion due to capsular perforators. The cortical rim sign may allow differentiation of infarction from infiltration. This is usually absent initially.
◉ Look for causes of renal infarction such as features suggestive of trauma or evidence of renal vein thrombosis.
◉ Embolic renal infarcts are usually multiple and bilateral. If this is a differential diagnosis, look for other areas of infarction, and remember to review the heart for a visible thrombus in the heart.
◉ It may not always be possible to differentiate between infarction and pyelonephritis. If this is the case, ask the examiner for any relevant clinical history, such as sepsis or atrial fibrillation.
◉ Ancillary findings are useful in narrowing the differential diagnosis:
  • Perinephric stranding or fluid, with an enlarged kidney and ill-defined areas of low density, are more suggestive of an inflammatory or an infective cause. Look for and comment on underlying causes, such as renal calculi.
  • Neoplasms (lymphoma, transitional cell carcinoma, renal leukaemia, or metastases) may also be infiltrative. Look for local invasion, locoregional enlarged lymph nodes, splenomegaly (in case of lymphoma), synchronous ureteric or renal lesions, or other primary tumours to support your diagnosis.

Differential Diagnosis

◉ Infiltrative neoplasm
◉ Vasculitis—often bilateral; look for evidence of aortitis, and for haemorrhage elsewhere (polyarteritis nodosa)
◉ Focal pyelonephritis—usually clinically evident

Notes

◉ The most common cause of renal infarction is thromboembolism from cardiovascular disease.

● It can also occur in trauma, as a manifestation of vasculitis (polyarteritis nodosa, systemic lupus erythematosus, or drug-induced), as a part of paraneoplastic syndrome, and due to septic emboli.
● It often clinically mimics renal colic.

Bibliography

Kawashima A, Sandler CM, Ernst RD, Tamm EP, Goldman SM, Fishman EK. CT evaluation of renovascular disease. Radiographics 2000;20(5):1321–1340

6 Introduction to Paediatric Imaging

Preena Patel and Maria E. K. Sellars

Paediatric imaging is part of the core radiology training curriculum[1]; therefore, it should come as no surprise to find a significant number of cases appearing in postgraduate radiology examinations. From our collective experience, some examiners may have predominantly paediatric films in the viva, so be prepared.

After clearing the hurdle of the examination, every radiologist is likely to encounter paediatric imaging regardless of their chosen radiological subspecialty. Furthermore, as paediatric imaging includes every organ system, a good grasp of both normal variants and common pathology will prove very useful for the future.

It is important to be aware of the major differences between paediatric and adult imaging. In children, ultrasound, plain radiographs, and fluoroscopy form the foundation of imaging. Plain radiographs are the cornerstone in the assessment of chest disease for children of all ages. Fluoroscopy is used extensively for abnormalities of the gastrointestinal and genitourinary tracts. Ultrasound is a very useful tool, especially for abdominal abnormalities—children normally have little body fat, allowing excellent visualisation of the solid organs. For a child presenting with abdominal pain or distension, ultrasound is the imaging modality of choice. Within the chest, ultrasound can detect pleural effusions and empyemas; it can also act as a problem-solving tool if there is, for example, concern on the plain radiograph regarding thymus versus an anterior mediastinal mass—thymic tissue has a distinctive appearance on ultrasound.

Children are more susceptible to the detrimental effects of radiation than adults, so every effort should be made to reduce the dose and apply the "as low as reasonably achievable" principle. There should be strict justification for performing studies involving radiation. However, if performed, paediatric-specific protocols should be used; this is especially true for CT and fluoroscopy. Other considerations include gonad, thyroid, and lens shielding, suitable collimation, added filtration, and grid removal. Movement artefact can ruin image quality, but this can be diminished with the use of short exposure times, immobilisation, sedation, or distraction techniques to reduce patient motion.[2]

CT and MRI are primarily used to problem-solve, with MRI being increasingly used more than CT, especially now high-resolution and isotropic sequences can give excellent anatomical detail. MRI is ideal for staging abdominal tumours and also for non-oncological pathology, such as congenital anomalies involving the genitourinary tract.

Nonaccidental injury must be on the examination candidate's awareness at all times. Always check the bones on every plain film for fractures; for example, fractures involving the ribs, scapulae, and sternum on a chest radiograph are more suspicious for nonaccidental injury. If nonaccidental injury is suspected, the appropriate paediatric clinician needs to be alerted immediately, and this must be documented in the report. Following discussion, a full skeletal survey may be performed; for standard views, see the report from the Royal College of Radiologist of the United Kingdom.[3]

There must be specific considerations for paediatric images in the examination:

1. State the imaging modality and body part.
2. Knowing the age of the patient can help narrow your list of differentials: neonate (less than 28 days old), infant (less than 1 year old), and then child can be used up to the age of 16 years. Look at the bones for clues to the age. For example, the proximal femoral epiphysis begins to ossify after 3 months of age, and the humeral head is not ossified in premature neonates.
3. The use of the various ossification centres of the elbow are important in the assessment of fractures, but can also help with ages:
   - Capitellum—8 months
   - Radial head—3–4 years
   - Internal (medial) epicondyle—5 years
   - Trochlea—7 years

- Olecranon—9 years
- Lateral epicondyle—11 years.

4 Be aware of associated findings and satisfaction of search. For example, if you do not realise that tracheo-oesophageal fistula is associated with the VACTERL syndrome, you will probably miss the vertebral abnormalities and you will definitely not ask for further renal imaging to get you those extra points.

5 Always ask for old films and review all of the available imaging.

6 Listen to the examiner: the clinical history is important and could be the deciding factor in determining your differential diagnosis.

References

1. Royal College of Radiologists. Specialty Training Curriculum for Clinical Radiology. May 2010. http://www.rcr.ac.uk/content.aspx?PageID=1805 (accessed June 2012)

2. Raissaki MT. Pediatric radiation protection. Eur Radiol 2004;14:74–83

3. Royal College of Radiologists and Royal College of Paediatrics and Child Health. Standards for Radiological Investigations of Suspected Non-Accidental Injury – March. 2008. Intercollegiate Report from the Royal College of Radiologists and Royal College of Paediatrics and Child Health. http://www.rcr.ac.uk/docs/radiology/pdf/RCPCH_RCR_final.pdf (accessed June 2012)

6.1 Choledochal Cyst

Clinical History

*A 2-month-old infant presents with jaundice (**Fig. 6.1.1**).*

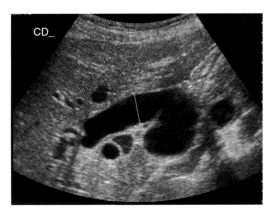

Fig. 6.1.1

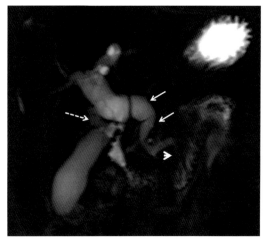

Fig. 6.1.2

Ideal Summary

This is a selected ultrasound image of the liver. There is a fusiform dilated structure in the region of the common hepatic duct, with no debris present (**Fig. 6.1.1**, between cursors). I would like to review further images to assess the remaining biliary system and gallbladder. This appearance is suggestive of a choledochal cyst, and I would recommend magnetic resonance cholangiopancreatography (MRCP) for further evaluation.

*This is the MRCP image (**Fig. 6.1.2**).*

This is a maximum-intensity projection image from an MRCP examination. There is fusiform dilatation of the common hepatic and common bile ducts (**Fig. 6.1.2**, arrows). There is an abrupt calibre change in the common bile duct just before the junction with the pancreatic duct (**Fig. 6.1.2**, arrowhead). The left and right hepatic ducts are also dilated. The gallbladder appears normal. The cystic duct originates from the abnormal dilated common duct (**Fig. 6.1.2**, dashed arrow). I cannot see any filling defects within the biliary tree. The pancreatic duct is not dilated. I would assess the other sequences for evidence of pancreatitis. The appearance of the common hepatic and the common bile duct are those of a choledochal cyst. I would inform the referring team.

Examination Tips

Ultrasound is the first-line investigation for jaundice in this group of patients, with even subtle changes in the calibre of the common or hepatic bile ducts warranting further investigation, as complications are substantial in the long term.

- Recommend MRI rather than CT as the next line of investigation in this age group.
- Check for any complications of a choledochal cyst:
  - Calculus formation. Ultrasound may depict echogenic stones with posterior acoustic shadowing in the choledochal cyst or biliary system. These will also be seen as filling defects on the MRCP.
  - There may be pancreatitis.
  - Cholangitis and hepatic abscess formation may be seen.
  - Choledochal cyst rupture. This may result in a collection or free fluid around the liver.
  - Biliary cirrhosis. Imaging features depend on the stage of the disease. If there is a late presentation, there will be an irregular, shrunken liver with signs of portal hypertension, ascites, and splenomegaly.
  - Cholangiocarcinoma. This may be subtle on imaging, but look for a mass or abnormal enhancement as a cause for focal intrahepatic duct dilatation.

Differential Diagnosis

There is no differential diagnosis for this appearance: any obstruction of the bile ducts will result in global dilatation of the bile ducts to the point of obstruction. Occasionally, on the ultrasound examination, other cystic structures may cause confusion.

- Hepatic cyst:
  - MRCP should not demonstrate any communication with the biliary system with no biliary dilatation.
  - No uptake of radiotracer will be seen on the technetium 99m DISIDA scan.

Notes

Choledochal cysts are an uncommon entity. They usually present early in life, and there is a classical triad of jaundice, an abdominal mass, and abdominal pain.
- Classification is based on site of the cyst or dilatation:
  - Type I: the most common variety (80 to 90%), involving saccular or fusiform dilatation of a portion of or the entire common bile duct (CBD), with normal intrahepatic ducts.
  - Type II: a true isolated diverticulum protruding from the CBD.
- Type III: a choledochocoele arising from dilatation of the duodenal portion of the CBD or where the pancreatic duct meets it.
- Type IV: characterised by multiple dilatations of the intrahepatic and extrahepatic biliary tree (IVa) or only the extrahepatic bile ducts (IVb).
- Type V: Caroli's disease, with cystic dilatation of the intrahepatic biliary ducts.
- In cases where the diagnosis is unclear, radionuclide studies will show tracer uptake into the choledochal cyst.
- Treatment depends on the type of choledochal cyst, and ranges from excision and biliary reconstruction to hepatic lobectomy (when there is stricture or stenosis).
- Biliary atresia is associated with choledochal cysts in neonates. Hepatobiliary scintigraphy with technetium 99m DISIDA scanning can be performed; lack of excretion into the small bowel is suggestive of biliary atresia.

Bibliography
Rozel C, Garel L, Rypens F, et al. Imaging of biliary disorders in children. Pediatr Radiol 2011;41(2):208–220

Kim OH, Chung HJ, Choi BG. Imaging of the choledochal cyst. Radiographics 1995;15(1):69–88

Chavhan GB, Babyn PS, Manson D, Vidarsson L. Pediatric MR cholangiopancreatography: principles, technique, and clinical applications. Radiographics 2008;28(7):1951–1962

6.2 Congenital Cystic Adenomatoid Malformation

Clinical History

*A neonate presents with respiratory distress (**Fig. 6.2.1**).*

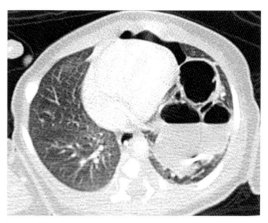

Fig. 6.2.2

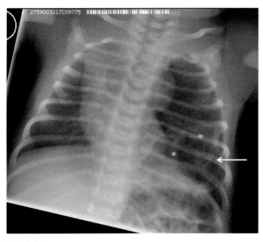

Fig. 6.2.1

of a communication with the bronchial tree. This is causing a mediastinal shift to the right, as seen on the radiograph. There are no anomalous vessels associated with the mass, and the diaphragm appears intact. The CT features confirm the diagnosis of CCAM.

Ideal Summary

This is a frontal chest radiograph of a neonate, with a prominent thymic shadow noted. There is an area of increased opacification with multiple lucencies occupying the lower aspect of the left lung (**Fig. 6.2.1**, arrow), which have the appearance of thin-walled cysts. The mediastinum is displaced to the right. The right lung appears normal. The abnormal area of left-sided opacification does not erode or scallop the posterior ribs. Two small metallic densities are seen in the left lower zone. Normal bowel gas is seen beneath the left diaphragm. These features are most likely to represent a congenital cystic adenomatoid malformation (CCAM). I would discuss these findings with the referring team and confirm the diagnosis with a chest CT.

*This is a chest CT image from the same patient (**Fig. 6.2.2**).*

This is an axial image on lung windows. There is a large multicystic mass centred on the left lower lobe, with air–fluid levels, raising the possibility

Examination Tips

When assessing lesions on CT in the neonate, you must check the following:
- Evaluate each lesion using both lung parenchymal and mediastinal window settings. If these are not initially available, the candidate will be expected to ask for them.
- Comment on the pattern of the abnormality: Is it soft tissue, cystic, nodular, or hyperexpanded lung parenchyma?
- Assess the distribution of abnormality: Is it confined to a particular lobe? Is it diffuse? Does it have an upper or lower zone predilection? Congenital cystic adenomatoid malformation is typically isolated to a single lobe with no lobar predominance.
- If the mass is responsible for significant mediastinal shift, comment upon compression of the bronchi, subsequent atelectasis, and even compression of the large vessels, as this assumes importance in a child.
- Carefully evaluate the tracheobronchial tree for areas of narrowing that could represent

tracheomalacia. Beware of the possibility of bronchial atresia.

- Evaluate the blood supply on mediastinal window settings: an arterial feeding vessel from the thoracic aorta and draining veins into the inferior pulmonary veins or inferior vena cava is seen in sequestration and should prompt the diagnosis.
- If the lesion erodes or scallops the posterior ribs, think of a thoracic neuroblastoma.

Differential Diagnosis

- Pulmonary sequestration:
  - Sequestration does not usually contain gas, unless there is concomitant infection.
  - Assessment of feeding and draining vessels is crucial to the diagnosis.
- Congenital lobar emphysema:
  - On plain radiographs, initially opacified areas may become progressively lucent on follow-up films.
  - The diagnosis is confirmed on CT imaging, which shows overexpansion of a single or multiple lung lobes, most frequently the left upper lobe.
- Congenital diaphragmatic hernia:
  - Look for lucencies within the chest that resemble bowel and are adjacent to the diaphragm.
  - There may be reduced bowel gas within the abdomen and low volumes in the chest.
  - The position of the nasogastric tube and intravenous lines may provide clues.

- Pulmonary interstitial emphysema:
  - This shows bubble-like or linear small lucencies within the lung that are classically uniform in size, unlike in CCAM.
  - On CT, a central arteriole is seen within each cystic area, compared with the empty cysts seen in CCAM.

Notes

CCAM is a congenital lung mass arising from disorganised hamartomas and adenomatoid proliferation of the primary bronchioles, which are in continuity with the bronchial tree. The majority are located within a single lobe and are rarely seen in the right middle lobe. There are three types of CCAM:

1. Type I (50%): single or multiple large cysts
2. Type II (40%): multiple small cysts
3. Type III (10%): solid with microscopic cysts

Type II and type III CCAMs are commonly associated with other congenital anomalies, such as cardiac abnormalities, renal agenesis, and jejunal atresia.

Bibliography

Lee EY, Boiselle PM, Cleveland RH. Multidetector CT evaluation of congenital lung anomalies. Radiology 2008;247(3): 632–648

Griffin N, Devaraj A, Goldstraw P, Bush A, Nicholson AG, Padley S. CT and histopathological correlation of congenital cystic pulmonary lesions: a common pathogenesis? Clin Radiol 2008;63(9):995–1005

6.3   Congenital Diaphragmatic Hernia

Clinical History

A neonate presents with severe respiratory distress from birth (**Fig. 6.3.1**).

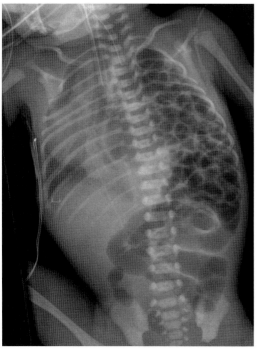

Fig. 6.3.1

Ideal Summary

This is a plain chest and abdominal radiograph of a neonate. The endotracheal tube is positioned low, and may be withdrawn slightly. The distal aspect of the nasogastric tube is at T2, and is incorrectly positioned. The tip of the left femoral line is deviated to the right of the midline. Multiple circular lucent areas with discernible walls fill the left hemithorax, extending into the left upper quadrant of the abdomen. The left hemidiaphragm is not visible. A larger lucent area is seen overlying the midline. There is marked mediastinal displacement to the right. Gas-filled loops of bowel are seen within the abdomen. No free intraperitoneal gas is evident. No bony abnormalities are seen. The most likely diagnosis is left-sided congenital diaphragmatic hernia (CDH), with bowel loops in the left hemithorax and possibly stomach overlying the mediastinum. I would recommend urgent referral to the paediatric surgical team.

Examination Tips

- The plain film appearances depend on the contents of the hernia: stomach and bowel are gas-filled, while liver is radiopaque.
- On the first film, before gas has entered the gastrointestinal tract, the affected hemithorax may be of increased opacification. On subsequent films, gas is usually seen within the bowel loops.
- The position of lines and tubes should be carefully assessed and commented upon as this may provide clues to the diagnosis:
  - The nasogastric tube may be curled within an intrathoracic stomach.
  - The tip of the umbilical venous catheter may be located within the left hemithorax, indicating that the liver has herniated into the left side of the chest; this is an uncommon but important observation to make as it is associated with a worse prognosis.
- Ultrasound can confirm loops of bowel, stomach, or solid viscera within the chest with CDH.
- If there is a small CDH, ultrasound may be able to depict the hemidiaphragm and the defect.
- The absence of the stomach bubble and small bowel in the abdomen supports the diagnosis of CDH.
- Always assess the positions of the umbilical arterial and venous catheters:
  - The umbilical arterial catheter passes from the umbilical artery into the internal iliac artery (where it is seen to "loop" on the plain film), and then into the aorta. On the plain film, the tip should be sited to the left of the midline between T6 and T10 or below L2, away from the major aortic branches. In the United Kingdom, it is usually positioned in the more cranial position.
  - The umbilical venous catheter passes from the umbilical vein to the left portal vein, ductus venosus, and finally the inferior vena cava. The tip should lie in the region of the cardiophrenic recess, that is, within the cephalad portion of the inferior vena cava.

Differential Diagnosis

Congenital cystic adenomatoid malformation (CCAM):
- Multiple cystic structures can be seen within the lung, with contralateral mediastinal displacement.
- There is a more stable position of the abnormality on serial films, whereas this may vary in CDH.
- Air–fluid levels are more likely in CCAM.
- If there is greater suspicion of CCAM, a CT examination may be performed, which will show the diaphragm to be intact and confirm the cystic abnormality in the lung.

Notes

- Hernias through the foramen of Bochdalek occur posterolaterally with a frequency of between 1 in 2,000 and 1 in 5,000 live births, and are more common on the left side (70%).
- Anterior retrosternal hernias through the foramen of Morgagni are right-sided in 90% of cases.
- Most neonates present at birth with severe respiratory distress. The sensitivity of ultrasound for the prenatal detection of CDH ranges from 18 to 87%, and appears to increase in the presence of associated, more easily observed anomalies and advancing gestational age.
- If detected antenatally, fetal endoscopic tracheal occlusion can be performed in selected cases. The procedure is based on the concept that lung growth can be triggered by tracheal occlusion. On the postnatal plain film, a radiodense marker is seen overlying the trachea if the residual balloon has not been removed.
- Abnormalities associated with CDH:
  - Cardiac anomalies are reported in up to 50% and include ventricular septal defects, transposition of the great vessels, and tetralogy of Fallot.
  - Oesophageal atresia may occur, with absence of bowel gas and opacification of the affected chest.

Bibliography

Taylor GA, Atalabi OM, Estroff JA. Imaging of congenital diaphragmatic hernias. Pediatr Radiol 2009;39(1):1–16

Deprest J, Nicolaides K, Done' E, et al. Technical aspects of fetal endoscopic tracheal occlusion for congenital diaphragmatic hernia. J Pediatr Surg 2011;46(1):22–32

6.4 Congenital Lobar Emphysema

Clinical History

A 3-week-old neonate presents with dyspnoea (**Fig. 6.4.1**).

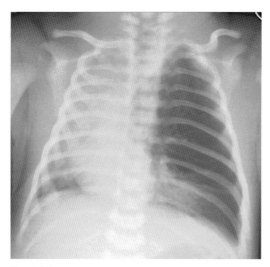

Fig. 6.4.1

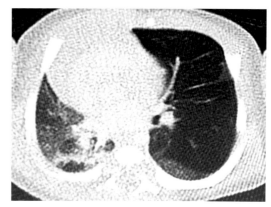

Fig. 6.4.2

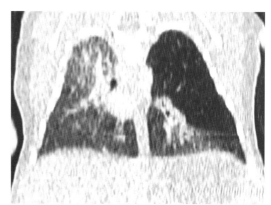

Fig. 6.4.3

Ideal Summary

This is a frontal chest radiograph of a neonate. There is a hyperlucent area with lung markings filling most of the left hemithorax. This is causing mediastinal shift to the right with increased opacification in most of the right lung as well as the left base, which may be due to collapse. The most likely differential diagnosis is congenital lobar emphysema (CLE), but other differentials include congenital cystic adenomatoid malformation (CCAM). I would like to check any previous imaging if available, and I would confirm the diagnosis with CT.

These are selected images from the CT chest examination (**Figs. 6.4.2** and **6.4.3**).

These are coronal and axial images on lung window settings through the chest. There is overexpansion of the left upper lobe, resulting in atelectasis of the left lower lobe and a portion of the right lung. I would like to assess the remainder of the study for bronchial atresia. If the bronchial tree is normal, the most likely diagnosis is CLE. I would refer the patient to the paediatric respiratory unit for further management.

Examination Tips

When dealing with hyperlucent lung on a plain film, assess the following:

- Distribution. Does it involve more than one lobe— the left upper lobe is most commonly affected in CLE.
- A mass effect can produce a variety of patterns. It is important to be aware of these and adjust your differential accordingly:
  - Congenital lobar emphysema in a single lobe may result in collapse and opacification of the ipsilateral lobe and contralateral lung.

- Congenital lobar emphysema in an entire lung may cause collapse and opacification of the contralateral lung.
- Volume loss of a single lobe causes opacification of that lobe, but lucency in the adjacent ipsilateral lobes and the contralateral lung.
- Volume loss of an entire lung (pulmonary agenesis or hypoplasia) causes opacification of that lung as well as lucency of the contralateral lung.
- Ancillary features:
  - Assess the bronchial tree and size of pulmonary vessels:
    - Attenuated pulmonary vessels in CLE
    - Hilar/tubular mass: this is suggestive of bronchial atresia with distended or plugged airways distal to the atretic segment
    - Small or absent bronchus and pulmonary artery in pulmonary hypoplasia.
  - The presence of cysts within the hyperlucent area may be due to CCAM or congenital diaphragmatic hernia (CDH). Look for varying size of the cysts in CCAM, and check for continuation of bowel loops below the level of the diaphragm in CDH.
  - CT may differentiate CLE (bronchovascular bundles at the periphery of lucent areas) from persistent pulmonary interstitial emphysema (bronchovascular bundles at the centre of cysts).

Differential Diagnosis

- Congenital hypoplasia of the lung:
  - The thoracic wall may be underdeveloped, with loss of volume on the affected side.
  - This is associated with cardiac abnormalities, scimitar syndrome, diaphragmatic abnormalities, gastrointestinal and genitourinary abnormalities (cystic renal disease), tracheo-oesophageal fistula, and imperforate anus.
- Reversible atelectasis:
  - Bronchial mucous plugs can be visualised on CT imaging.
  - Appearances typically resolve on follow-up imaging.
- Bronchial atresia:
  - The characteristic CT finding is a central opacity that may have a tubular shape or may contain an air–fluid level representing the obstructed, dilated, and mucoid-filled segmental or subsegmental bronchus.
  - Hyperinflation due to collateral air drift and a relative dearth of vessels due to obstructed or nonexistent blood supply in the involved segment of lung are also frequently seen on CT imaging.

Notes

- Congenital lobar emphysema should be considered when an opacified lobe becomes progressively hyperlucent and hyperinflated just after birth on serial radiographs.
- The left upper lobe is the most commonly affected, followed by right middle lobe, right upper lobe, and lower lobes. Occasionally, more than one lobe is involved.
- Surgical resection of the affected lobe is indicated, especially in patients with progressive hyperinflation of CLE, which can be life-threatening.

Bibliography

Lee EY, Boiselle PM, Cleveland RH. Multidetector CT evaluation of congenital lung anomalies. Radiology 2008;247(3):632–648

6.5   Hepatoblastoma

Clinical History

*A 2-year-old child presents with increasing abdominal girth (**Fig. 6.5.1**).*

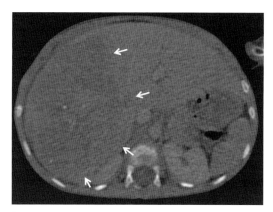

Fig. 6.5.1

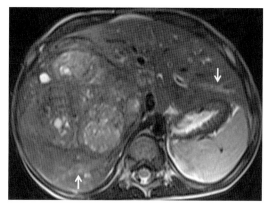

Fig. 6.5.2

Ideal Summary

This is a noncontrast axial CT image through the upper abdomen of a young child. There is a large predominantly low-attenuation lesion in the right lobe of the liver (**Fig. 6.5.1**, arrows). This contains a few small foci of high density, likely to be calcification. No biliary dilatation or ascites is seen. I would like to review the remainder of the study and ask for contrast-enhanced images. Any further evaluation of this abnormality should be performed with MRI.

*These are selected images from an MRI examination of the same patient (**Figs. 6.5.2** and **6.5.3**).*

These are selected axial T2-weighted MRI scans through the upper abdomen. In the right lobe of the liver, there is a large multilobulated lesion that is well circumscribed and demonstrates mixed signal intensity. I cannot see any biliary duct dilatation. There is a mass effect with displacement of the inferior vena cava to the left of midline. I cannot see the right hepatic or portal vein, but I am able to identify the left and right hepatic veins (**Fig. 6.5.2**, arrows). I would like to review all the images to assess for vascular occlusion and the presence of a separate intra-abdominal mass, and to confirm that this is a solitary liver lesion. The findings in a child of this age are likely to represent a

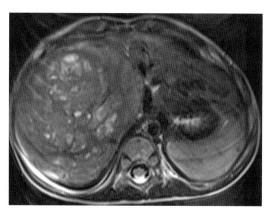

Fig. 6.5.3

primary hepatic tumour, such as a hepatoblastoma. I would recommend referral to a specialist paediatric oncology centre and correlation with serum alphafetoprotein levels.

Examination Tips

The assessment of a liver mass may be difficult due to the lack of pathognomonic imaging characteristics. However, careful identification of following features will narrow the differential diagnosis:

- Listen to the examiner for the patient's age. Hepatoblastoma peaks at 1 to 2 years, with hepatocellular carcinoma (HCC) rare below the age of 3.
- Hepatoblastoma is typically large at presentation and is usually single.
- Calcification is not a differentiating feature, being present in 50%.

Hepatoblastoma is classically of low density on CT and low T1/high T2 signal on MRI, although the degree of haemorrhage and necrosis will alter these characteristics.

Look for mass effect: hepatoblastoma is more likely to displace rather than invade the hepatic structures.

Serum alphafetoprotein is positive in hepatoblastoma (70 to 90% of cases) and HCC (80% of cases), and is negative in haemangioendothelioma.

Differential Diagnosis

HCC: This is the most common liver tumour in children over 5 years.

Metastatic disease: This is most commonly from other intra-abdominal primary tumours such as Wilms' tumour, neuroblastoma, or rhabdomyosarcoma.

Notes

Hepatoblastoma is the most common primary malignant hepatic tumour and accounts for 79% of all liver tumours in children.

Typically, the tumour enhances heterogeneously with intravenous contrast medium, but enhancement is less than the normal liver.

High survival rates are seen in those who have complete surgical clearance of the tumour at diagnosis, followed by adjuvant chemotherapy.

If performing an ultrasound examination:
- Always check the patency of the portal and hepatic veins, hepatic artery, inferior vena cava, and aorta with colour Doppler imaging.
- Look carefully for other subtle hepatic lesions.
- Always assess for biliary dilatation as decompression may be necessary depending on the patient's clinical status.

Abnormalities associated with hepatoblastoma:
- Beckwith–Weidemann syndrome. There is likely to be hepatomegaly, in addition to hypertrophy of other solid abdominal and pelvic viscera.
- Familial adenomatosis polyposis coli. Look at the bowel for large polyps.

Bibliography
Das CJ, Dhingra S, Gupta AK, Iyer V, Agarwala S. Imaging of paediatric liver tumours with pathological correlation. Clin Radiol 2009;64(10):1015–1025

6.6 Hirschsprung's Disease

Clinical History

*A neonate that has failed to pass meconium (**Fig. 6.6.1**).*

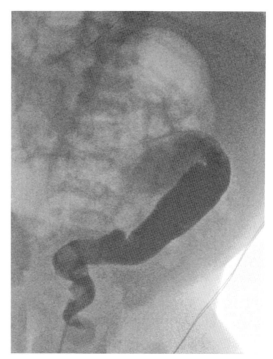

Fig. 6.6.2

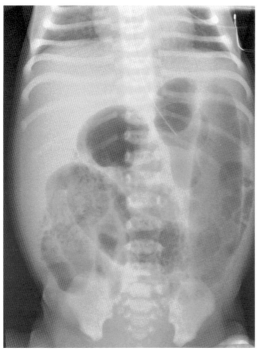

Fig. 6.6.1

Ideal Summary

This is a supine abdominal radiograph of a neonate. There are multiple, markedly dilated loops of bowel within the abdomen with a paucity of bowel gas seen in the pelvis. A nasogastric tube is correctly positioned. There is no free gas. The appearances are those of a distal bowel obstruction. The differential diagnosis includes Hirschsprung's disease and meconium plug syndrome. If the neonate is not septic, I would perform a water-soluble contrast enema to assess the extent and cause of obstruction.

*This is an image from the contrast examination (**Fig. 6.6.2**).*

This is a selected anteroposterior image from a contrast enema study. The sigmoid and descending colon are dilated, and there is a transition point in the region of the rectosigmoid junction. The rectum is abnormally narrowed. I would like to view the rest of the series. The most likely diagnosis is Hirschsprung's disease, and I would inform the paediatric surgeons.

Examination Tips

When shown a contrast enema, comment on the following:
- Ask for all available views. Early filling anteroposterior and lateral views are essential.
- The rectum is normally bigger than the sigmoid colon. A rectum:sigmoid ratio of less than 1 is suggestive of Hirschsprung's disease.
- The rectum is always involved, but it is important to assess the extent of colonic involvement:
  - Hirschsprung's disease may involve the entire colon, producing a "microcolon" appearance.
  - Other causes of microcolon include meconium ileus and ileal atresia.

Differential Diagnosis

- Meconium plug syndrome (also known as functional immaturity of the colon):
  - Meconium plug syndrome demonstrates a normal rectosigmoid ratio with a small left colon and transition point at the splenic flexure. This may be difficult to differentiate from a long segment of Hirschsprung's disease.
  - A contrast enema should demonstrate intraluminal colonic filling defect (meconium plugs).
  - This condition is often self-limiting, and contrast enema can be therapeutic by washing out the meconium plugs.
- Colonic stenosis:
  - The majority of cases are acquired, as a complication of necrotising enterocolitis (NEC).
  - Contrast enema will show focal narrowing with varying degrees of dilated bowel proximal to the stricture, depending on the degree of stenosis.
  - The history is very important, as a colonic stricture after NEC is not likely to be Hirschsprung's disease.

Notes

- Hirschsprung's disease is defined by the absence of ganglion cells within a portion of colon.
- The rectum is most commonly affected; however, any part of the bowel can be involved.
- The diagnosis is made by rectal biopsy.
- Surgical resection of the aganglionic segment of colon is the definitive treatment.
- In the long term, 75% of children will suffer from some form of continence or constipation problem.
- There are many anomalies associated with Hirschsprung's disease, divided into neural crest-related anomalies, cardiovascular skeletal and limb anomalies, cleft palate, and trisomy 21.

Bibliography

Kenny SE, Tam PK, Garcia-Barcelo M. Hirschsprung's disease. Semin Pediatr Surg 2010;19(3):194–200

Fotter R. Imaging of constipation in infants and children. Eur Radiol 1998;8(2):248–258

6.7 Intussusception

Clinical History

*An 8-month-old infant presents with increasing irritability and a lack of feeding (**Fig. 6.7.1**).*

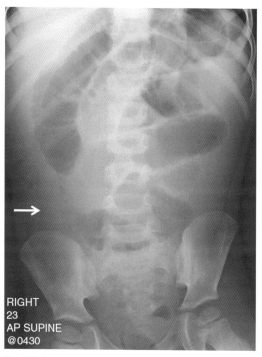

Fig. 6.7.1

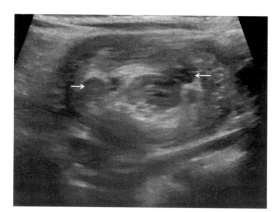

Fig. 6.7.2

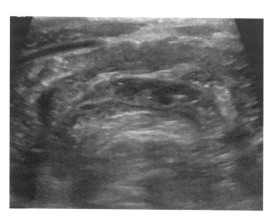

Fig. 6.7.3

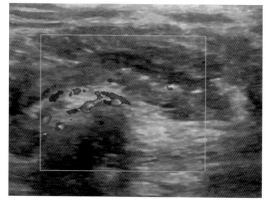

Fig. 6.7.4

Ideal Summary

This is a supine abdominal radiograph. A nasogastric tube is in a satisfactory position. There are loops of dilated proximal bowel, with a paucity of bowel gas seen in the right iliac fossa. There is a suggestion of a soft tissue abnormality in the right iliac fossa, with a paucity of gas in the ascending colon (**Fig. 6.7.1**, arrow). No free intraperitoneal gas is evident. In this age group and with these symptoms, I think an intussusception is very likely, and I would perform an immediate ultrasound examination.

*These are the images from the subsequent ultrasound examination (**Figs. 6.7.2–6.7.4**).*

These are transverse and longitudinal ultrasound images, depicting a soft tissue mass with layers of alternating reflectivity. A few lymph nodes are also seen within this mass (**Fig. 6.7.2**, arrows). The mass shows some vascularity on Doppler ultrasound. There is no free fluid. This confirms the diagnosis of intussusception, with enlarged lymph nodes probably acting as the lead point. I would contact the paediatric surgeons and discuss with them air reduction with fluoroscopy.

Examination Tips

- On the plain film, dilated loops of bowel should always alert the observer to seek out a soft tissue abnormality, with the distended loops proximal to the mass indicating the presence of an intussusception.
- Ultrasonography is the ideal method for diagnosis. The incidence of perforation with air enema reduction is approximately 1%.
- Contraindications to air reduction include bowel perforation, peritonitis, and shock. It is important to identify free fluid on the ultrasound examination as this raises the possibility of bowel perforation.
- Air enema reduction should only be attempted in the presence of a paediatric surgeon, with prior patient hydration with intravenous fluids if needed.
- During the procedure, the intussusception mass should be seen to move proximally and then disappear as air enters the small bowel. This indicates a successful reduction.
- The recurrence rate after enema reduction is around 10%. These cases can be treated nonsurgically even if they occur several times, with enema reduction.

Differential Diagnosis

There are no differential diagnoses for the above imaging appearances.

Notes

- Ileocolic intussusception typically affects the 3 month to 1 year age group.
- Intussusception is the most common cause of acute bowel obstruction in neonates, and usually involves both the small and large bowel.
- The most frequently seen location of intussusception is in the right upper quadrant, due to idiopathic ileocolic intussusception.
- Pathological lead points are present in around 5 to 6% of children with intussusception; these include lymph nodes, Meckel's diverticulum, duplication cysts, polyps, and, less commonly, lymphoma.
- Ultrasound examination has a high accuracy in diagnosis, with a sensitivity of 98 to 100% and a specificity of 88 to 100%.

Bibliography

Ko HS, Schenk JP, Tröger J, Rohrschneider WK. Current radiological management of intussusception in children. Eur Radiol 2007;17(9):2411–2421

6.8 Malrotation

Clinical History

A 2-day-old neonate presents with bilious vomiting (**Fig. 6.8.1**).

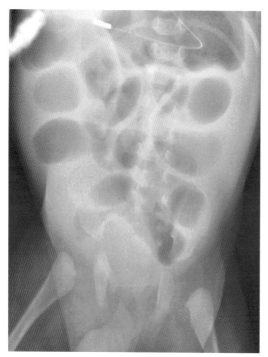

Fig. 6.8.1

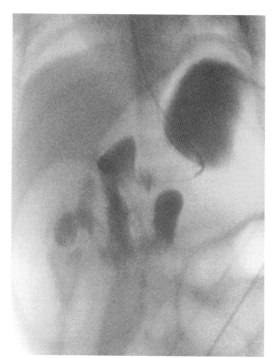

Fig. 6.8.2

Ideal Summary

This is a plain abdominal film with the tip of the nasogastric tube projected over the stomach. There are multiple loops of distended bowel sited within the abdomen that are gas-filled, in keeping with bowel obstruction. No distal bowel loops or gas in the rectum can be seen. There is no bowel gas in the hernial orifices, and I can see no free gas. Given the clinical symptoms, I would be concerned about malrotation, and I would discuss the case with the paediatric surgeons with a view to an upper gastrointestinal contrast study.

*These are images from an upper gastrointestinal contrast study of the same patient (**Figs. 6.8.2** and **6.8.3**).*

These are selected images from an upper gastrointestinal contrast study. The duodenojejunal flexure is low-lying to the left of the L3 vertebra, and below the level

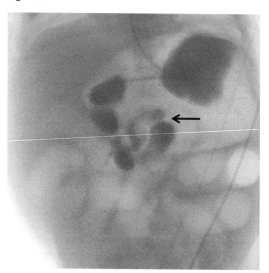

Fig. 6.8.3

of the pylorus (**Fig. 6.8.3**, arrow). Furthermore, the opacified jejunal loops are located in the right upper quadrant. I would like to review the remainder of the series, but these appearances are strongly suggestive of malrotation. While there is no obvious volvulus of the proximal small bowel loops, the cause of the bowel obstruction may be due to volvulus distally. I would urgently discuss the case with the paediatric surgeons.

Examination Tips

- Always think of malrotation in a patient with bowel obstruction as the consequence is bowel necrosis.
- If there are multiple dilated loops of bowel within the abdomen and you are "stuck" between small bowel and colonic pathology, make sure you exclude important causes first. The examiner will be more lenient if you are safe and logical.
- The presence of bilious vomiting plus features consistent with malrotation constitutes a surgical emergency.
- The normal duodenojejunal flexure lies in the transpyloric plane on the left side (commonly to the left of the L1 pedicle).
- On a lateral view, the duodenum should course posteriorly before diving inferiorly. The posterior course may be absent in malrotation.
- In borderline cases, it is important to identify the caecum on a small bowel follow-through; it should be located in the right lower quadrant.
- If the contrast study is equivocal, an ultrasound may help confirm that the superior mesenteric artery lies to the left of the vein. If these are reversed in position, this would support the diagnosis of malrotation.
- The "corkscrew" appearance of the small bowel twisting around the superior mesenteric artery on an upper gastrointestinal contrast study is associated with the presence of midgut volvulus.
- Always assess for complications:
  - Intra-abdominal free gas (perforation)
  - Portal venous gas (bowel ischaemia).

Differential Diagnosis

No differential diagnoses should be offered in a case with the above findings.

Notes

- Around 30 to 40% present within the first 10 days of life, the majority within the first month.
- Malrotation is commonly seen in gastroschisis and omphalocoele, but also in patients with duodenal and jejunoileal atresia.
- Malrotation is associated with Hirschsprung's disease, intussusception, cloacal anomalies, and imperforate anus.
- Malrotation is defined as the abnormal rotation and fixation of the small bowel mesentery, resulting in a short mesenteric root, which then allows the bowel to twist and cause a volvulus.
- When performing an upper gastrointestinal contrast series, water-soluble contrast should be used as barium could cause a severe peritonitis if perforation were to occur or if there were intraoperative spill of contrast from the bowel.
- The Ladd's procedure is performed to treat malrotation, this consists of:
  - Reduction of the volvulus, if present
  - Dissection of mesenteric bands
  - Positioning the small bowel on the right and the large bowel on the left of the abdomen
  - Appendicectomy

Bibliography

Long FR, Kramer SS, Markowitz RI, Taylor GE. Radiographic patterns of intestinal malrotation in children. Radiographics 1996;16(3):547–556, discussion 556–560

6.9 Meconium Aspiration Syndrome

Clinical History

A neonate presents with intrauterine distress (**Fig. 6.9.1**).

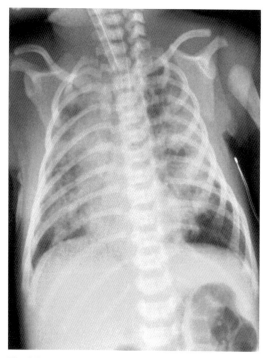

Fig. 6.9.1

Ideal Summary

This is a frontal chest radiograph of a neonate. The tip of the endotracheal tube is high in position and should ideally lie at the T2 to T3 level. The distal end of the nasogastric tube is in the region of the gastro-oesophageal junction and should be advanced further. There is hyperinflation of the lungs. There are coarse opacities throughout both lungs, which are asymmetrical in distribution. No pleural fluid is present. There is increased lucency at the left base, but no definite pneumothorax is present on this frontal view. I would like to see a lateral view to confirm the absence of a pneumothorax. Given the history, the lung appearances are most likely due to meconium aspiration syndrome (MAS). I would discuss these findings with the neonatal team, after reviewing any previous imaging.

Examination Tips

Plain film findings do not correlate with severity of clinical symptoms and may appear much worse than the clinical picture or vice versa. Other radiographic features seen in MAS include the following:
- There are high lung volumes, areas of hyperinflation being mixed with areas of atelectasis, usually asymmetrically.
- Pleural effusions are uncommon.
- Pneumothorax is common and, together with pneumomediastinum, must be excluded.
- The chemical pneumonitis may show progressive air-space opacification on successive films.
- New areas of focal consolidation on serial films may be due to superadded infection, as there is increased susceptibility to pneumonia.

Differential Diagnosis

- Neonatal pneumonia:
  - The plain film appearance is of patchy perihilar air-space opacification and hyperinflated lungs. Pleural fluid may be present.
  - Distinction from MAS is difficult on a plain film, and it may be necessary to ask the examiner for the relevant clinical history. Blood and sputum cultures may yield the diagnosis.
- Transient tachypnea of the newborn:
  - This is due to late clearance of fetal lung fluid, and hence is more common with caesarian deliveries as the "compression" effect of vaginal delivery is absent.
  - The plain film will show features similar to those of pulmonary oedema, that is, perihilar opacities, interstitial lines, pleural effusions, and cardiomegaly.
  - Lung volumes may also be increased.
  - There is a benign course, with improving symptoms and plain film appearances by 2 to 3 days.

Notes

During delivery, approximately 9% of term babies pass meconium, and 20% of these will become symptomatic. The treatment is supportive, with oxygen therapy, ventilation, and extracorporeal membrane oxygenation needed in severe cases. The inhaled meconium is toxic in several ways:

- Meconium occupying the distal airways can have a "ball-valve" effect causing air-trapping and air leaks.
- Meconium causes irritation of the lung parenchyma resulting in pneumonitis, which predisposes to infection.

An echocardiogram is necessary to evaluate the cardiac structure and function, in addition to assessing the degree of pulmonary hypertension and right-to-left shunting.

Bibliography

Cleveland RH. A radiologic update on medical diseases of the newborn chest. Pediatr Radiol 1995;25(8):631–637

6.10 Necrotising Enterocolitis

Clinical History

*A premature neonate presents with increasing abdominal distension and unstable blood pressure (**Fig. 6.10.1**).*

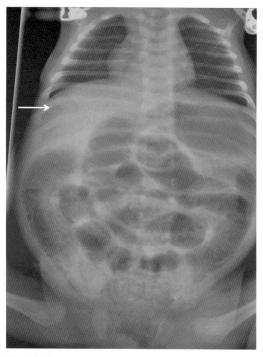

Fig. 6.10.1

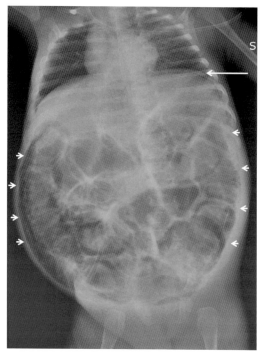

Fig. 6.10.2

Ideal Summary

This is a supine radiograph of the chest and abdomen of a neonate. There are dilated loops of bowel throughout the abdomen. Multiple "mottled" lucencies are seen overlying the distended bowel, which are highly suspicious for intramural gas. In addition, there are linear lucencies projected over the liver (**Fig. 6.10.1**, arrow) that reach the periphery of the liver, likely to represent portal venous gas. I cannot see any free intraperitoneal gas. No other abnormality is seen in the chest. Given the clinical history, the appearances are consistent with necrotising enterocolitis (NEC) with portal venous gas, but without evidence of perforation. I would immediately inform the referring team and recommend an urgent paediatric surgical review.

*This is another neonate in the intensive care unit (**Fig. 6.10.2**).*

This is a supine radiograph of the chest and abdomen of a neonate. The nasogastric tube and umbilical vein catheter are adequately sited. The abdomen is grossly distended. There are multiple loops of very dilated bowel, with lucencies overlying the bowel wall, consistent with intramural gas. In addition, there is a "football sign" (**Fig. 6.10.2**, short arrows) and gas seen under the left hemidiaphragm (**Fig. 6.10.2**, long arrow), in keeping with free intraperitoneal gas. The diagnosis is NEC with perforation. This is a surgical emergency, and I would immediately inform the paediatric surgeons.

Examination Tips

- The candidate must have a high index of suspicion for NEC in a premature neonate.
- The following signs must be identified and commented upon:

Pneumatosis. This is diagnostic of NEC, but may not always be present:
- It may produce a bubbly appearance, mimicking stool (which is not present in premature neonates), or curvilinear lucencies.
- Portal venous gas is usually not identified unless the candidate specifically looks for this:
  - Beware—the most frequent cause of portal venous gas in neonates is small quantities of air passing through an umbilical venous catheter in the absence of NEC.
- Free gas:
  - If you are not sure, ask for a lateral decubitus view to show you are a safe radiologist.
  - Free intraperitoneal gas on the plain film is the only universally accepted radiological finding for surgical intervention.

Generalised bowel dilatation occurs during the early phase of NEC. However, the development of focal bowel dilatation with a persistent asymmetrical pattern indicates the development of full-thickness bowel infarction.

CT imaging is not needed as the plain film findings are unequivocal.

Differential Diagnosis

No differential diagnosis should be offered with these imaging findings.

Notes

- Necrotising enterocolitis is one of the most common acquired, life-threatening gastrointestinal conditions in premature neonates, affecting up to 10% of neonates with a birth weight under 1,500 g.
- The overall mortality rate lies between 20 and 40%.
- High-frequency ultrasound can assess bowel wall thickness, peristalsis, perfusion, intramural gas, free fluid, and intra-abdominal collections.
- Enemas are contraindicated in acute NEC.

Bibliography

Epelman M, Daneman A, Navarro OM, et al. Necrotizing enterocolitis: review of state-of-the-art imaging findings with pathologic correlation. Radiographics 2007;27(2):285–305

6.11 Osteogenesis Imperfecta

Clinical History

A child presents with pain in the right leg for 2 days (**Fig. 6.11.1**).

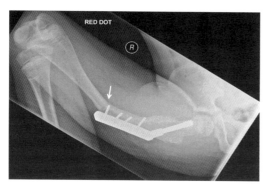

Fig. 6.11.1

Ideal Summary

This is radiograph of the right femur of a child. There is a dynamic hip screw on the proximal femur. The bones are osteopaenic and gracile. Old fractures at the femoral neck and proximal shaft are seen. There is a transverse fracture of the midfemoral shaft just distal to the dynamic hip screw plate (**Fig. 6.11.1**, arrow). There are also multiple transverse sclerotic lines at the distal femoral and proximal tibial metaphyses. The appearances are consistent with an acute fracture on a background of osteogenesis imperfecta (OI); the sclerotic bands are most likely to be secondary to bisphosphonate therapy or growth arrest lines. I would inform the referring clinician and review any other available imaging.

These are some images from a different patient; an 8-week-old infant (**Figs. 6.11.2** and **6.11.3**)

These are plain anterior–posterior radiographs of a skull and the left femur. There is bony deformity of the right skull vault with bony expansion and a lucent centre (**Fig. 6.11.2**, arrow), which does not cross the midline. This is in keeping with a cephalohaematoma. There is no evidence of acute fractures and there are no wormian bones. There is also a bony deformity of the left femur that appears bowed and there is periosteal reaction along the medial diaphysis (**Fig. 6.11.3**, arrow). Furthermore, the left femoral head is abnormal and appears flattened, most likely

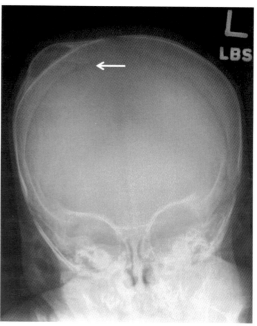

Fig. 6.11.2

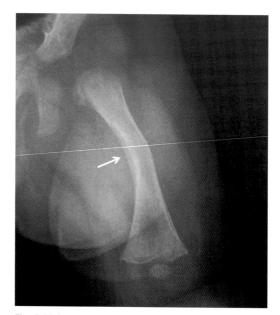

Fig. 6.11.3

representing avascular necrosis. Again, I can see no signs of acute fractures. There is no convincing evidence of osteopaenia.

The two main differentials I would be concerned about are nonaccidental injury and OI. I would like to review any other available images to look for any specific features to narrow my differentials, such as metaphyseal corner fractures or posteromedial rib fractures. At our institution, I would urgently inform the paediatric team.

Examination Tips

Depending on the bones visible on the film, look for the following where OI is suspected:
- Long bones:
  - Gracile bones with a thin cortex and osteopaenia
  - Thin metaphyseal bands parallel to the physis after bisphosphonate treatment
  - Exuberant callus formation
  - Fractures of different ages
  - Pseudoarthrosis
  - Coxa vara and protrusio acetabuli
  - Growth arrest lines are often present
- Skull:
  - Wormian bones
  - Platybasia is also seen
- Spine:
  - Platyspondyly with either wedged vertebral bodies or complete collapse
  - Kyphoscoliosis

Differential Diagnosis

Nonaccidental Injury

If nonaccidental injury (NAI) is suspected from the plain film findings then the referring clinician and paediatric consultant on call need to be immediately notified. To differentiate OI from NAI:
- Classic metaphyseal corner fractures are strongly suggestive of NAI, as opposed to OI where diaphyseal fractures are primarily seen.
  - Although classic metaphyseal corner fractures have been described in severe forms of OI, they have been associated with osteopaenia and/or wormian bones, so look for or ask for these features when presented with this case.
  - Furthermore, classic metaphyseal corner fractures are rare in children below 1 year of age.
- Posteromedial rib fractures are highly specific for NAI with rib fractures more likely to occur in the severe forms of OI and usually laterally. Again, look for signs of osteopaenia to suggest OI.
- Skull fractures are occasionally seen in OI, but are appropriately related to trauma.
- When reviewing an image with either classic metaphyseal corner fractures or posteromedial rib fractures, NAI must be top of your differential unless you have clear evidence of OI. In these cases, it is important to show you are safe:
  - If not given, ask for the patient's age
  - Say you would like to correlate with any relevant clinical history. This shows you are looking for mechanism of injury and if this is appropriate to the case.
  - If you are still unsure, ask to look at further imaging to help.
- A history and clinical examination by a paediatrician with experience of OI is always required before establishing the diagnosis.

Notes

- Osteogenesis imperfecta is a broad group of disorders.
- Initial classification involved four types based on abnormalities in type 1 collagen.
- However, there are now further types of OI that are not identifiable by investigations aimed at collagen 1, leading to potential difficulties with diagnosis.
- The most common form is type 1 OI, which causes mild to moderate disease, with blue sclera and wormian bones in the skull.
  - Hearing loss is common due to otosclerosis—the otic capsule is under-mineralised.
  - Neonatal fractures can occur during delivery and 10% have fractures in utero.
- The diagnosis can be made using collagen culture, which is positive in approximately 80% of patients with OI. However, this test should only be performed after meticulous history-taking and examination by specialists in this field.

Bibliography

Ablin DS. Osteogenesis imperfecta: a review. Can Assoc Radiol J 1998;49(2):110–123

Dwek JR. The radiographic approach to child abuse. Clin Orthop Relat Res. 2011;469:776-789.

6.12 Osteomyelitis

Clinical History

A 4-year-old boy presents with a painful ankle (**Fig. 6.12.1**).

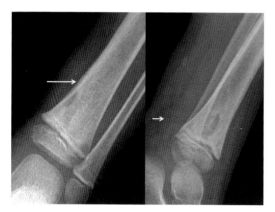

Fig. 6.12.1

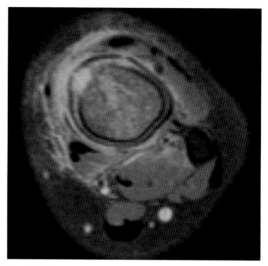

Fig. 6.12.2

Ideal Summary

These are anteroposterior and lateral radiographs of the distal tibia and fibula of a child. There is irregular lucency within the metaphysis of the distal tibia. I can also see a single layer periosteal reaction along the medial aspect of the distal tibia (**Fig. 6.12.1**, long arrow). There is associated soft tissue swelling posterior to the distal tibia (**Fig. 6.12.1**, short arrow) on the lateral view. There is no cortical destruction. The fibula and imaged talus look normal. These appearances are those of an aggressive process, such as osteomyelitis or malignancy. I would arrange for MRI of the ankle.

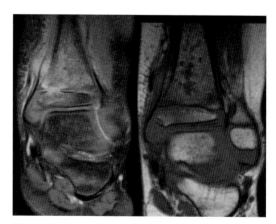

Fig. 6.12.3

These are the MR images from the same patient (**Figs. 6.12.2** and **6.12.3**).

These are selected axial and coronal short T1 inversion recovery (STIR) and T1-weighted images through the distal tibia and fibula. The periosteum is elevated at the medial distal tibial metaphysis. The STIR images show a medial subperiosteal collection in the tibia. There is also marrow oedema predominantly involving the metaphysis, but also crossing the physis to involve the epiphysis. Associated oedema of the surrounding tissues is present. On the T1-weighted image, multiple foci of low signal intensity are seen within the metaphysis and epiphysis. The appearances most likely represent acute osteomyelitis involving the distal tibial metaphysis and epiphysis. I would like to review further images of the series to identify any associated tibiotalar joint effusion, but no obvious effusion is present on the available images. I would advise an urgent referral to the orthopaedic team.

Examination Tips

In all cases of suspected osteomyelitis, comment on the following:

- Describe the location and extent of the abnormality clearly, and whether it crosses the physis.

- Is the abnormality permeative and is there cortical destruction?
- Comment on the zone of transition: a wide zone of transition implies an aggressive process.
- Look specifically for and characterise the type of periostitis.
- Check the soft tissues: look for soft tissue swelling and obliteration of the fat planes.

All patients with aggressive features should be inspected for the following, suggestive of osteomyelitis:
- An abscess can form within the bone; this is classically ring-enhancing on postcontrast T1-weighted MR images.

Differential Diagnosis

- Eosinophilic granuloma:
  - The plain film appearance depends on the phase of disease. In the acute phase, eosinophilic granuloma often has an aggressive, permeative, and lytic appearance.
  - Lytic lesions may contain a sequestrum, which can help in distinguishing them from malignancy, but not from osteomyelitis.
- Metastases:
  - The most frequent primary tumours to metastasise to bone are neuroblastoma (under 5 years of age) and leukaemia (above 5 years of age).
  - In a child under 3 years, metastasis of a neuroblastoma is much more likely than a primary bone tumour.

- Leukaemia can infiltrate the metaphyses and cause bone lysis; lucent metaphyseal bands are frequently seen.
- An abdominal ultrasound should identify a retroperitoneal neuroblastoma, which is the most common location. A white blood cell count and bone marrow aspirate or biopsy will help make the diagnosis of leukaemia.

Notes

- *Staphylococcus aureus* is responsible for osteomyelitis in children.
- Around 70% of osteomyelitis cases occur in the long bone metaphyses, particularly the distal femur and proximal tibia.
- Most cases of paediatric osteomyelitis occur secondary to haematogenous spread.
- Plain film features of osteomyelitis lag behind the onset of infection by at least 10 days. Initial radiographs are likely to appear normal.
- After around 10 to 14 days, lucencies appear in the metaphysis, with varying degrees of cortical destruction and periosteal reaction.
- After 10 to 12 weeks, sclerotic areas may be seen on radiographs, suggesting regenerative changes.

Bibliography

McCarville MB. The child with bone pain: malignancies and mimickers. Cancer Imaging 2009;9 (Spec No A): S115–S121

6.13 Osteosarcoma

Clinical History

*An 8-year-old boy presents with pain in his right leg after playing football (**Fig. 6.13.1**).*

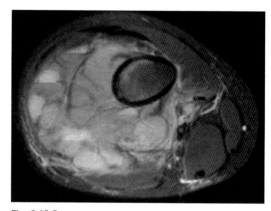

Fig. 6.13.2

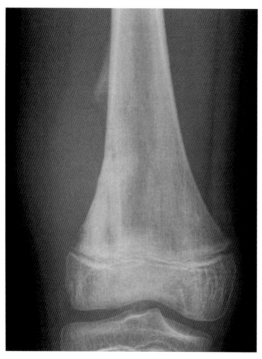

Fig. 6.13.1

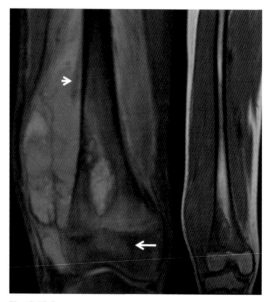

Fig. 6.13.3

Ideal Summary

This is a plain anteroposterior radiograph of the distal right femur. There is a mixed sclerotic and lytic lesion involving the distal femoral metadiaphysis. This has a permeative appearance. The lesion has a wide zone of transition, and I can also see cortical destruction. A Codman's triangle is present proximally. There is a soft tissue mass lateral to the distal femur, adjacent to the bone changes. No fracture is seen. These features are of an aggressive lesion and, if solitary, osteosarcoma is the most likely diagnosis. I would advise urgent MRI and referral to a bone tumour unit.

*These are the MR images from the same patient (**Figs. 6.13.2** and **6.13.3**).*

These are selected axial and coronal short T1 inversion recovery (STIR) plus coronal T1 images of the right distal femur. There is a large soft tissue mass completely surrounding the distal femur, with fluid–fluid levels present on the axial image. The abnormality in the femoral metaphysis is high signal on STIR and low signal on T1-weighted imaging. There is also increased STIR signal within the epiphysis (**Fig. 6.13.3**, long arrow), which may represent oedema, although transphyseal spread of tumour is possible. However, there is no obvious focal destruction of the physis. Some fluid is present in the knee joint. Periosteal elevation is also seen at the lateral femur as on the plain film (**Fig. 6.13.3**, short arrow). The presence of fluid–fluid levels is suggestive of telangiectatic osteosarcoma. I would recommend a staging CT chest and referral to a specialist paediatric bone tumour unit.

neurovascular bundle, features that impact surgical management.

- A CT chest is needed to assess for pulmonary metastases. The lungs are the preferential site for osteosarcoma metastases, which are often ossified.

Differential Diagnosis

No differential diagnosis should be offered in this case.

Examination Tips

- Osteosarcoma classically exhibits new bone formation beyond the area of normal bone.
- The telangiectatic subtype accounts for less than 5% of osteosarcomas and does not demonstrate new bone formation, but fluid–fluid levels may be seen on MRI.
- On plain film, the sunburst and spiculated type of periosteal reaction is the most commonly seen. This is almost pathognomonic of osteosarcoma; however, this may also be seen with osteoblastic metastases.
- Beware that a Codman's triangle can also be seen in osteomyelitis—look for the sequestrum in osteomyelitis. Ask if there is a history of sepsis.
- Skip lesions can occur with osteosarcoma, so assess the entire affected bone.
- Bone scan or whole-body MRI should be performed to look for further lesions.
- MRI is key to evaluating transphyseal spread of the tumour into the epiphysis, intra-articular extension of tumour, and involvement of the

Notes

- Osteosarcoma is the most common primary malignant bone tumour in children. It is most common in the 10- to 15-year age group.
- Osteosarcoma has a predilection for involving the metaphysis of the long bones, most frequently the distal femur, proximal tibia, and proximal humerus. Around 55 to 80% are located around the knee.
- The majority of patients present with pain.
- The mainstay of treatment is resection of the lesion. Limb-salvaging procedures can often be performed to preserve function. Chemotherapy is also required to treat micrometastases, which are present but are not detectable in the majority of patients at the time of diagnosis.

Bibliography

McCarville MB. The child with bone pain: malignancies and mimickers. Cancer Imaging 2009;9 (Spec No A): S115–S121

6.14 Perthes Disease

Clinical History

A 7-year-old boy presents with right hip pain (**Fig. 6.14.1**).

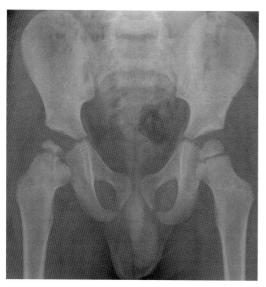

Fig. 6.14.1

Ideal Summary

This is an anteroposterior pelvic radiograph of a child. The right proximal femoral epiphysis is small, sclerotic, and irregular. The adjacent metaphysis is also irregular, splayed, and osteopaenic. There is widening of the right hip joint. The left hip appears normal. The most likely diagnosis is Perthes disease, and I would advise an orthopaedic referral.

Examination Tips

- If the anteroposterior film looks normal, a frog-leg lateral view is useful as the subchondral lucency (thought to represent a fracture) in the femoral epiphysis may be easier to detect.
- Assess:
  - Size and shape of the epiphysis
  - Presence of fragmentation and sclerosis
  - Amount of the epiphysis that is involved (> 50% involvement = worse prognosis)
  - Irregularity and splaying of the metaphysis

- Degree of widening of the joint space, and loss of contour of the acetabulum.
- As Perthes disease is a form of avascular necrosis, the imaging features are indistinguishable from those of other causes, although they are more commonly bilateral:
  - In leukaemia and lymphoma, the bones may have a generalised permeative appearance or lucent lesions.
  - In sickle cell anaemia, look for H-shaped vertebrae.
  - Sacroiliitis and bowel wall thickening may be seen in inflammatory bowel disease.

Differential Diagnosis

- Septic arthritis:
  - Septic arthritis may be indistinguishable from Perthes disease. Ultimately, a history of sepsis is key to making the diagnosis.
  - In the acute stage, the plain film may look normal.
  - There should be bone changes on both sides of the joint in the chronic phase, such as sclerosis, irregularity, modelling deformity. Asymmetrical epiphyseal growth can be seen if the physis has been damaged.
  - If there is clinical suspicion of septic arthritis, ask if there is a history of sepsis. The presence of a joint effusion may be demonstrated on ultrasound.
- Other causes of avascular necrosis include:
  - Trauma
  - Radiation
  - Sickle cell disease
  - Gaucher's disease
  - Steroid therapy.

Notes

- Perthes disease is an idiopathic avascular necrosis of the femoral epiphysis, usually affecting 4- to 10-year-olds, and peaking between 5 and 7 years.
- Four times as many boys are affected as girls.
- Bilateral disease is seen in 10%.
- If the diagnosis is unclear, MRI is helpful. In early Perthes disease, this would show low T1 signal in the femoral epiphysis corresponding to a loss of

normal fatty marrow, and an increased signal on T2, reflecting marrow oedema.

- A bone scan would show a reduction of uptake of tracer on the affected side; this is usually seen before plain film signs appear.
- Treatment consists of rest to reduce weight-bearing on the femoral head. Sometimes orthoses such as an abduction brace can help lessen stress on the femoral head.

- Older children (> 6 years) have a poorer prognosis than younger children.

Bibliography

Houghton KM. Review for the generalist: evaluation of pediatric hip pain. Pediatr Rheumatol Online J 2009;7:10

6.15 Respiratory Distress Syndrome

Clinical History

A neonate presents with shortness of breath (**Fig. 6.15.1**).

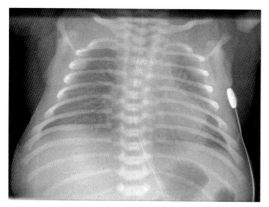

Fig. 6.15.1

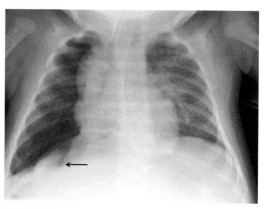

Fig. 6.15.2

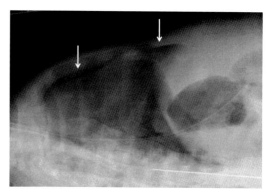

Fig. 6.15.3

Ideal Summary

This is a frontal chest radiograph of a neonate. I note the absence of the humeral head ossification centres, suggesting this is a premature neonate. The distal end of the nasogastric tube is projected beyond the edge of the film. There is diffuse ground-glass opacification throughout both lungs, and the lung volumes are normal. No pneumothorax or pleural effusion is present. The heart and mediastinal contours look normal. Assuming this is a premature neonate, the most likely diagnosis is respiratory distress syndrome (RDS).

*These are some images of the same neonate a few days later, without improvement (**Figs. 6.15.2** and **6.15.3**).*

These are frontal and high-beam lateral radiographs of the chest. The endotracheal tube is in a satisfactory position. The distal nasogastric tube is beyond the lower edge of the film. There is hyperlucency of the right hemithorax with a "deep sulcus sign" (**Fig. 6.15.2**, arrow) consistent with a right pneumothorax. Although the trachea is deviated to the right, the nasogastric tube and heart are sited centrally. The diagnosis is confirmed on the lateral film with pleural gas anteriorly (**Fig. 6.15.3**, arrows). There is diffuse ground-glass opacification in the left lung, in keeping with an underlying diagnosis of RDS. I would urgently inform the clinical team for consideration of a chest drain insertion.

Examination Tips

- Respiratory distress syndrome occurs in preterm infants. Look for an absence of the humeral head ossification centre, or the examiner may tell you in the history.
- Lung volumes are typically low in RDS due to collapsed alveoli, although this is increasingly absent with the use of surfactant therapy.
- Pleural effusions are rare. Consider pneumonia or transient tachypnea of the newborn if this is present.
- Check specifically for an air leak, which is a complication of therapy:
  - Pneumothorax. Infants are imaged in the supine position, and the signs of pneumothorax are

often more subtle, with increased lucency on one side.

- A pleural edge is often not seen in infants, and the diagnosis may be made by identifying a well-defined costophrenic recess (the "deep sulcus sign") or increased lucency adjacent to the mediastinum, where there is anterior pleural air.
- The presence of the anterior junctional line, which is not normally seen on chest radiographs of healthy infants, can suggest bilateral pneumothorax.

- Pneumomediastinum. Mediastinal gas may elevate the lobes of the thymus ("angel wing sign") or track within the mediastinal pleural, outlining both parietal and visceral pleural surfaces. Gas can also pass into the retroperitoneum, so always check below the diaphragm on a chest film.
- Pneumopericardium. Pericardial gas outlines the heart, but is restricted superiorly by the pericardial reflection at the great vessels.
- Pulmonary interstitial emphysema:
  - This usually occurs secondary to barotrauma and is also related to the sequelae of an air leak.
  - On the plain radiograph, there are tubular and cystic lucencies that do not correspond to the branching nature of air bronchograms.
  - Lung volumes are static in the affected areas, which may be highlighted on serial films.
  - On CT, there is a characteristic central arteriole (dots) seen within each cystic area in pulmonary interstitial emphysema, compared with the empty cysts seen in congenital cystic adenomatoid malformation.
- Another feature on the chest radiograph, related to prematurity, is bone disease of prematurity, which usually manifests as poorly mineralised bones.

Differential Diagnosis

- Pneumonia:
  - Plain film findings are nonspecific. There may be ground-glass opacification with or without

consolidation. The radiographic findings may be indistinguishable from those of RDS, so a history of sepsis should be sought.

- Pulmonary oedema:
  - Assess for cardiomegaly.
  - On the plain film, there is diffuse or perihilar opacification. Pleural effusions may also be seen.
  - An echocardiogram is needed to assess the heart for congenital anomalies and function of the heart.

Notes

- Respiratory distress syndrome is a common entity seen in premature neonates and is related to the inability of type II pneumatocytes to produce surfactant. Inadequate surfactant leads to alveolar deficiency and pulmonary interstitial thickness, which impede normal gas exchange.
- There is a higher risk of lung injury in these premature neonates secondary to prolonged mechanical ventilation.
- Initially, lung volumes are low, and they usually increase following surfactant administration, indicating a response to treatment.
- Chronic lung disease, also known as bronchopulmonary dysplasia, was originally believed to be consequent to positive-pressure mechanical ventilation and oxygen toxicity. Before using surfactant replacement therapy, chest radiographs of infants with chronic lung disease showed coarse reticular lung opacities, cystic lucencies, areas of fibrosis, and hyperinflation. However, with the advent of surfactant replacement, chronic lung disease is predominantly seen only in low-birth-weight neonates.

Bibliography

Agrons GA, Courtney SE, Stocker JT, Markowitz RI. From the archives of the AFIP. Lung disease in premature neonates: radiologic-pathologic correlation. Radiographics 2005;25(4):1047–1073

6.16 Sequestration

Clinical History

A neonate presents with a persistent infection (**Fig. 6.16.1**).

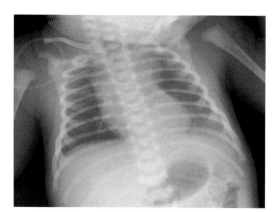

Fig. 6.16.1

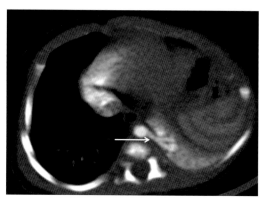

Fig. 6.16.2

Ideal Summary

This is a frontal chest radiograph of a neonate. There is ill-defined "hazy" opacification in the left lower zone. I cannot see any other focal lung abnormality. The heart and mediastinal contours are normal. This appearance is nonspecific, and the differential diagnosis includes segmental left lower lobe consolidation or a pleural effusion. A review of previous films would be helpful, as it may show this abnormality to be present on earlier radiographs. I would perform an ultrasound to assess for pleural fluid, and identify any underlying lung consolidation.

An ultrasound was performed, and CT imaging was then undertaken. These are the CT images (**Figs. 6.16.2–6.16.5**).

These are axial CT images through the chest. The images demonstrate a soft tissue abnormality in the left hemithorax with an arterial supply originating from a direct branch of the descending thoracic aorta (**Figs. 6.16.2** and **6.16.3**, long arrow). There is also venous drainage from the lesion (**Figs. 6.16.4** and **6.16.5**, short arrow) that leads into the left inferior pulmonary vein. No obvious pleural covering to the mass is evident. The diagnosis is that of sequestration,

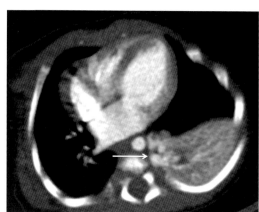

Fig. 6.16.3

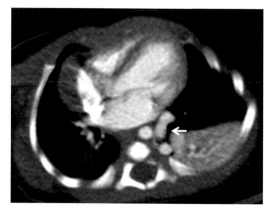

Fig. 6.16.4

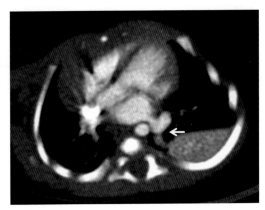

Fig. 6.16.5

which favours the intralobar type due to its venous drainage. I would inform the clinical team for further management.

Examination Tips

- Differentiating between intralobar and extralobar sequestration is difficult and not always possible on imaging:
  - In intralobar sequestration, the anomalous venous drainage usually flows into the inferior pulmonary vein.
  - In extralobar sequestration, the anomalous venous drainage is frequently systemic, but this is variable and it may also drain into the inferior pulmonary vein.
- The arterial supply is via a vessel from the descending aorta in both types of sequestration. The origin may be from the abdominal aorta in 20%.
- Gas is not usually found within the abnormal lung, unless it is associated with infection.
- Pulmonary sequestration may occasionally be found in association with congenital cystic adenomatoid malformation.
- Intralobar sequestration is not associated with congenital abnormalities.

- Extralobar sequestration is associated with up to 60% of other congenital anomalies, including congenital heart disease and diaphragmatic abnormality.
  - The chest radiograph may show an enlarged heart or abnormal mediastinal contour depending on the cardiac abnormality. An echocardiogram should be performed if there is suspicion of congenital heart disease.

Differential Diagnosis

No differential diagnosis should be offered in this case.

Notes

- Pulmonary sequestration denotes a congenital abnormal region of lung not connected to the bronchial tree or pulmonary arteries.
- For further evaluation, cross-sectional imaging is needed:
  - MRI or MR angiography provides information similar to that obtained from CT.
  - Ideally, MRI or MR angiography should be used as this has no radiation burden.
  - Isotropic MRI sequences mean that 1 mm slices can be obtained, which can be easily reconstructed into axial, sagittal, and coronal planes.
- Suspicion for sequestration should be raised when there is a history of recurrent infections in the left lower lobe in children.
- CT angiography with three-dimensional reconstruction is useful for evaluating anomalous vessels associated with sequestration, which helps in surgical planning.

Bibliography

Lee EY, Boiselle PM, Cleveland RH. Multidetector CT evaluation of congenital lung anomalies. Radiology 2008;247(3):632–648

6.17 Slipped Upper Femoral Epiphysis

Clinical History

A 12-year-old girl presents with pain in left hip (**Fig. 6.17.1**).

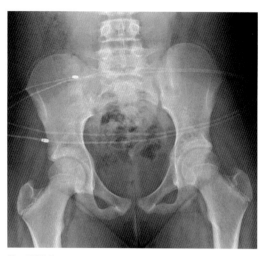

Fig. 6.17.1

Ideal Summary

This is a pelvic radiograph of a girl. Both hips appear normal. Klein's line intersects the epiphyses normally, and there is no widening of the physis. There is no evidence of sclerosis of the femoral head to suggest avascular necrosis. There is no evidence of an apophyseal injury that could account for the left hip pain. I would like to see a frog-leg lateral view to exclude a slipped upper femoral epiphysis (SUFE).

This is the view you requested (**Fig. 6.17.2**).

This is a frog-leg view. The left proximal femoral epiphysis has slipped medially, and there is lucency related to the physis. The right hip looks normal. The diagnosis is left SUFE. I would advise an urgent orthopaedic referral.

Examination Tips

- Normal radiographs do not always exclude a SUFE.

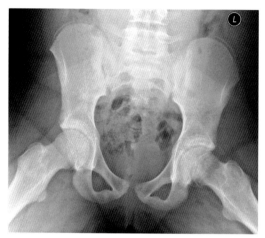

Fig. 6.17.2

- A slipped upper femoral epiphysis may be secondary to previous developmental dysplasia of the hip, so look for a shallow acetabulum.
- Avascular necrosis occurs in approximately 15%, and its presence or absence should be commented upon.
- Do not just look for asymmetry as SUFE may be bilateral in 20 to 40%. Use the radiological devised lines of normality.
- If the diagnosis is unclear, MRI can be performed, and you may ask for these images if uncertain.
- In pre-slip, there is widening of the physis with a variable degree of increased signal on T2 in the epiphysis and metaphysis, reflecting marrow oedema. No slippage of the epiphysis is seen at this stage.
- Later findings of SUFE on MRI would be similar to radiographs, but with posteromedial migration of the femoral epiphysis.

Differential Diagnosis

Acute trauma:
- A slipped upper femoral epiphysis is thought to be a Salter–Harris type 1 fracture from repetitive microtrauma. However, a single episode of trauma could cause the same fracture.
- An appropriate history of trauma and an acute presentation would point to this diagnosis.

Notes

- A slipped upper femoral epiphysis usually affects 11- to 14-year–olds.
- It is more prevalent in overweight children and boys.
- The vascular supply to the femoral head can be disrupted and cause avascular necrosis; therefore, all cases warrant urgent orthopaedic referral.
- Surgical treatment consists of pinning the epiphysis to preclude further slippage.
- Other complications include premature osteoarthritis, chondrolysis, and leg length discrepancy.

Bibliography

Boles CA, el-Khoury GY. Slipped capital femoral epiphysis. Radiographics 1997;17(4):809–823

Lalaji A, Umans H, Schneider R, Mintz D, Liebling MS, Haramati N. MRI features of confirmed "pre-slip" capital femoral epiphysis: a report of two cases. Skeletal Radiol 2002;31(6):362–365

6.18 Wilms' Tumour

Clinical History

A 4-year-old boy presents with abdominal discomfort (**Figs. 6.18.1–6.18.4**).

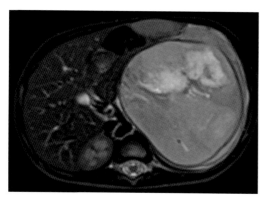

Fig. 6.18.1

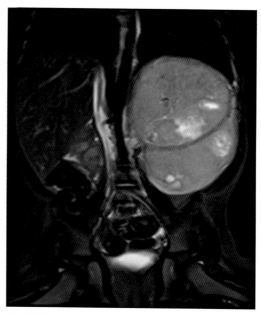

Fig. 6.18.3

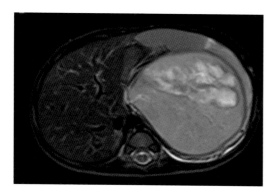

Fig. 6.18.2

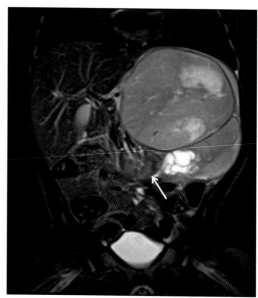

Fig. 6.18.4

Ideal Summary

These are selected axial and coronal short T1 inversion recovery images of the abdomen. There is a large multilobulated left flank mass, which is predominantly of intermediate T2 signal with focal areas of high signal. The aorta and coeliac axis are displaced to the right, and the spleen has been pushed anteriorly. The left kidney has been displaced inferiorly (**Fig. 6.18.4**, arrow) and is stretched, described as the "claw sign." The liver and right kidney appear normal. I would assess the renal vessels and inferior vena cava for thrombus or invasion, and review the remaining solid viscera and the lungs for metastatic disease on the whole series of images. The imaging findings are in keeping with a Wilms' tumour. I would advise urgent referral to a paediatric oncology centre, and I would discuss this with the paediatric team.

Examination Tips

In a case with suspected malignant nephroblastoma, comment on the following:

- Location. If the mass is centred on the flanks, renal pathology must be considered if the normal kidney cannot be identified.
- Size. There is usually a large mass at presentation that displaces, rather than encases, adjacent organs.
- Signal. It is classically heterogeneous with high T2 signal due to haemorrhage.
- Enhancement. There is less contrast enhancement than for the adjacent renal parenchyma.
- Margins:
  - There are well-defined margins, but look for the presence of invasion into the perinephric fat.
  - Always check the relationship of the mass with the aorta. In Wilms' tumour, extension across the midline typically passes anterior to the aorta, while neuroblastomas tend to encase the aorta, lifting it anteriorly.
  - Tumour thrombus. Check the renal vein, inferior vena cava, and right atrium.
- Look for homogeneous nephroblastomatosis on postcontrast T1-weighted images as approximately one-third will develop a Wilms' tumour.
- Contralateral kidney. Always check the other kidney: Wilms' tumours are bilateral in 5%, and are associated with nephroblastomatosis.
- Metastases. Lung metastases are present in 20% at time of diagnosis and must be excluded.

Differential Diagnosis

- Neuroblastoma:
  - This commonly demonstrates calcification.
  - It encases adjacent structures.
- Renal lymphoma:
  - This is a less common cause of renal malignancy.
  - Ultrasound may show solitary or multiple renal masses of low reflectivity, enlarged kidneys, and perirenal soft tissue masses.
  - On contrast-enhanced MRI, lymphoma tends to enhance less than normal renal tissue.

Notes

- There is a peak incidence of a nephroblastoma at around 3 years of age, with 80% occurring under 5 years of age.
- Syndromes with an increased predisposition to Wilms' tumour include Beckwith–Wiedemann syndrome and aniridia.
- Patients may experience pain if there is intratumoural haemorrhage; otherwise, this is commonly an asymptomatic abdominal mass.
- The prognosis is generally good. The overall 4-year survival rate is between 86 and 96% for those without metastatic disease outside the abdomen.

Bibliography

McHugh K. Renal and adrenal tumours in children. Cancer Imaging 2007;7(7):41–51

6.19 Developmental Dysplasia of the Hip

Clinical History

A 12-month-old infant presents with an abnormal gait (**Fig. 6.19.1**).

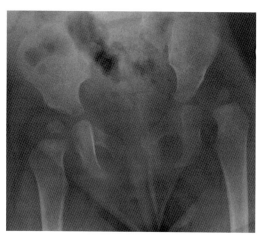

Fig. 6.19.1

*This is the same X-ray with Hilgenreiner's and Perkin's lines drawn on it (**Fig. 6.19.2**).*

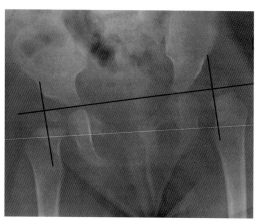

Fig. 6.19.2

Ideal Summary

This is a pelvic radiograph of an infant. The identical plain film of the pelvis has Perkin's and Hilgenreiner's lines overlaid. The left acetabular roof is very shallow. The left proximal femoral epiphysis is also small; it is located superolaterally, and does not lie within the hip joint. Using Perkin's and Hilgenreiner's lines, the left proximal femoral epiphysis is not located within the inner lower quadrant, where it should be normally. The right hip is normal. The most likely diagnosis is developmental dysplasia of the hip (DDH).

Examination Tips

- Various imaging modalities are used to investigate DDH:
  - Ultrasound is the investigation of choice in infants up to 8 months of age to monitor acetabular development and hip alignment. Sonography is also able to assess both the static and dynamic appearances of the hip joints, and thus can comment on instability.
  - Ideally, ultrasound should not be performed before 6 weeks as the hip is immature and may give a false-positive result.
  - The femoral head usually ossifies by 3 months and plain films are the modality of choice after 8 months.
  - CT and MRI may be performed to accurately assess the femoral head position postsurgically. MRI is preferred due to lack of ionising radiation, but this depends on local availability.
- Know your lines:
  - Hilgenreiner's line is a horizontal line along the superolateral aspect of triradiate cartilage.
  - Perkin's line is a perpendicular line drawn along the lateral edge of the acetabulum bisecting Hilgenreiner's line.
  - The femoral head should be located in the lower medial quadrant.
  - Always check Shenton's line, as it is discontinuous in the presence of hip subluxation or dislocation.

Differential Diagnosis

Proximal focal femoral deficiency:
- This is a developmental defect of the proximal femur. The abnormality varies from hypoplasia of the entire femur to complete absence of the proximal portion.
- There can be associated severe dysplasia of the acetabulum, with the femoral head being present, delayed in ossification, or absent altogether.

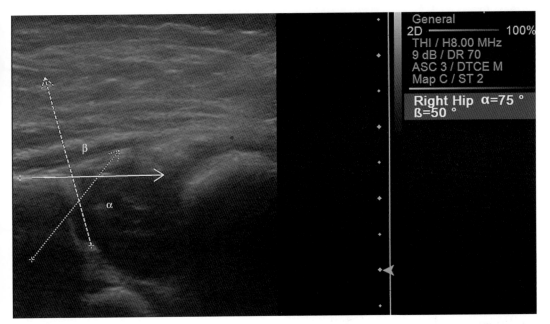

General
2D ────────── 100%
THI / H8.00 MHz
9 dB / DR 70
ASC 3 / DTCE M
Map C / ST 2

Right Hip α=75 °
ß=50 °

Fig. 6.19.3

○ The diagnosis is made by the presence of an abnormal proximal femur; this is usually already suspected clinically. In DDH, there may be a delay in femoral head ossification, but the remainder of the femur is not shortened.

Notes

○ The incidence of DDH is around 1 to 1.5 cases per 1,000 live births.
○ Risk factors for DDH include family history, breech presentation, Down's syndrome, and associated orthopaedic problems such as clubfoot deformity.
○ Early detection and intervention is paramount to prevent long-term disability.
○ Nonsurgical treatment keeps the hip in a flexed and abducted position using a harness.
○ For infants less than 6 to 8 months old, ultrasound is the imaging examination of choice to monitor acetabular development and hip alignment (**Fig. 6.19.3**).

● The Graf classification system is widely used to grade DDH. Three lines are drawn on the coronal hip ultrasound image:
1. Through the plane of the ilium
2. From the lateral end of the acetabulum to the labrum
3. Along the plane of the bony acetabulum.

In a normal hip, the α angle should be over 60 degrees, and the β angle should be less than 55 degrees.

Bibliography

Graf R, Scott S, Lercher K. Hip Sonography, Diagnosis and Management of Infant Hip Dysplasia. Berlin, Germany: Springer Verlag;2006

6.20 Neuroblastoma

Clinical History

A 4-year-old child presents with increased abdominal distension (Fig. 6.20.1).

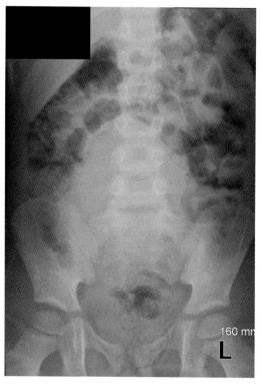

Fig. 6.20.1

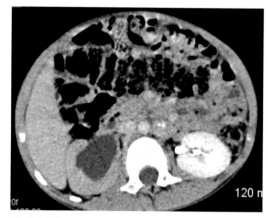

Fig. 6.20.2

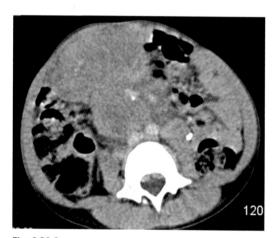

Fig. 6.20.3

Ideal Summary

This is a plain abdominal film of a child. There is increased density over the centre of the abdomen, with displaced bowel loops around the mass. No calcification is seen. There is no underlying bone destruction. I cannot clearly see the outline of the kidneys. The differential diagnosis for this soft tissue abnormality in a child of this age would include a malignant cause, including neuroblastoma, Wilms' tumour, and lymphoma. I would like to arrange for CT to further evaluate the mass.

These are the CT images of the same patient (Figs. 6.20.2 and 6.20.3).

These are selected delayed contrast-enhanced CT images through the upper abdomen. There is a large soft tissue mass occupying the central abdomen and retroperitoneum, and displacing bowel around it. The mesenteric vessels appear to be encased by the mass. High density is seen within the mass, but I would like to review a precontrast image to confirm calcification. The adrenal glands are not seen on the two images provided. There is right hydronephrosis and poor enhancement of the right kidney. No liver lesions are seen on the images provided. The most likely diagnosis is neuroblastoma, but lymphoma is also possible. Given the age, the patient is at high risk for metastatic disease, and I would like to assess this by reviewing the remainder of the chest and abdomen, as well as on bone windows for skeletal secondaries. I would recommend referral to a paediatric oncology centre and further evaluation with MIBG imaging.

Examination Tips

- A neuroblastoma is most commonly located in the adrenal gland (35%) or extra-adrenal retroperitoneum (30 to 35%), so it is important to check if the mass involves either of these areas.
- Comment on the presence of calcification as this is seen in 85% on CT, compared with 15% in Wilms' tumours.
- Neuroblastoma is an invasive tumour, so it is important to look at the following regions:
  - Neuroblastoma surrounds and encases vessels, such as mesenteric arteries and aorta (compare with Wilms' tumour).
  - Both kidneys need to be identified and assessed for the possibility of Wilms' tumour and obstruction.
  - Check the spine for evidence of invasion via the neuroforamina.
- Children over 18 months of age are at high risk of metastatic disease, with 70 to 80% presenting with distant spread. As such, you must specifically check for liver and bone lesions, and ask for the appropriate images or window settings if these are not available.
- Pulmonary metastases are uncommon in neuroblastoma, but are seen in approximately 20% with Wilms' tumour.

Differential Diagnosis

- Wilms' tumour
  - There is a peak incidence at around 3 years of age.
  - In approximately 15% of cases, there are associated congenital anomalies such as horseshoe kidney or cryptorchidism.
  - The mass typically has both solid and cystic components.
- Lymphoma:
  - Non-Hodgkin's disease can involve the mesentery and retroperitoneum.
  - It occurs in an older age group.
  - Imaging findings are nonspecific; however, lymph node enlargement elsewhere will raise suspicion for lymphoma.
  - Tissue may be needed to confirm the diagnosis.

Notes

- Neuroblastoma is the most common extracranial solid tumour in the paediatric population, and is most common before the age of 2 years.
- It accounts for 8 to 10% of all childhood malignancies.
- The levels of urinary catecholamines, such as vanillylmandelic acid, are raised in 95% of children with neuroblastoma.
- MIBG scanning can help identify the primary and metastatic disease.
- Prognosis for low- and intermediate-risk tumours is favourable, with a 3-year survival of 75 to 90%.

Bibliography

McHugh K. Renal and adrenal tumours in children. Cancer Imaging 2007;7:41–51

7   Introduction to Radionuclide Imaging

Simon M. Y. Wan and Nicola Mulholland

A working knowledge of radionuclide imaging is important for success in the FRCR 2B examination and beyond. The 2010 specialty training curriculum of the Royal College of Radiologists has listed "interpretation of normal and abnormal results of commonly performed [radionuclide] investigations across all clinical systems" as a core skill.[1] Anecdotal experience suggests that candidates are usually confronted with at least one radionuclide study, either in the long case or in the viva section. Beyond the FRCR 2B examination, radiologists in the United Kingdom are likely to be involved in radionuclide imaging regardless of subspecialty interest, often by being asked to review studies in a multidisciplinary meeting or in making recommendations for further imaging options. Furthermore, a U.K. national survey demonstrated that radiologists have been major providers of the nuclear medicine service in the country.[2]

Bone scans are the most common general radionuclide examination performed in the United Kingdom, with lung, kidney, thyroid, and cardiac studies constituting the majority of non-positron emission tomography (PET) radionuclide examinations performed.[3] PET/computed tomography (CT), specifically with fluorine 18-fluorodeoxyglucose (FDG), is increasingly available and used particularly in oncological application. It is difficult to predict what would be shown in the FRCR 2B examination, but it is likely to reflect the relative "prevalence" of examinations normally reviewed by the radiologist. Other radionuclide examinations may only be presented during discussion of cases (e.g., candidates may be expected to be aware of the use of MIBG studies to complete the staging of neuroblastomas shown on a CT, ultrasound, or MRI sequence), and a limited knowledge pertaining to the significance of the examination may be all that is required of the candidate.

Like other cases selected for the examination, the radionuclide cases shown may represent an uncommon presentation of common pathology or a common presentation of unusual diseases. Some cases may demonstrate a constellation of apparently disparate findings that relate to an underlying unifying diagnosis, for example:

① A bone scan in a teenager with prosthesis or amputation and lung uptake points to treated osteosarcoma with lung metastases.

② A "standing column" in the ureters with hepatic uptake may suggest a pelvic tumour causing outflow obstruction and liver metastases.

Basic Principles of Radionuclide Imaging

An in-depth review of the techniques of radionuclide imaging is beyond the scope of this chapter. A brief overview is presented here.

① Radionuclide imaging begins with the administration of a *radiolabelled tracer*. The tracer contains a radioactive isotope bound to a complex or molecule, which determines its kinetics and distribution in the body, and hence the type of physiological process studied. For instance, technetium 99m when bound to MAG3 is used for a renogram, whereas when it is bound to sestamibi, it can be used for cardiac or parathyroid imaging.

② Image acquisition is by positioning the patient under a gamma camera or a PET scanner depending on the radioisotope. The radiation emitted from the radioisotope in the patient is captured and analysed to construct an image.

③ Imaging can be *dynamic*, with the counts over seconds to minutes collated into "frames" and displayed as a cine sequence (e.g., renogram or gastric emptying study) or displayed as a sequence of summed images (e.g., in gastrointestinal bleeding studies). Alternatively, it may be *static*, with an accumulation or summation of counts over a longer time to form a single image (e.g., a standard bone scan).

④ Images acquired at different time points following tracer administration may give different clinically useful information. For example, a three-phase bone scan with dynamic acquisition at the time of injection, followed by static acquisition at 5 minutes and then at 3 to 4 hours, results in vascular, blood pool, and delayed-phase images, which reflect regional blood flow, blood volume (correlates with tissue oedema), and osteoblastic activity, respectively.

5 *Planar* images may be a "whole-body sweep" or spot views showing a specific anatomical region. Spot views may be done on their own if the clinician is interested in only one particular body part or as additional dedicated views to supplement a whole-body study. Single-photon emission CT (SPECT) and PET imaging captures the radiation emitted from different angles around the patient to reconstruct cross-sectional images, in a fashion similar to CT image formation. The resultant image may be co-registered with CT or MRI scans for enhanced synergistic diagnostic power.

6 The radiation dose to the patient is related to the activity of the administered tracer. Unlike in CT or fluoroscopy, the duration of image acquisition, volume scanned, and number of views obtained does not alter the patient's radiation burden.

Specific Examination Technique for the FRCR 2B

1 When presented with a radionuclide examination, begin by establishing the type of study shown. Some of the radionuclide examinations have specific or limited indications (as shown by some of the cases later). Awareness of these often focuses the candidate on the abnormalities.

2 From the images, try to work out what has been done. Is it a whole-body study? Has dynamic imaging been done, or are they just static views? Has the patient been imaged at multiple phases? What is the distribution of tracer in the body? It is usually apparent if the study shown is a PET, as supposed to a general radionuclide study. PET imaging results in higher spatial resolution, and hence images appear to be of "higher quality." FDG is a glucose analogue and has a normal blood pool distribution in the brain, liver, and mediastinum, with variable uptake in the heart and bowel.

3 There is a large variation in the way images are displayed across centres. It is important to review the labels on the image carefully:

- The image often states the agent used and indicates what examination has been performed.
- Other nonimaging parameters would carry important information necessary for the interpretation of the case (e.g., renogram curve, "total thyroid uptake," "split renal function").

- Pay attention to the surface and side markers (e.g., "SSN" in thyroid or parathyroid imaging showing the suprasternal notch). Images with markers are usually acquired over a short time, with low counts and an appearance of noise. Posterior planar views are not "flipped," and the laterality is reversed to that of conventional radiographic display (e.g., a posterior view of a bone scan; renograms are often imaged with camera head at the patient's back). Axial SPECT and PET images are displayed as per CT/MRI in this regard.

4 Unless stated on the image, it is sensible to state the type of examination rather than the specific tracer; for example, different centres may use HDP or MDP for bone scans, MAG3 or DTPA for renograms, and krypton or aerosols for ventilation scans, which may have subtly different behaviour not apparent to nonspecialists.

5 If the diagnosis is still unsure, suggest reviewing the clinical history or other previous imaging. Examiners may offer hints.

6 Examination technique for the detection of abnormalities, providing a differential diagnosis, formulation, and management plan, should then follow approaches similar to those of the other radiological systems.

References

1. Royal College of Radiologists. Specialty training curriculum for clinical radiology. May 2010. http://www.rcr.ac.uk/content.aspx?PageID=1805 (accessed March 2012)
2. Nuclear medicine and radionuclide imaging, a strategy for provision in the UK: A report of the Intercollegiate Standing Committee on Nuclear Medicine. Jan 2003. http://bookshop.rcplondon.ac.uk/contents/6dbefc58-0f7b-4f16-8341-a307de45e338.pdf (accessed March 2012)
3. Heath Protection Agency. Review of national surveys of population exposure from nuclear medicine examinations in eight European countries. 2008. http://ddmed.eu/_media/background_of_ddm1:dd_report_1_a_.pdf (accessed March 2012)

7.1 Cold Spot

Clinical History

*A 76-year-old man presents with back pain. He has previously had a documented left ninth rib fracture, but this is not relevant to the current examination (**Fig. 7.1.1**).*

Ideal Summary

These are whole-body planar images of a bone scan of an adult patient. There is a photopenic area in the L1 vertebral body. No other significant abnormality is present in the rest of the skeleton or soft tissues, apart from a presumed inadvertent subcutaneous injection in the right elbow and the left ninth rib fracture given in the history.

The main diagnosis to consider in an elderly patient with back pain and a "cold spot" in the spine is

malignancy such as multiple myeloma, plasmacytoma, or a metastatic deposit from either a renal or thyroid cancer. Artefact, avascular necrosis, and osteomyelitis are other considerations. I would review any other imaging studies and recommend further evaluation with MRI of the spine.

*These are further imaging studies (**Figs. 7.1.2–7.1.4**).*

These are dedicated views of the bone scan, plain film, and coronal MR images. The spot views of the bone scan confirm a photopenic area in the left of midline of L1 (**Fig. 7.1.2**, arrow). The frontal lumbar spine radiograph shows a left-sided lateral wedge deformity of the L1 vertebral body with destruction of the left pedicle (**Fig. 7.1.3**, arrow), which is replaced by enhancing soft tissues on the coronal MR image (**Fig. 7.1.4**, arrow), potentially threatening the spinal canal. I would review the rest of the

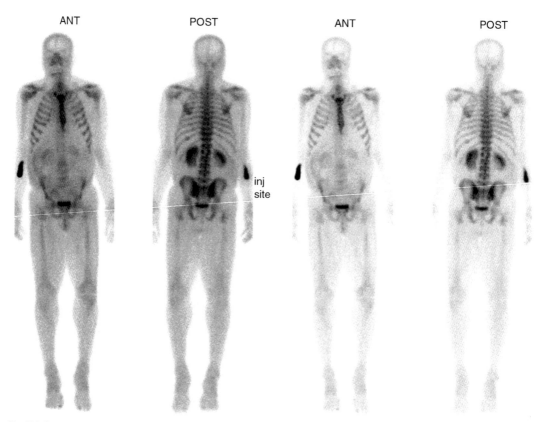

ANT　　　　POST　　　　ANT　　　　POST

inj
site

Fig. 7.1.1

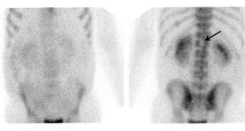

ANT ABDO   POST L–SPINE

Fig. 7.1.2

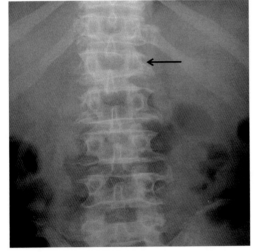

Fig. 7.1.3

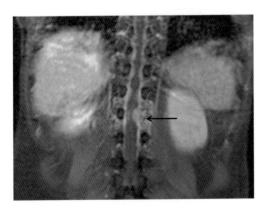

Fig. 7.1.4

MR images to evaluate for this. The findings would be consistent with my diagnosis of a neoplastic process.

Examination Tips

- "Cold spots" are uncommon findings on bone scans, and are often difficult to identify.
- Check that all the bones are present and "complete" to identify any cold spot.
- Review uptake by the kidneys. If there is also a photopenic area in the kidneys, a potential unifying diagnosis may be metastatic renal cell carcinoma.

Differential Diagnosis

The differential diagnosis of a cold spot may include:
- Neoplastic/metastatic lesions:
  - These are relatively common—myeloma, renal cell carcinoma, thyroid cancer, chordoma in the spine, Ewing's sarcoma, and aneurysmal bone cysts.
- Metallic artefact at characteristic sites, for example:
  - Coins or keys in trouser pockets (cold spots in the lower pelvis or proximal femur on anterior views)
  - Pacemaker in the upper chest anteriorly
  - Belt buckle overlying the lower spine on an anterior view
  - Joint prosthesis and orthopaedic implant.
- Haemangioma:
  - Less common, and most often affects the thoracic spine.
- Avascular necrosis
- Osteomyelitis, especially in children

Notes

- The traditional bone scan agent (e.g., technetium 99m MDP or HDP) equilibrates with the extravascular space and eventually binds to hydroxyapatite in bones, with excess excreted in the urine.
- Uptake depends on regional blood flow, tissue extraction, and the balance between osteoclastic and osteoblastic activity stimulated by the local pathology.
- Predominantly lytic lesions produce photopenic defects, which are difficult to appreciate. Some may incite osteoblastic activity at their leading edge, which improves visualisation.

Bibliography

Brooks ME. The skeletal system. In: Sharp PF, Gemmell HG, Murray AD, eds. Practical Nuclear Medicine. 3rd ed. London: Springer-Verlag;2005:143–161.

Sopov V, Liberson A, Gorenberg M, Groshar D. Cold vertebrae on bone scintigraphy. Semin Nucl Med 2001;31(1):82–83

7.2   Gastrointestinal Bleeding

Clinical History

*A 50-year-old man presents with melaena and anae-mia (**Figs. 7.2.1** and **7.2.2**).*

Ideal Summary

These are images of the abdomen from a radio-labelled red blood cell study, acquired over the first

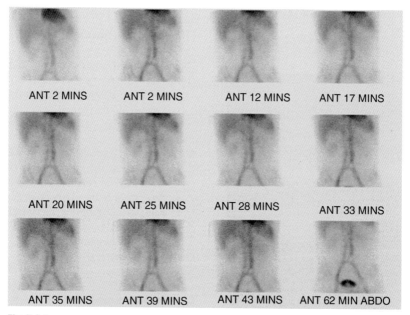

ANT 2 MINS	ANT 2 MINS	ANT 12 MINS	ANT 17 MINS
ANT 20 MINS	ANT 25 MINS	ANT 28 MINS	ANT 33 MINS
ANT 35 MINS	ANT 39 MINS	ANT 43 MINS	ANT 62 MIN ABDO

Fig. 7.2.1

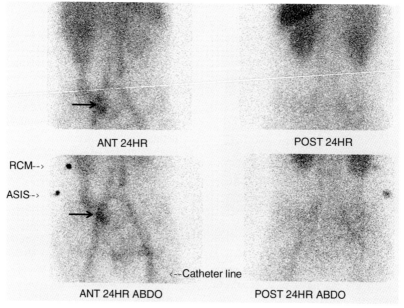

ANT 24HR   POST 24HR

RCM-->

ASIS->

<--Catheter line

ANT 24HR ABDO   POST 24HR ABDO

Fig. 7.2.2

hour and then at 24 hours. There is no abnormal activity in the images over the first hour. On the 24-hour images, there is tracer accumulation in the right abdomen (**Fig. 7.2.2**, arrows), in an area conforming to the caecum and ascending colon. There is no further abnormal activity elsewhere. The findings are in keeping with a focal area of haemorrhage (bleeding point) proximal to or at the caecum. I would recommend a CT angiogram specifically looking at this to try and identify a cause for the haemorrhage. I would also discuss this with the clinical team in view of the findings, with colonoscopy, a possible useful investigation.

Examination Tips

- Intraluminal accumulation of tracer, increasing intensity with time, and movement of the tracer with time in a pattern conforming to the intestinal anatomy are the criteria necessary to identify the site of haemorrhage. Therefore, comment on:
  - When and where the abnormal activity is first seen?
  - How the abnormal area "behaves" with time?
- Look carefully for more than one haemorrhage point.
- Subtle abnormality may sometimes be difficult to identify: exact localisation of the site of haemorrhage may be complicated by retrograde transit of extravasated blood within the bowel. If in doubt, offer to review any raw dynamic data in the movie (cine) mode.
- Delayed images up to 18 to 24 hours may help, as in this case.

Differential Diagnosis

- Causes of gastrointestinal bleeding from the large bowel include:
  - Angiodysplasia
  - Diverticular disease

- Tumours
- Colitis.
- These cannot be distinguished on the basis of the radiolabelled red blood cell study, and would require further imaging or endoscopic evaluation.

Notes

The technique of radiolabelled red blood cell study involves labelling the red blood cells of a patient in vitro and subsequently reinjecting these back into the patient's bloodstream. Normal vascular and blood pool activity is seen in the great vessels, spleen, liver, and kidneys.

- Advantages:
  - The most sensitive modality—it can detect haemorrhage down to a rate of 0.1 mL/min.
  - Can identify arterial and venous haemorrhage, but cannot differentiate the two.
  - Imaging over a period of time allows the detection of intermittent haemorrhage.
- Disadvantages:
  - The procedure is lengthy, not available "out of hours," and not suitable for acute episodes of brisk haemorrhage.
  - Does not provide information about the cause of the haemorrhage.

Bibliography

Graça BM, Freire PA, Brito JB, Ilharco JM, Carvalheiro VM, Caseiro-Alves F. Gastroenterologic and radiologic approach to obscure gastrointestinal bleeding: how, why, and when? Radiographics 2010;30(1):235–252

Laing CJ, Tobias T, Rosenblum DI, Banker WL, Tseng L, Tamarkin SW. Acute gastrointestinal bleeding: emerging role of multidetector CT angiography and review of current imaging techniques. Radiographics 2007;27(4):1055–1070

7.3 Hypertrophic Osteoarthropathy

Clinical History

A 50-year-old man complains of bilateral ankle pain (**Fig. 7.3.1**).

Ideal Summary

These are whole-body planar bone scan images of a skeletally mature patient. They show bilateral and symmetrical irregular cortical uptake along the femur and tibia on both sides (**Fig. 7.3.1**, arrows), where there is an early "double-stripe" appearance near the ankles. The only other abnormality on the remainder of the images is mild lumbar scoliosis with areas of focal uptake compatible with degenerative changes. There is no abnormal extraosseous uptake. The most likely diagnosis is that of hypertrophic osteoarthropathy (HOA). I would like to review any old images and suggest ankle and thoracic radiography if these have not been performed recently.

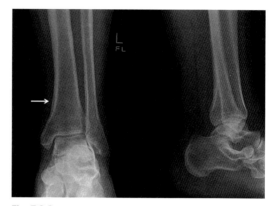

Fig. 7.3.2

These are the plain X-rays of the ankles (**Fig. 7.3.2**).

These are frontal and lateral radiographs of the left ankle. There is a periosteal reaction seen along the distal tibia and fibula, which confirms the diagnosis of HOA (**Fig. 7.3.2**, arrow).

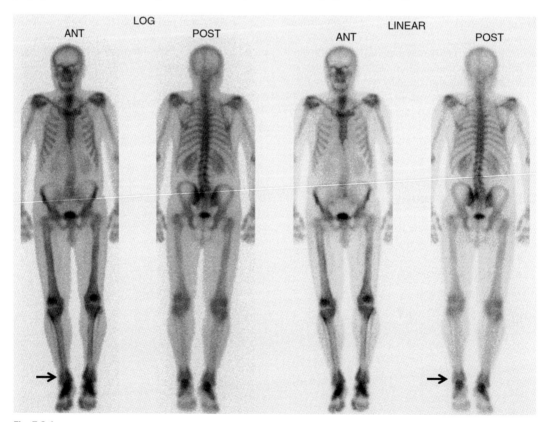

Fig. 7.3.1

Examination Tips

- Look at the long bones and at the periarticular regions for the "double stripe" or "rail track" sign.
- Look carefully to confirm that the uptake is predominantly at the cortex or periosteum rather than the medullary cavity. If there is abnormal increased uptake in the medullary cavity, consider metastases.
- Comment on extraosseous activity. Diagnosis of the underlying disease association is usually not possible from a bone scan. However, possible indicators include:
  - Diffuse increased activity in the thorax or hemithorax, pointing to a malignant pleural effusion
  - Signs of previous thoracotomy, chest wall resection, or sternotomy for lung or breast cancer surgery
  - "Cold spots" in the kidneys suggestive of renal lesions
  - Obstructed renal collecting systems from an abdominal or pelvic mass

Differential Diagnosis

Consider other causes of diffuse cortical hyperostosis:
- In adult patients:
  - Venous stasis
  - Thyroid acropachy

- In younger patients:
  - Caffey's disease
  - Engelmann's disease
  - Hypervitaminosis A

Notes

- Hypertrophic osteoarthropathy is characterised by periostitis and periosteal new bone formation, clinically manifesting with bone and joint pain and digital clubbing. A bone scan is more sensitive in detecting early disease.
- Primary HOA or pachydermoperiostosis is a rare hereditary disease, whereas secondary HOA is much more common.
- Hypertrophic osteoarthropathy is most commonly associated with bronchogenic carcinoma.
- Other causes of secondary HOA include other benign and malignant intrathoracic tumours, cystic fibrosis, bronchiectasis, lung abscess, *Pneumocystis* infection, and cyanotic heart disease.
- Extrathoracic disease is less often implicated, but includes Hodgkin's disease, inflammatory bowel disease, cirrhosis, and biliary atresia.

Bibliography

Love C, Din AS, Tomas MB, Kalapparambath TP, Palestro CJ. Radionuclide bone imaging: an illustrative review. Radiographics 2003;23(2):341–358

7.4   Malignant "Super Scan"

Clinical History

*A 52-year-old man presents with weight loss, polydipsia, and polyuria (**Fig. 7.4.1**).*

Ideal Summary

These are whole-body planar images of a bone scan showing a "super scan" appearance. The kidneys are not visualised. There is general increased activity in the axial and proximal appendicular skeleton, with random distribution of more focal increased uptake. The findings are those of widespread osteoblastic bony metastases. In a male patient, the primary is likely to be from prostate or lung cancer. In the absence of a known malignancy, I would like to review any previous imaging and recommend further clinical evaluation with a CT chest, abdomen, and pelvis, serum prostate-specific antigen evaluation, and calcium measurement.

Examination Tips

- Comment on the absence of renal uptake.
- The heterogeneous activity in this case points towards a malignant rather than a metabolic cause of the "super scan." Metabolic causes are more homogenous on the bone scan.

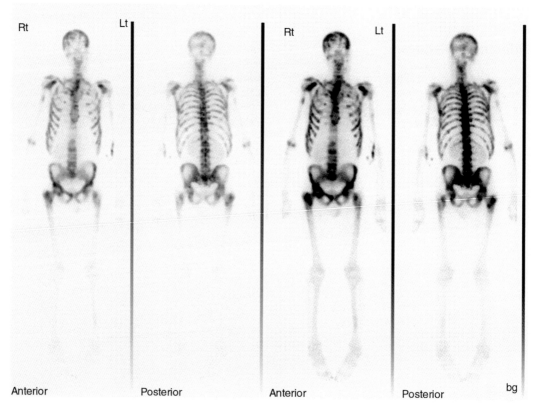

Rt   Lt   Rt   Lt

Anterior   Posterior   Anterior   Posterior   bg

Fig. 7.4.1

Differential Diagnosis

Commonly implicated malignancies include:
- Prostate
- Breast
- Lung
- Transitional cell carcinoma

Notes

- A bone scan is sensitive for the detection of metastatic disease and can detect lesions before there is any radiographic change.

- A response to therapy evaluation is, however, difficult with a bone scan and may not be possible, especially in patients with a "super scan." Increased activity in the known lesions and apparently new lesions may be due to a flare response within the first 3 months for hormonal and chemotherapy, and peaking at 3 months for radiotherapy.

Bibliography

Love C, Din AS, Tomas MB, Kalapparambath TP, Palestro CJ. Radionuclide bone imaging: an illustrative review. Radiographics 2003;23(2):341–358

7.5 Meckel's Diverticulum

Clinical History

A 28-year-old patient presented with two episodes of lower gastrointestinal haemorrhage. Gastroscopy, colonoscopy, capsule endoscopy, and CT imaging of the abdomen have not identified a cause for the symptoms (Fig. 7.5.1).

Ideal Summary

This is an isotope study with images acquired up to 1 hour 40 minutes postinjection. The distribution of tracer and the clinical story would suggest a per-technetate scan for Meckel's diverticulum. There is a focus of activity below the aortic bifurcation on the 20-minute image, coinciding with the appearance of intense activity in the stomach (arrow). This is a positive study for a Meckel's diverticulum containing gastric mucosa, which would explain the patient's symptoms. I would inform the clinical team. I would like to review the previous CT images to correlate with these findings.

Examination Tips

- Pertechnetate is normally taken up by the gastric mucosa, thyroid tissue, and salivary glands.
- Haemorrhage secondary to Meckel's diverticulum is associated with ectopic gastric mucosa. This forms the basis of using pertechnetate for the identification of a Meckel's diverticulum.
- The diffuse gastric activity in this example distinguishes this from a labelled red blood cell study for a source of haemorrhage. However, gastric activity in a labelled red blood cell study may occur if:
  - There is haemorrhage in the stomach.
  - There is imperfect labelling, with contamination of the injected tracer by free pertechnetate.

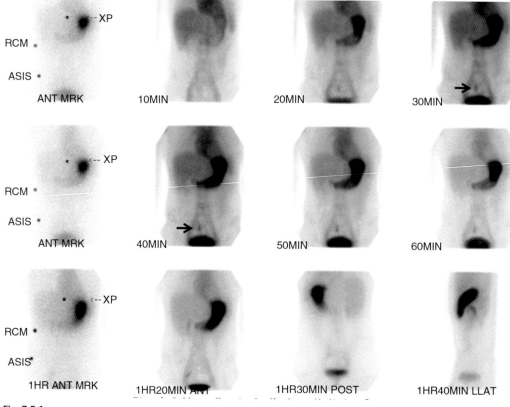

Fig. 7.5.1

If in doubt when performing a red blood cell study, image the head and neck looking for thyroid and salivary gland uptake, which would suggest the presence of free pertechnetate.

- A positive study for a Meckel's diverticulum would show an abnormal focal area of activity in the abdomen, appearing at about the same time as the gastric activity.

Differential Diagnosis

The imaging appearance of a positive Meckel's study is characteristic.

Notes

- Meckel's diverticulum is present in 2% of the population. It is an embryological remnant of the omphalomesenteric duct that has failed to regress.

- Heterotopic mucosa is found in up to 60% of cases, many of which contain gastric mucosa (62%). Others may contain pancreatic mucosa, small bowel mucosa, or Brunner's glands.

- It is typically asymptomatic, but there is a 4 to 40% lifetime risk of developing complications, which may include:
  - Haemorrhage secondary to ectopic gastric mucosa
  - Bowel obstruction
  - Enterolith formation
  - Inflammation/diverticulitis
  - Rarely, perforation and neoplasm (most frequently carcinoid).

Bibliography
Elsayes KM, Menias CO, Harvin HJ, Francis IR. Imaging manifestations of Meckel's diverticulum. AJR Am J Roentgenol 2007;189(1):81–88

7.6 Carcinoid Tumour

Clinical History

*A 70-year-old woman presented with diarrhoea. These images were taken 24 hours after tracer injection (**Figs. 7.6.1** and **7.6.2**).*

Ideal Summary

These are whole-body planar and coronal SPECT/CT images of an indium 111 octreotide study. The planar images show multiple foci of abnormal activity in the liver, with further foci in the central abdomen and in the left supraclavicular region. The SPECT/CT image confirms the hepatic lesions and shows additional foci in the retroperitoneum, likely from lymphadenopathy. The findings are those of metastatic

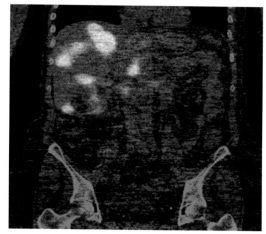

Fig. 7.6.2

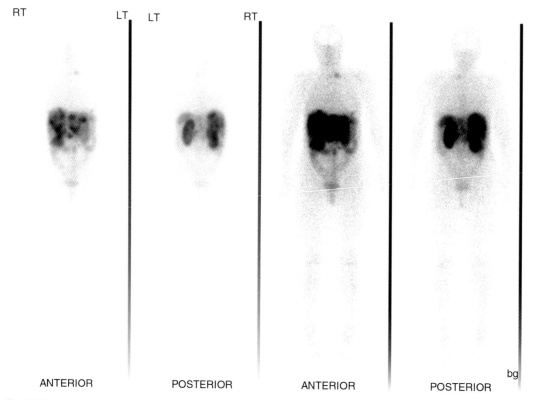

RT   LT   LT   RT

ANTERIOR   POSTERIOR   ANTERIOR   POSTERIOR

bg

Fig. 7.6.1

neuroendocrine tumours. I would review the rest of the dataset and recommend a CT of the neck, chest, abdomen, and pelvis to fully stage the disease and to locate a primary tumour. Referral to a dedicated neuroendocrine centre would be prudent for further management.

Examination Tips

- Octreotide is a somatostatin peptide analogue that, when radiolabelled with indium, is useful in the localisation and staging of neuroendocrine tumours.
- Normal uptake is present in the spleen and kidneys, with lesser uptake in the liver (in contrast to an MIBG study, where hepatic uptake is higher).
- Images are usually obtained at 4 hours and then between 18 and 24 hours. The earlier images allow visualisation of the abdomen before biliary excretion obscures abdominal lesions. The later images provide a better tumour-to-liver ratio.

Differential Diagnosis

- The findings are characteristic of a metastatic neuroendocrine tumour in this case.
- Octreotide uptake may also be present in:
  - Carcinoid tumour
  - Glucagonoma
  - Gastrinoma
- Vasoactive intestinal peptide tumour (VIP-oma)
- Insulinomas and poorly differentiated neuroendocrine tumours are not generally octreotide avid.

Notes

- Regarding carcinoid tumours (small bowel-derived gastroenterohepatic neuroendocrine tumours), 40% of patients have metastases at time of presentation. A third of patients will develop carcinoid syndrome.
- Most originate from the gastrointestinal tract, followed by the lungs.
- Primary resection is the treatment of choice. Even in the presence of metastases, there is some evidence that debulking of disease, if possible, will increase survival. Medical therapy is useful for symptom control.
- FDG PET/CT imaging usually has little role for primary staging, unless with poorly differentiated tumours. During the course of the disease, loss of octreotide uptake and increase in FDG uptake is associated with "dedifferentiation" of the tumour and is a poor prognostic sign.

Bibliography

Intenzo CM, Jabbour S, Lin HC, et al. Scintigraphic imaging of body neuroendocrine tumors. Radiographics 2007; 27(5):1355–1369

7.7 Osteomalacia

Clinical History

A 50-year-old Asian woman presents with bone pain (**Fig. 7.7.1**).

Ideal Summary

These are whole-body planar bone scan images of a skeletally mature patient. There is an increased target-to-background ratio with very good visualisation of the skull, mandible, and rest of the skeleton, and poor visualisation of the kidneys. There are numerous areas of focal uptake in the ribs bilaterally in a linear configuration across several ribs. Two symmetrical foci are present at the neck of femur bilaterally. Foci of activity in the lumbar spine and cervical spine are compatible with degeneration. There is some bladder activity but no abnormal soft tissue uptake. The findings are those of a metabolic "super scan," with areas of uptake in the ribs compatible with numerous fractures and the uptake in the femoral neck being typical locations of Looser's zones. The most likely diagnosis is osteomalacia, and I would correlate the bony abnormalities with the plain films. Biochemical correlation of vitamin D deficiency would confirm the diagnosis.

*This is the plain X-ray of the pelvis (**Fig. 7.7.2**).*

There are linear lucencies with surrounding sclerosis at the medial aspect of the femoral necks bilaterally (**Fig. 7.7.2**, arrows), characteristic of Looser's zones.

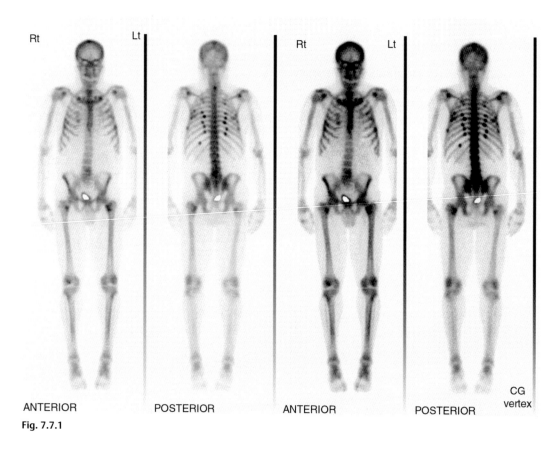

ANTERIOR   POSTERIOR   ANTERIOR   POSTERIOR

CG vertex

Fig. 7.7.1

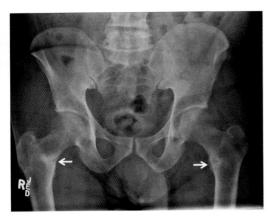

Fig. 7.7.2

Examination Tips

- A "super scan" occurs when there is increased tracer activity in the skeleton with reduced uptake in the soft tissues and kidneys. These can be broadly grouped into:
  - Metabolic "super scan": these have a more homogenous appearance
  - Malignant "super scan": diffuse bone metastases with increased but slightly heterogeneous activity throughout the affected skeleton
  - Haematological causes: lymphoma, mastocytosis, and myelofibrosis.
- Bone scans are sensitive but nonspecific. Nevertheless:
  - Uptake across several ribs in a "linear" configuration would be compatible with rib fractures; metastatic deposits are more randomly distributed.
  - Uptake in the spine with activity apparently outside the expected contours of the vertebral bodies points to a degenerative cause (osteophytes).
- Comment on:
  - Soft tissue uptake. Ectopic calcification in the soft tissues or microcalcification in the lungs are sometimes seen in severe hyperparathyroidism, often as part of renal osteodystrophy.

- Bladder activity. Lack of bladder activity may be a clue to renal osteodystrophy in the presence of renal failure.
- Any focal bone activity. Depending on the location, they may represent Looser's zones in osteomalacia (a typical location in the proximal femur, scapula, pubic rami, and ribs), pathological fractures, or a brown tumour in hyperparathyroidism.

Differential Diagnosis

Differential diagnosis of "super scan":
- Metabolic
  - Hyperparathyroidism
  - Osteomalacia
  - Renal osteodystrophy
- Malignancy
  - Prostate
  - Breast
- Haematological
  - Lymphoma
  - Myelofibrosis
  - Mastocytosis

Notes

- Osteomalacia results in weakened bone from reduced mineralisation.
- Causes of osteomalacia may include reduced dietary intake of vitamin D, reduced sun exposure, malabsorption syndromes, malnutrition, chronic renal impairment, and long-term anticonvulsant use. Uncommonly, it may be tumour-induced.
- The bone scan appearance can be normal in early osteomalacia. The bone scan is more sensitive in identifying pseudofractures than plain films. The mechanism of increased bone scan uptake in later disease is unclear but probably relates to associated hyperparathyroidism.

Bibliography

Cook GJR, Gnanasegaran G, Chua S. Miscellaneous indications in bone scintigraphy: metabolic bone diseases and malignant bone tumors. Semin Nucl Med 2010;40(1):52–61

7.8 Paget's Disease

Clinical History

A 78-year-old man is having a bone scan for the staging of newly diagnosed prostate cancer (Fig. 7.8.1).

Ideal Summary

These are whole-body planar bone scan images. They show a skeletally mature adult with multiple areas of increased tracer activity involving the right scapula, humerus, hemipelvis, distal femur, and distal tibia. The affected bones either show whole-bone involvement or have the abnormal activity extending from an articular surface. They also appear expanded, and there is bowing deformity of the right tibia. There is absence of the entire left lower limb. The most likely unifying diagnosis would be polyostotic Paget's disease, complicated by sarcomatous transformation in the left lower limb, subsequently treated by amputation. I would like to review any previous imaging for confirmation if these are available. Radiographs of any symptomatic areas should be obtained and compared with old films, as metastatic disease within Pagetic bones are difficult to identify on bone scan.

Examination Tips

- Look for the age of the patient on the images—Paget's disease typically occurs in elderly patients.
- Look carefully to compare the two sides to assess for enlargement of the affected bones.
- Check for focal areas of photopenia within the affected bones as these may represent areas of aggressive bone destruction from sarcomatous transformation or metastatic deposits.

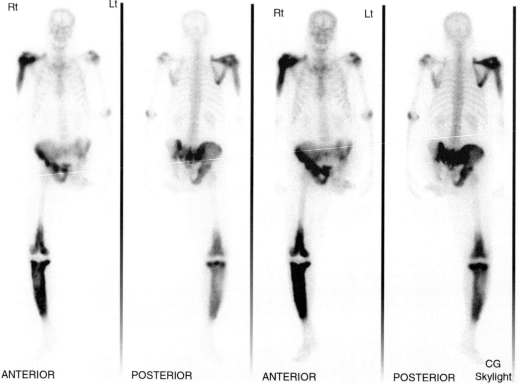

ANTERIOR POSTERIOR ANTERIOR POSTERIOR Skylight CG

Fig. 7.8.1

Look for evidence of previous treatment for Paget's sarcoma, such as amputation in this example or prostheses for shafts of the long bones or joints.

Differential Diagnosis

- Appearances of Paget's disease on bone scans are usually characteristic, with expansion and increased activity involving the entire bone or in a "flame shape" extending from an articulation surface. Bone expansion may be subtle on a bone scan.
- Diagnosis may not be straightforward with monostotic disease or disease at less typical sites.
- Imaging differential diagnosis with polyostotic regions of increased tracer activity may include:
  - Metastatic disease, the main differential diagnosis in elderly patient. There are multiple randomly distributed areas of increased uptake of varying size, shape, and intensity.
  - Polyostotic fibrous dysplasia. This typically affects young patients who show affected bones predominantly on one side of the body.
  - Chronic recurrent multifocal osteomyelitis. This affects young patients. This history is different from that of Paget's disease.

Notes

- The aetiology of Paget's disease is unclear. A viral cause has been postulated.

- It affects approximately 10% of the population over the age of 80 years in Europe, America, and Australia. It is unusual in those below 40 years of age.
- It commonly affects the pelvis, skull, spine, and proximal long bones.
- Tracer is avid in all the three phases (lytic phase, mixed phase, and osteoblastic phase) due to increased vascularity initially and increased osteoblastic activity in the late phases. It is recognised that quiescent late-phase disease may show normal activity.
- Non-neoplastic complications of Paget's disease include fracture, deformity, arthritis, osteomyelitis, and neurological complications secondary to basilar invagination, encroachment on the spinal canal or neural foramen in the spine or skull.
- There is a 10% risk of sarcomatous transformation in severe polyostotic Paget's disease (usually osteosarcoma but it can be chondrosarcoma). There is also an association with giant cell tumour. It is usually difficult to identify on a bone scan and would require cross-sectional imaging for diagnosis.

Bibliography

Smith SE, Murphey MD, Motamedi K, Mulligan ME, Resnik CS, Gannon FH. From the archives of the AFIP. Radiologic spectrum of Paget disease of bone and its complications with pathologic correlation. Radiographics 2002;22(5): 1191–1216

7.9 Parathyroid Adenoma

Clinical History

A 47-year-old woman presents with weakness (**Figs. 7.9.1** and **7.9.2**).

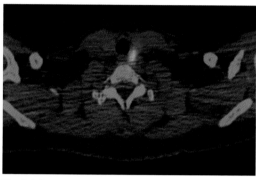

Fig. 7.9.2

Ideal Summary

This is a dual-phase isotope study with technetium sestamibi obtained at 20 minutes and at 3 hours. There is a focus of increased activity in the region of the lower pole of the left thyroid gland in the early images, which shows delayed washout

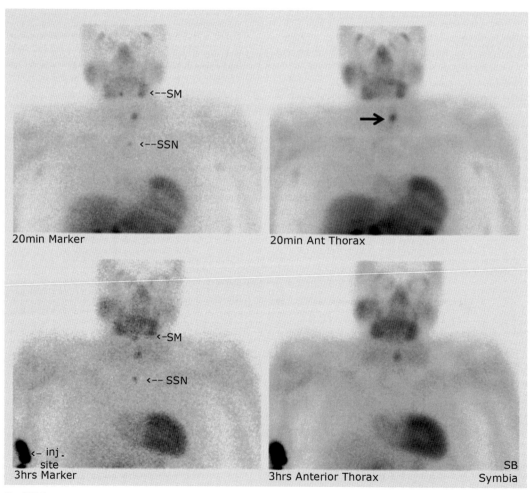

Fig. 7.9.1

(**Fig. 7.9.1**, arrow). The SPECT/CT image localises this to a posterior position to the left lobe of the thyroid in the tracheo-oesophageal groove (**Fig. 7.9.2**). There is no ectopic focus of activity. The findings are be in keeping with a parathyroid adenoma close to the inferior lobe of the left thyroid gland. Correlation with biochemical markers and ultrasound examination should be recommended. Referral to an endocrine surgeon would be appropriate.

These are the ultrasound images (**Figs. 7.9.3** and **7.9.4**).

The gray-scale ultrasound image demonstrates an oval-shaped abnormality at the lower aspect of a lobe of the thyroid gland (**Fig. 7.9.3**, arrow), which is likely to represent a parathyroid adenoma. The second image using colour Doppler ultrasound demonstrates colour Doppler flow within the adenoma. The pattern of colour Doppler flow is unlike that of an enlarged lymph node, establishing the abnormality as that of a parathyroid adenoma.

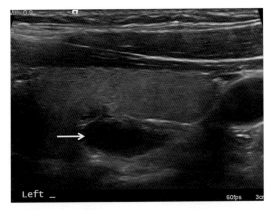

Fig. 7.9.3

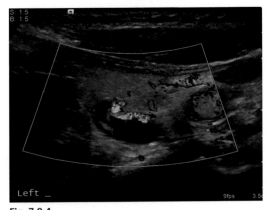

Fig. 7.9.4

Examination Tips

- Sestamibi is taken up normally by the salivary glands and heart, in addition to thyroid and parathyroid glands.
- Look for focal areas of increased uptake in the early images, which persists in the late images—a typical finding for a single parathyroid adenoma.
- Comment on the location of the abnormal focus in relation to the thyroid gland, especially if it appears to be ectopic.
- If the thyroid uptake is heterogeneous, it may be relevant as a thyroid adenoma and may also show delayed washout. Conversely, an intrathyroid parathyroid adenoma may occur, and both SPECT/CT and ultrasound would be necessary to suggest the diagnosis.

Differential Diagnosis

- A single parathyroid adenoma shows early increased uptake and delayed washout on scintigraphy. It accounts for 90% of cases of primary hyperparathyroidism.
- A single parathyroid adenoma may not be responsible for hyperparathyroidism. A double adenoma (4%) may be present, or there may be hyperplasia of multiple glands (6%).
- Parathyroid carcinoma (1%) can occur.
- A thyroid nodule may also show delayed washout and is a recognised false positive on scintigraphy.

Notes

- Hyperparathyroidism is a clinical and biochemical diagnosis, so measure serum calcium and parathyroid hormone levels.
- Surgery is considered to be the definitive treatment for symptomatic disease. Historically, this would have been bilateral surgical exploration.
- Preoperative localisation allows a more focused approach to surgery, reducing surgery time and complications.
- Ultrasound and scintigraphy are commonly used for this purpose. MRI or PET (e.g., carbon 11-methionine) may be useful for recurrent disease or difficult cases.

Bibliography

Eslamy HK, Ziessman HA. Parathyroid scintigraphy in patients with primary hyperparathyroidism: 99mTc sestamibi SPECT and SPECT/CT. Radiographics 2008;28(5):1461–1476

7.10 Pulmonary Embolism

Clinical History

*A 23-year-old previously healthy person who now presents with shortness of breath (**Fig. 7.10.1**).*

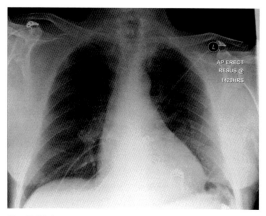

Fig. 7.10.1

Ideal Summary

This is a well-centred frontal radiograph of an adult patient obtained in the emergency department.

There is increased lucency in the right upper zone, with reduced vascular markings. There is no focal consolidation or pleural effusion on either side. No abnormality is identified on the remainder of the image. In the context of a previously healthy patient, the findings may be in keeping with Westermark's sign, which is suggestive of a pulmonary embolism. I would recommend further clinical evaluation and imaging in the form of either a CT pulmonary angiogram or ventilation/perfusion (V/Q) scan depending on local policy and provision.

*Here are the images from the V/Q scan (**Fig. 7.10.2**).*

These are planar ventilation/perfusion images of this patient. They show multiple areas of focal and peripheral segmental mismatch defects, consistent with pulmonary embolism.

Examination Tips

- A normal planar ventilation/perfusion (V/Q) study would have similar ventilation and perfusion images, with homogenous tracer distribution and smooth contours around the anatomical

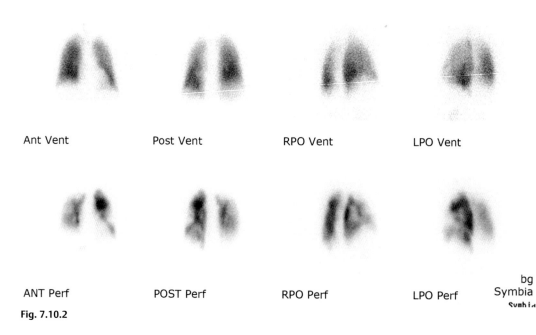

Ant Vent   Post Vent   RPO Vent   LPO Vent

ANT Perf   POST Perf   RPO Perf   LPO Perf

bg
Symbia
Svnhia

Fig. 7.10.2

boundaries of the lungs, such as in the ventilation images.
- The hilum can often be seen as mildly photopenic areas centrally. There may be some gradation of counts depending on how close the body parts are to the camera (e.g., apices appear less "dense"; and the lung bases are more "dense" on the oblique views). The trachea and main bronchi may sometimes be seen on the ventilation images.
- Look carefully at the images to identify peripheral wedge-shaped areas of mismatch defect (areas of photopenia on the perfusion images where ventilation is normal). Many of the lung segments are represented on several views and can be correlated with each other if the diagnosis is uncertain. Do not stop looking, as multiple defects are often present.
- Visualisation of the brain and kidneys on the perfusion images suggest a right-to-left shunt. Beware of the V/Q scan with this pattern and a photopenic area in the lung (pulmonary arteriovenous malformation).

Differential Diagnosis

- V/Q mismatch may also be uncommonly caused by:
  - Congenital vascular abnormalities
  - Veno-occlusive disease
  - Vasculitis
  - Lung cancer or mediastinal lymph node enlargement.
- The clinical presentation and initial plain film may provide helpful clues to raise suspicion.

Notes

- It is accepted that V/Q scanning has a high negative predictive value. However, historically, it suffers from a high indeterminate rate.

- There is emerging evidence that, with modern camera and cross-sectional techniques (SPECT), the indeterminate rate can be markedly reduced. Current European guidelines have moved away from probability-based reporting.
- Advantages of CT pulmonary angiogram over V/Q scanning:
  - More widely available, especially out of hours
  - Often identifies an alternative reason for the patient's symptoms if there is no pulmonary embolus
- Advantage of V/Q scanning over CT pulmonary angiogram:
  - Can be used in patients with contrast allergy or renal failure
  - Where radiation dose is a concern (e.g., in pregnant patients, the protocol may be modified, such as with a low dose and with a perfusion study only).
- Relative contraindications for V/Q scanning:
  - Right-to-left cardiac shunt
  - Known pulmonary hypertension
  - Known airways disease (asthma, chronic obstructive pulmonary disease) and cardiac disease are associated with an increased indeterminate rate.

Bibliography

Bajc M, Neilly JB, Miniati M, Schuemichen C, Meignan M, Jonson B; EANM Committee. EANM guidelines for ventilation/perfusion scintigraphy: Part 1. Pulmonary imaging with ventilation/perfusion single photon emission tomography. Eur J Nucl Med Mol Imaging 2009;36(8):1356–1370

Bajc M, Neilly JB, Miniati M, Schuemichen C, Meignan M, Jonson B. EANM guidelines for ventilation/perfusion scintigraphy: Part 2. Algorithms and clinical considerations for diagnosis of pulmonary emboli with V/P(SPECT) and MDCT. Eur J Nucl Med Mol Imaging 2009;36(9):1528–1538

7.11 Phaeochromocytoma

Clinical History

*A 46-year-old woman with hypertension (**Figs. 7.11.1** and **7.11.2**).*

Ideal Summary

The upper image is taken to be planar views of an iodine 123 MIBG study obtained at 24 hours. There is focal tracer accumulation in the left upper abdomen, probably in the suprarenal region (**Fig. 7.11.1**, arrow). Tracer uptake elsewhere is within normal limits. The SPECT/CT fusion image (**Fig. 7.11.2**) localises the focus of abnormal activity to the left adrenal region. Taken with the clinical history, the imaging

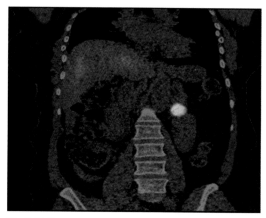

Fig. 7.11.2

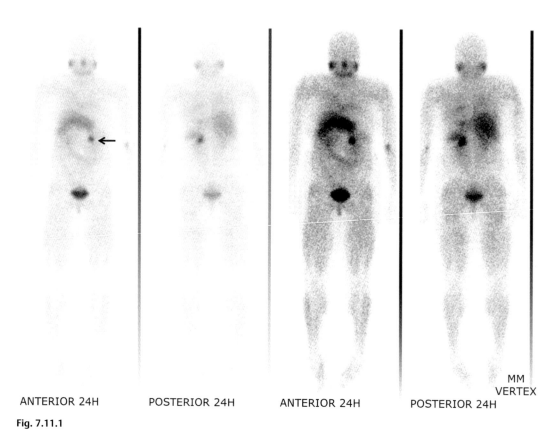

| ANTERIOR 24H | POSTERIOR 24H | ANTERIOR 24H | POSTERIOR 24H |

MM
VERTEX

Fig. 7.11.1

findings are that of a phaeochromocytoma. I would recommend biochemical correlation and endocrinology referral.

Examination Tips

- Normal tracer distribution in a MIBG study would include salivary glands, liver, and heart. Brown fat may sometimes show an uptake.
- MIBG can be radiolabelled with iodine 123 or iodine 131. Iodine 123 MIBG produces better quality images and allows SPECT imaging. Iodine 131 is used for MIBG therapy.
- Images are acquired at 24 hours for maximal target-to-background ratio. Earlier images may be obtained depending on individual practise.
- Look carefully for abnormal MIBG uptake elsewhere in the body as other areas may be affected:
  - Extra-adrenal phaeochromocytoma or paraganglioma
  - Other neural rest tumours, such as carcinoid or medullary thyroid cancer

Differential Diagnosis

- The appearances are characteristic of a phaeochromocytoma in the left adrenal gland. SPECT/CT helps confirm the adrenal location.

- In children, MIBG study forms part of routine staging for neuroblastoma.

Notes

- Phaeochromocytomas are rare catecholamine-secreting tumours; 90% are in the adrenal glands and often part of the multiple endocrine neoplasia II syndrome.
- Clinical presentation may include arrhythmia or hypertension; 10% are asymptomatic and generally thought to be less secretory.
- Iodine 123 MIBG study has a sensitivity of 83 to 100%, and a specificity of 100% for the diagnosis of phaeochromocytoma.
- Appearances on CT and MRI can be variable, but it typically appears as a hyperenhancing adrenal lesion, which has density higher than 10 HU on CT and a high T2/low T1 signal on MRI. MRI may show "salt and pepper" appearances due to signal void from florid tumour vessels. Degenerate lesions may have cystic, calcified, or haemorrhagic components.

Bibliography
Blake MA, Kalra MK, Maher MM, et al. Pheochromocytoma: an imaging chameleon. Radiographics 2004;24(Suppl 1): S87–S99

7.12 Pelviureteric Junction Obstruction

Clinical History

A 32-year-old woman presents with right-sided abdominal pain (Figs. 7.12.1 and 7.12.2).

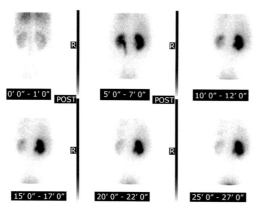

Fig. 7.12.1

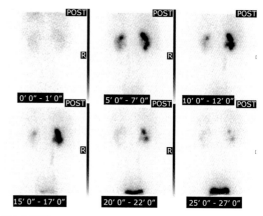

Fig. 7.12.3

Kings	Right kidney	Left kidney	Right parenchyme	Left parenchyme
Function (%)	53	47		
Integral 1 2(min)	6772	5989		
Mean Transit Time (MTT)(min)	9.6	4.3	5.6	3.3
Outflow efficiency (%)	77	94		

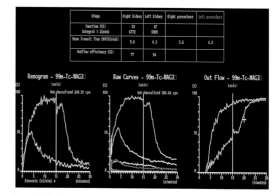

Fig. 7.12.4

Kings	Right kidney	Left kidney	Right parenchyme	Left parenchyme
Function (%)	51	49		
Integral 1 2(min)	9533	9189		
Mean Transit Time (MTT)(min)	14.7	4.6	14.0	4.3
Outflow efficiency (%)	56	95		

Fig. 7.12.2

Ideal Summary

This is a MAG3 renogram study demonstrating the symmetrical size and perfusion of the kidneys. No obvious cortical defect is seen on the images displayed. There is rapid transit of tracer into the collecting systems bilaterally. The right kidney shows tracer retention within a dilated collecting system and a continuously rising renogram curve. There is little response to the diuretic administration (furosemide diuresis) at 15 minutes. The left kidney shows

normal drainage. Split renal function is symmetrical. The appearances are those of a pelviureteric junction obstruction. An ultrasound examination would be useful to confirm and assess the degree of hydronephrosis. I would refer the patient to a urologist.

This is a renogram of the same patient at a later date. (**Figs. 7.12.3** and **7.12.4**). *What does it show?*

Compared with the previous examination, the drainage of the right kidney is no longer obstructed and now shows a good response to diuretic administration, the renogram curve shows a fall after the diuretic administration; this did not occur on the earlier renogram. The patient is likely to have undergone a corrective procedure following the previous renogram.

Examination Tips

- The renogram provides:
  - Structural and anatomical information
  - Functional information in the form of:
    - Renogram curve
    - Numerical indices such as split renal function and other parameters.
- It is important to review and comment on all these components.
- The renogram curve is a time–activity curve showing the number of counts within the region of interest of the individual kidneys. The left kidney in this example shows a normal renogram curve.

Differential Diagnosis

- A continuously rising renogram curve is usually indicative of obstruction.
- Other differential diagnosis for a continuously rising renogram would include:
  - Parenchymal retention: acute tubular necrosis; no tracer is seen in the collecting system on the images.
  - False "positive": dehydration, a massively dilated upper tract, full bladder, and poor renal function.

Notes

- The cause and natural history of pelviureteric junction obstruction is poorly understood. Intrinsic pelviureteric junction muscle, or collagen abnormality, or crossing renal vasculature have all been implicated as a cause.
- Adults classically present with the symptoms of intermittent flank pain at times of high urine output, for example, after alcohol consumption.
- Accepted indications of surgical treatment include pain symptoms, infection, stone formation, or progressive worsening renal function. A MAG3 study provides objective functional information to allow for patient selection and evaluation of treatment response.

Bibliography

Cosgriff PS. The urinary tract. In: Sharp PF, Gemmell HG, Murray AD, eds. Practical Nuclear Medicine. 3rd ed. London: Springer-Verlag;2005:205–229.

Tan BJ, Smith AD. Ureteropelvic junction obstruction repair: when, how, what? Curr Opin Urol 2004;14(2):55–59

7.13 Renal Laceration

Clinical History

*A 15-year-old boy undergoing this investigation a few months after an acute hospital admission (**Fig. 7.13.1**).*

Ideal Summary

This is a DMSA study. The kidneys are symmetrical in size and position. There is a photopenic area in the interpolar region of the left renal cortex (**Fig. 7.13.1,** arrow). No further focal defect is present in the rest of the kidneys. There is no feature suggestive of hydronephrosis. The split renal function is symmetrical, with the left kidney contributing 49% and the right kidney 51% to total renal function. The differential diagnosis for the appearance would include a focal renal scar, a cystic abnormality, or a focus of infection. I would review the images from the previous admission, as this may be relevant, to identify a cause for this.

*This image was acquired shortly after the boy attended the emergency department on his earlier admission (**Fig. 7.13.2**).*

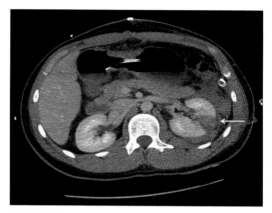

Fig. 7.13.2

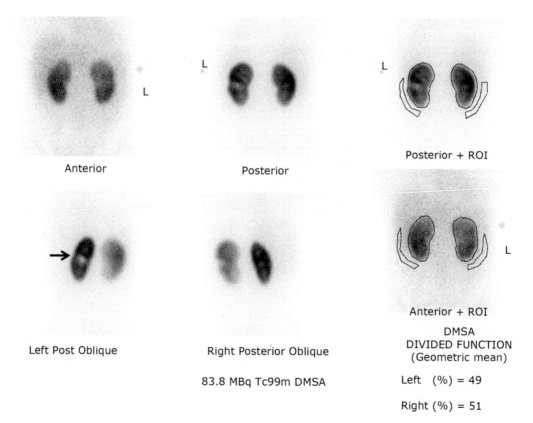

Anterior

Posterior

Posterior + ROI

Left Post Oblique

Right Posterior Oblique

Anterior + ROI

83.8 MBq Tc99m DMSA

DMSA
DIVIDED FUNCTION
(Geometric mean)

Left (%) = 49

Right (%) = 51

Fig. 7.13.1

This is an axial image of a contrast-enhanced CT examination at the mid-abdominal level. There is a focal wedge-shaped, low-density area in the interpolar region of the left kidney extending from the cortex to the collecting system (**Fig. 7.13.2,** arrow). There is surrounding blood in the perinephric space and left paracolic gutter. There is no evidence of contrast extravasation on this image. There has been recent surgery with superficial surgical clips anteriorly in the midline, a surgical drain, and a nasogastric tube. There is a further skin defect and fat stranding in the left lateral abdominal wall; the musculature at this site is thickened. I would like to review the rest of the images. Overall, the findings would be consistent with a renal laceration from a penetrating injury. This would have been a surgical emergency at the time of imaging.

The DMSA study would be in keeping with the subsequent development of a focal scar with no loss of renal function. The prognosis is likely to be good, with no risk of future development of hypertension.

Examination Tips

- DMSA is a renal cortical imaging agent.
- Comment on the location, size, and shape of the kidneys. DMSA scanning is often performed to locate and assess ectopic renal tissue.
- Comment on split renal function. This may sometimes not be possible to measure in cases of crossfused ectopia or horseshoe kidneys where the two moieties overlap.

- Take note of background activity. If it is prominent in relation to renal uptake, it would suggest poor overall renal function.

Differential Diagnosis

- Causes of focal cortical photopenia include:
  - Scars: peripheral, wedge-shaped, often multiple
  - Space-occupying lesion: cystic lesions, or benign or malignant solid renal lesions
  - Focal infection: may take 6 months to resolve, and may result in scars.
- Clinical presentation and cross-sectional imaging would help distinguish between these.

Notes

- DMSA may be a prognostic indicator in the context of paediatric renal trauma, and can be useful in the early diagnosis of scar and hypertension if injury is severe.
- Grade IV renal injury usually commands surgical exploration, whereas conservative management may be used in less severe injury.
- Penetrating renal injury can be complicated by the development of urinoma, pseudoaneurysm, or arteriovenous fistula.

Bibliography

European Association of Urology. Guidelines on urological trauma: pocket guideline. http://www.uroweb.org/gls/pockets/english/17%20Urological%20Trauma.pdf (accessed March 2012)

7.14 Spondylolysis

Clinical History

A 14-year-old tennis player presents with back pain (**Figs. 7.14.1** and **7.14.2**).

Ideal Summary

The first image shows a whole-body planar bone scan of a skeletally immature patient. There are two foci of increased tracer uptake at the lower lumbar spine, one on each side at the level of L5 posteriorly. Tracer distribution elsewhere is within normal limits. The second image is an axial SPECT image of the lumbosacral spine, showing areas of increased

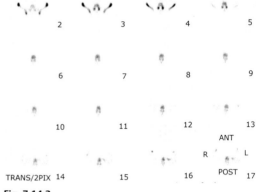

Fig. 7.14.2

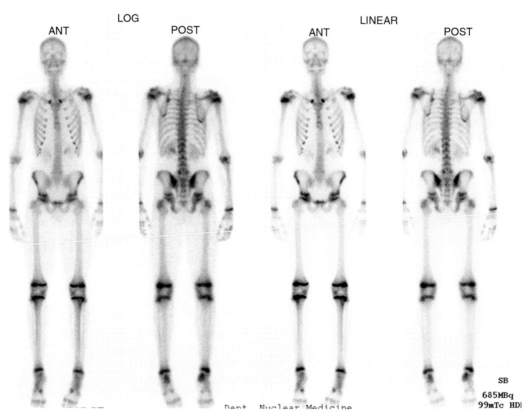

Fig. 7.14.1

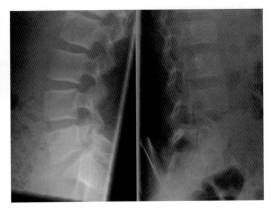

Fig. 7.14.3

uptake at the posterior elements of the vertebral body. The findings would be most compatible with bilateral spondylolysis. I would suggest plain films in the first instance to confirm this and to assess for spondylolisthesis.

These are two X-rays from the same patient (**Fig. 7.14.3**).

These are plain films in the oblique and lateral projections, confirming the presence of spondylolysis at L5/S1, with bilateral L5 pars interarticularis defects. There is no significant spondylolisthesis. I would recommend orthopaedic referral.

Examination Tips

- Bone scan findings may be subtle, especially in the young skeleton, but carefully consider the history and think of the area likely to be affected—the lower lumbar spine in an athlete.
- Growth plates show avid uptake of the bone scan agent. These may distract candidates from prompt identification of any abnormality. More importantly, they are not uncommonly the site of

pathology where they may be masked (e.g., osteomyelitis or bone tumours). Growth plates should be scrutinised for asymmetry.

Differential Diagnosis

- The finding of bilateral posterior elements uptake in an adolescent skeleton is characteristic of spondylolysis.
- When unilateral, differential diagnosis in this age group would include:
  - Osteoid osteoma: < 2 cm, a radiolucent nidus with central sclerosis on CT imaging
  - Osteoblastoma: > 2 cm, can have mixed sclerotic and lytic features
  - Aneurysmal bone cyst: expanded lobulated radiolucent lesion on CT imaging; may show septation and a fluid level on MRI.

Notes

- The pars interarticularis is the weakest part of the vertebral body.
- The typical patient is a young athletic male, in whom the pars are subjected to continued increased stress.
- When bilateral, spondylolysis (pars defect) can lead to spondylolisthesis with an anterior slip of a vertebral body over the one inferiorly.
- Bone scanning is sensitive for its diagnosis, and specificity can be improved with SPECT imaging, which can now be acquired with a localisation CT, further improving diagnostic accuracy.

Bibliography

Afshani E, Kuhn JP. Common causes of low back pain in children. Radiographics 1991;11(2):269–291

De Maeseneer M, Lenchik L, Everaert H, et al. Evaluation of lower back pain with bone scintigraphy and SPECT. Radiographics 1999;19(4):901–912, discussion 912–914

7.15 Autonomous Toxic Thyroid Nodule

Clinical History

A 38-year-old man with hyperthyroidism (**Fig. 7.15.1**).

Ideal Summary

This is a pertechnetate thyroid scan. There is a focal hot nodule in the right lobe of the thyroid. The rest of the gland shows markedly reduced activity. The total thyroid uptake is at the upper limit of normal at 4% of the total injected activity, 20 minutes postinjection. The findings are that of a toxic autonomous nodule. Endocrinology referral and an ultrasound examination would be advised.

Examination Tips

- The normal uptake value is usually in the range of 1 to 4% of the total injected activity at 20 minutes.
- A "hot" nodule can be defined as a nodule with increased uptake on a nuclear medicine study, with suppression of the remaining gland.

Differential Diagnosis

Possible causes for an apparent single area of uptake on thyroid scan may include:

- Non-autonomous hyperplastic nodule. Typically, the patient would be euthyroid and there would be less "suppression" of the rest of the gland.

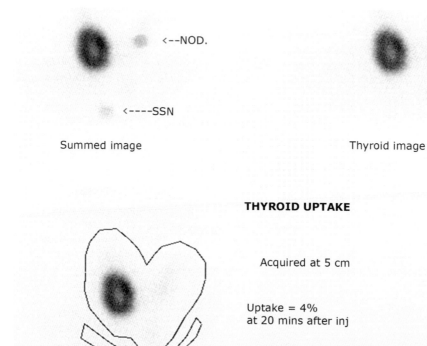

<--NOD.

<----SSN

Summed image

Thyroid image

THYROID UPTAKE

Acquired at 5 cm

Uptake = 4%
at 20 mins after inj

Thyroid image + ROI

Fig. 7.15.1

- Unilateral uptake may be seen with previous hemithyroidectomy or hemiagenesis. The remaining lobe would have a bulbous appearance.

Notes

- The radionuclide thyroid scan serves two purposes in the management of solitary thyroid nodules:
  - Distinction of a benign versus malignant nodule. Malignancy is rare in a "hot" nodule. Fine-needle aspiration for cytological diagnosis is not necessary.
  - Confirmation of diagnosis and increased uptake in a patient with a palpable nodule and hyperthyroidism, in anticipation of radioiodine therapy. The differential diagnosis here would include a toxic autonomous nodule, a toxic multinodular goitre or a nodule with Graves' disease.
- Radioiodine therapy for a single hot nodule less commonly results in hypothyroidism compared with treatment for other entities such as Graves' disease.

Bibliography

Cooper DS, Doherty GM, Haugen BR, et al; American Thyroid Association (ATA) Guidelines Taskforce on Thyroid Nodules and Differentiated Thyroid Cancer. Revised American Thyroid Association management guidelines for patients with thyroid nodules and differentiated thyroid cancer. Thyroid 2009;19(11):1167–1214

Index